Governing Health Systems in Africa

Governing Health Systems in Africa

Edited by
Martyn Sama and Vinh-Kim Nguyen

CODESRIA

Council for the Development of Social Science Research in Africa

ISBN: 2-86978-182-2
ISBN 13: 9782869781825

Typeset by Sériane Camara Ajavon
Cover image designed by Ibrahima Fofana
Printed by Graphiplus, Dakar, Senegal

Distributed in Africa by CODESRIA
Distributed elsewhere by the African Books Collective
www.africanbookscollective.com

The Council for the Development of Social Science Research in Africa (CODESRIA) is an independent organisation whose principal objectives are facilitating research, promoting research-based publishing and creating multiple forums geared towards the exchange of views and information among African researchers. It challenges the fragmentation of research through the creation of thematic research networks that cut across linguistic and regional boundaries.

CODESRIA publishes a quarterly journal, *Africa Development*, the longest standing Africa-based social science journal; *Afrika Zamani*, a journal of history; the *African Sociological Review; African Journal of International Affairs* (AJIA); *Africa Review of Books;* and the *Journal of Higher Education in Africa.* It copublishes the *Africa Media Review* and *Identity, Culture and Politics: An Afro-Asian Dialogue.* Research results and other activities of the institution are disseminated through 'Working Papers', 'Monograph Series', 'CODESRIA Book Series', and the *CODESRIA Bulletin.*

CODESRIA would like to express its gratitude to the Swedish International Development Cooperation Agency (SIDA/SAREC), the International Development Research Centre (IDRC), Ford Foundation, MacArthur Foundation, Carnegie Corporation, NORAD, the Danish Agency for International Development (DANIDA), the French Ministry of Cooperation, the United Nations Development Programme (UNDP), the Netherlands Ministry of Foreign Affairs, Rockefeller Foundation, FINIDA, CIDA, IIEP/ADEA, OECD, OXFAM America, UNICEF and the Government of Senegal for supporting its research, training and publication programmes.

Contents

Contributors vii

I: Introduction

1   Governing the Health System in Africa 3
    Martyn T. Sama and Vinh-Kim Nguyen

II: Governance and Health System Reforms

2   Governance and Primary Health Care Delivery in Nigeria 15
    Omar Massoud

3   Governing Traditional Health Care Sector in Kenya:
    Strategies and Setbacks 25
    Kibet A. Ngetich

4   Corruption et crise des hôpitaux publics à Douala:
    Le schémas d'une organisation tripolaire 34
    Victor Bayemi

5   Health Sector Reforms in Kenya: User Fees 44
    Alfred Anangwe

6   Decentralisation of Health Care Spending and HIV/AIDS
    in Cameroon 60
    Christopher Sama Molem

7   Another Look at Community-Directed Treatment (ComDT) in
    Cameroon: A Quality Challenge to Health System Development 82
    Martyn T. Sama and Richard Penn

III: Health Systems and HIV in the Maghreb

8   Le Système de santé au Maghreb 95
    Sofiane Bouhdiba

9   La Lutte contre le SIDA en Afrique du Nord 116
    Sofiane Bouhdiba

IV: Health Systems and Chronic Diseases

10 Les Maladies chroniques non transmissibles dans le système
de santé au Sénégal: Le cas du diabète dans la ville de Dakar 133
Oupa Diossine Loppy

11 La Gestion de maladies chroniques en Algérie: Le Cas du cancer 146
Farida Mecheri

12 Situation des malades tuberculeux perdus de vue en cours de
traitement au centre antituberculeux de Brazzaville (Congo):
Une Revue 155
Mbou André

V: Priority Setting and Policy Making

13 Retirement Stress in Nigeria: A Psycho-political Analysis 163
Jane-Frances Agbu

14 Préfinancement communautaire des soins de santé pour
un meilleurs accès des populations rurales aux services de santé
de base: Une estimation du consentement à pre-payer
des ménages au Centre du Cameroun 177
Joachim Nyemeck Binam et Valère Nkelzok

15 The Impact of Structural Adjustment Programmes (SAPs)
on Women's Health in Kenya 191
Damaris S. Parsitau

16 Should We 'Modernise' Traditional Medicine? 201
Mugisha M. Mutabazi

17 Empowering Traditional Birth Attendants in the Gambia: A Local
Strategy to Redress Issues of Access, Equity and Sustainability 225
Stella Nyanzi

VI: Conclusion

18 Social Context and Determinants of HIV Transmission:
Lessons from Africa 237
Vinh-Kim Nguyen and Martyn T. Sama

References 256

Contributors

Alfred Anangwe: AIDS Focus, Ministry of Health Nairobi, Kenya.

Christopher Sama Molem: Department of Economic and Management, Faculty of Social and Management Sciences, University of Buea, Cameroon.

Martyn T. Sama: Tropical Medicine Research Center, Kumba SW Province, Cameroon.

Vinh-Kim Nguyen: Department of Social and Preventive Medicine, University of Montréal, Québec, Canada.

Richard Penn: TEYEN Research Foundation, Yaoundé, Cameroon.

Kibet A. Ngetich: Department of Sociology & Anthropology, Egerton University, Njoro Kenya.

Mugisha M. Mutabazi: Department of Economics, Faculty of Arts & Social Sciences, Kyambogo University, Uganda.

Stella Nyanzi: MRC Laboratories, Faranni Field Station, Banjul, The Gambia.

Jane-Frances Agbu: Department of Psychology, University of Lagos, Lagos, Nigeria.

Damaris S. Parsitau: Department of Philosophy & Religious Studies, Egerton University, Njoro, Kenya.

Omar Massoud: Department of Local Government Studies, Faculty of Administration, Ahmadu Bello University, Zaria, Nigeria.

Victor Bayemi: Chargé de Cours FSGA Université de Douala, Cameroun.

Christopher Sama Molem: Department of Economic and Management Faculty of Social and Management Sciences, University of Buea, Cameroon.

Richard Penn: Department of neurology, The University of Chicago Medical Center.

Sofiane Bouhdiba: Human and Social Sciences Faculty of Tunis, Tunisia.

Oupa Diossine Loppy: Amnesty International 303, Résidence Arame Siga Sacré-Coeur II Dakar (Senegal).

Farida Mecheri: Département de sociologie, Université Mostaganem, Groupe de recherche en anthropologie de la santé, Algérie.

Mbou André: Chargé de Cours, Ecole nationale d'administration et de Magistrature, Brazzaville, Congo.

Damaris Parsitau: Department of Philosophy and Religious Studies, Egerton University, Kenya.

Joachim Nyemeck Binam: Institut de Recherche Agricole pour le Développement (IRAD/ASB), Yaoundé, Cameroun.

Valère Nkelzok: Département de Philosophie-Sociologie, Faculté des Lettres et des Sciences Humaines, Université de Douala.

I

Introduction

1

Governing the Health System in Africa

Martyn T. Sama & Vinh-Kim Nguyen

Today, health systems in all countries, rich and poor, play a bigger and more influential role in people's lives than ever before. Health systems of some sort have existed for as long as people have tried to protect their health and treat diseases. Traditional practices, often integrated with spiritual counselling and providing both preventive and curative care, have existed for thousands of years and often co-exist today with modern medicine.

Years ago, organised health systems in the modern sense barely existed. Few people alive then would ever visit a hospital. Most were born into large families and faced an infancy and childhood threatened by a host of potentially fatal diseases – measles, smallpox, malaria and poliomyelitis among them. Infant and child mortality was very high as were maternal mortality rates. Life expectancy was short.

Health systems have undergone overlapping generations of reforms in the past years, including the founding of national healthcare systems, and the extension of social insurance schemes. Later came the promotion of primary health care as a route to achieving affordable universal coverage - the goal of health for all. Despite its many virtues, a criticism of this route has been that it gave too little attention to people's demand of health care, and instead concentrated almost exclusively on their perceived needs.

Primary health care became a core policy for WHO in 1978, with the adoption of the declaration of Alma-Ata and the strategy of 'Health for all by the year 2000'. Over twenty-five years later, international support for the values of primary health care remains strong. Preliminary results of a major review suggest that many in the global health community consider primary health care orientation to be crucial for equitable progress in health.

No uniform, universally applicable, definition of primary health care exists. Ambiguities were present in the Alma-Ata documents, in which the concept was discussed as both a level of care and an overall approach to health policy and service provision. In high income and middle income countries, primary health care is mainly understood to be the first level of care. In low income countries where significant challenges in access to health care persist, it is seen more as a system-wide strategy.

The institutional context of health policy-making and health care delivery has changed. Government responsibilities and objectives in the health sector have been redefined, with private sector entities, both for profit and not-for profit, playing an increasingly visible role in health care provisions. The reasons for collaborative patterns vary, but chronic under-funding of publicly financed health services is often an important factor. Processes of decentralisation and health sector reforms have had mixed effects on health care system performance.

The growth of private health insurance markets and private clinics are pointers to a growing stratification of the health market in line with the intensified income and social differentiation that has occurred over the last two decades; it is, however, also a development which poses new policy-making, managerial and regulatory challenges to which governments and professional associations have to respond. Similarly, the growth of the popular market for alternative medicines and the rediscovery and popularisation of the institutions of the 'traditional'/faith healer point to the crisis in the formal health sector and popular coping strategies that are being adopted. They also open new terrains of power, rights and standards which elicit regulatory responses of their own. The increase in the illegal production and distribution of fake and sub-standard drugs points to an opportunistic entrepreneurial logic, seeking to profit from the African health crises and the problems of the health system.

Changes in the health system brought about by the explosion of the HIV/ AIDS pandemic, the persistence of malaria as a major killer, and the resurgence of diseases like tuberculosis which were previously under control, have implications for the governance of health systems in so far as they are correlated with the diminished capacity of the public health facilities to cope with a complex range of expanded needs. This diminished capacity proliferates through all spheres of the health systems, ranging from the drain of talents to the collapse of personnel management training structures designed to produce and reproduce critical human resources.

The various participants of this Institute on Health, Politics and Society in Africa have from their various disciplinary perspectives addressed some of those aspects of health system governance in Africa. At a time when the African continent is faced with one of the most severe health crisis in its history, most symbolic of the crisis is the challenge of HIV/AIDS. Today, the average life expectancy in sub-Saharan Africa is forty-seven years, without AIDS, it would be sixty-two. As more adults perish, the education of children is compromised. In Swaziland, school enrolment has fallen by 36 percent, mainly because girls have left school to care for sick relatives. The ILO estimates that in SSA, 200,000 teachers will die from AIDS by 2010. A report from the Ivory Coast indicated that during the1996-97 academic year, more than fifty percent of deaths among elementary school teachers were from AIDS, and 280 teaching hours a year were lost because of teachers being absent.

The Concept of Stewardship in Health Policy

Stewardship can be defined as a function of a government responsible for the welfare of the population, and concerned about the trust and legitimacy with which its activities are viewed by the citizenry. It requires vision, intelligence and influence, primarily by the Health Ministry, which must oversee and guide the working and development of the nation's health actions on the government's behalf.

Outside the government, stewardship is also a responsibility of purchasers and providers of health services who must ensure that as much health as possible results from their spending. In terms of effective stewardship, government's key role is one of oversight and trusteeship.

What Is Wrong with Stewardship Today

Ministries of Health in LMIC have a reputation for being among the most bureaucratic and least effectively managed institutions in the public sector. The ministries are fragmented with vertical programmes, or ritual chiefdoms, dependent on uncertain international donor funding.

The notion of stewardship over all health actors and actions deserves renewed emphasis. Much conceptual and practical discussion is needed to improve the definition and measurement of how well stewardship is actually implemented in different settings. However, several basic tasks can already be identified:

(i) Formulating Health Policy – Defining the Vision and Directions.
(ii) Exerting influence – approaches to regulations.
(iii) Collection and using intelligence.

The first function encompasses a range of activities intended to ensure that the health research system demonstrates quality leadership, is productive, has strategic directions and operates in a coherent manner rather than as a collection of fragmented and uncoordinated activities. It should aim at creating or promoting a 'research culture', that recognises the need for evidence-based decision making and the importance of health research as a vital component of health development. In this way, it has a fundamental influence on all the other functions since it establishes the framework for their implementation.

Stewardship

Stewardship can be divided into a number of distinct sub-functions. These include: strategic vision, overall system design and policy formulation; priority-setting, performance and impact assessment; promotions and advancing; and setting of norms, standards and ethical frameworks.

At country-level, these functions include the development of rational health research policy, translating it into a rational plan and priorities, and overseeing its implementations. These functions also include improving links and coordination with the initiatives of various and the creation of a supportive environment that fosters dialogue and networking among the various stakeholders.

Government Stewardship, Community Involvement

Responsible health sector oversight and pro-equity commitments by the state are essential to building and maintaining health systems based on primary health care. However, government must engage with and respond to communities in a two-way relationship if they are to perform their stewardship role effectively. Community involvement – including the dimensions of participation, ownership and empowerment – is a key demand-side component of the health system, necessary to promote accountability and effectiveness.

As stewards of the health system, ministries of health are responsible for protecting citizens' health and ensuring that quality health care is delivered to all who need it. This requires making the best choices given the available evidence, and systematically privileging the public interest over other competing priorities. The responsibilities ultimately rest with governments, even in the context of decentralisation where lines of accountability may be blurred. When the right structures are in place, effective governance and vigorous community involvement support each other.

Financing

Financing for health research comes from a number of sources. If the resources available are to be used effectively and efficiently, consistent with research priorities, mechanisms are needed to ensure coordination and to monitor resource flows over time, both within and between levels. Financing refers to financial resources for health research, resource mobilisation, and the national capacity to monitor where and how research funds are being spent.

Knowledge Generation

This function encompasses the production of scientifically validated research. Each country needs to be able to generate knowledge relevant to its own situation, to allow it to determine its particular health problems, appraise the measures available for dealing with them, and choose the actions likely to produce the greatest improvement in health. This should not be seen as the exclusive preserve of universities or research institutes, but equally public/health services and non-governmental organisations.

Utilisation and Management of Knowledge

The generation of new knowledge is only a part of the research process; for knowledge to be used, it should be shared with other researchers and communicated, in a suitable format, to the different users/stakeholders. It needs to be translated into policy or action or absorbed into the existing knowledge/technology base. Low income countries, in particular, need to ensure that health research brings tangible benefits to the health status of their people. This implies a need to strengthen the link between researchers, policy-makers, health and communities. A critical aspect is the need to improve interactions and connectedness, both horizontally and vertically, through accelerated and creative use of new information technologies.

Activities include promoting an information culture, constructing closer links and fostering communication amongst stakeholders, ensuring that research results are retrievable, generating demand for research, converting research results into user friendly end products, promoting use of information and communications technologies, and developing databases of national exports.

Capacity Development

A long-term, system approach to the development and maintenance of research capacity is needed, addressing such issues as the depth and range of research competencies, gender disposition in education and training, institutional mix and capacity, and the fostering of sustained collaboration, along with clear plans that include provision for monitoring and evaluation. Efforts need to focus on both the quantity and quality of skills available, not just in research techniques, but also over a broad range of related areas.

The Politics of Health in Africa Before and After Aids

The AIDS epidemic challenges the very notion that even rudimentary public health can be achieved in Africa. A litany of statistics testifies that the epidemic continues to spread largely unchecked, erasing hard-gotten gains in public health. In the hardest hit countries, decreasing life expectancy raises the spectre of demographic decline. Flare-ups in HIV incidence in groups in the North that had succeeded in controlling the epidemic suggest that successes in curbing the epidemic (such as in Senegal and Uganda) are fragile, temporary advances in a long war.

It would be a mistake to view AIDS as an isolated case, an exception that confirms the rule. Rather, AIDS should be taken as symptomatic of historically deep social conditions that have provided a ripe environment for infectious diseases on the continent. (Nor is Africa an exception in this regard, as indicated by burgeoning epidemics in China, Central Asia, and Eastern Europe). While the notion of 'tropical diseases' obscures the political nature of the ecology of disease in Africa, which first took root in the inequalities of the colonial period, the particular conditions under which AIDS emerged - in the North and the South, among rich and poor – challenged easy geographic determinism. Indeed, simple determinisms of any sort – cultural or economic – have not withstood scrutiny. Just as there is no 'African sexual system' rooted in African culture, HIV prevalence does not demonstrate a linear relationship with economic variables. The fastest growing epidemic was in the richest country (South Africa), and there are no differences in sexual behaviour between high and low prevalence cities.

Not coincidentally, the AIDS epidemic surged throughout the continent at the same time as deep cuts, mandated by structural adjustment programmes, were being made to public health services, a gap that was largely replaced by a proliferating private sector comprising a vast range of actors drawn from the biomedical and various other healing traditions. This only added to the epidemic's bio-social complexity: breakdowns in public health may have unwittingly amplified epidemics by diminishing control of other sexually transmitted infections or by increasing unsafe use of injection equipment, both of which intensify HIV transmission. Current attempts to dramatically expand access to lifesaving treatments for the disease have called attention to the inadequacy of public health systems in Africa, and heralded yet more calls for health sector reform.

Thus, the AIDS epidemic has raised the stakes of health sector reform in a continent grown too used to bearing a heavy burden of preventable and treatable infectious diseases. Indeed, the inability of health services in Africa to deliver improved health for all has been known, debated, and addressed since the first flush of post-colonial optimism dissipated in the 1970s. Primary health care and the Bamako initiative have been succeeded by a series of reforms: cost-recovery, sustainability, decentralisation, empowerment etc. To this list of reforms must be added a long list of experiments for delivering health, piloted by a broad range of non-state actors ranging from grass-roots community groups to trans-national NGOs whose own budgets dwarf those of African states. Nothing much seems to have worked. Why has it been so difficult to deliver the goods in Africa? Does this mean that African health systems just might be ungovernable? Is the economic situation so dire, the politics so messy and corrupt, the biological terrain so pathogenic, the culture so recalcitrant?

Clearly, we do not think so. Nor do we believe that the failure to deliver health for Africans can be easily pinpointed to a definite cause. Certainly it is by now quite clear that health in Africa is dramatically under-funded and that there are insufficient resources for health to be a sustainable option for Africa if it is expected to pay for it by itself (Commission on Macro-economics and Health). But the economic determinant of ill health in Africa should not blind us to the fact that economic policies are the result of political processes. This only confirms countless other examples from the past century that demonstrate that health is above all a political matter, of which biology and epidemiology are the expression. Epidemics of cholera, tuberculosis or HIV are the embodiment of politics: wars that spread refugees across the land, breakdowns in public health, policy failures. Governing the health system in Africa is an eminently political affair. The truism that politics is always local in many ways does not hold in Africa, where economic and Bretton Woods' institutions largely decide social policy and agencies are run from distant capitals on other continents. While it is tempting to view the current focus on 'good governance' as a Bretton Woods' flavour of the month that is, as usual, predicated on some idea of deficiency on the part of recipients, the focus on governance has the advantage of putting politics front and centre and provides a unique vantage point for addressing both the global and local politics of health. It draws attention to the processes that lead to policy, and that refract how policy plays out at the local level.

If African health systems are ungovernable, it may be in large part because powerful international donors work at cross-purposes, setting competing agendas, cycling policies at a rate that defies bureaucratic assimilation, fragmenting health efforts, and undermining local systems of accountability. This hypothesis remains to be verified, as curiously little attention has been paid to how global forces constrain and shape local governance, but it is an example of the kind of exploration the focus on governance allows. Too much emphasis has been placed on policies and their eventual failures, rather than on the broader social processes – global and local – by which policies are developed and enacted. Thus, we propose to use governance as a lens onto the politics of health in Africa in the broadest sense, to explore the practices that shape the conduct of individuals, families, communities, organisations, and governments with the goal of improving health.

For instance, in the case of AIDS, initial efforts to combat the epidemic failed largely because raising awareness did not translate into changes in sexual behaviour, particularly given the structural constraints on individuals living in poverty to which policy makers in Northern countries, steeped in an individualistic health promotion ideology, were blind. Emerging evidence indicates that the epidemic's spread was not, in fact, due to behavioural factors but was mediated by concurrent epidemics of sexually transmitted infections and, perhaps, improper use of injection equipment. This suggests that the focus on sexual behaviour may have been a massive policy failure, and implicates global policies that cut back health services in the spread of the epidemic. Others have argued that the focus on human rights, while laudable, has weakened attempts to control the epidemic, particularly by insisting on voluntary testing. Current attempts to expand access to treatment are long overdue, but concern has been expressed that this risks overwhelming what little health care infrastructure is left in Africa and undermining fledgling attempts to reinforce primary health care. Finally, the emergence of a transnational AIDS activism in Africa has been significantly able to shift policy, but it remains to be seen whether this dynamism can be used to leverage meaningful additional resources and harnessed to implement needed health sector reforms. AIDS has fundamentally called into question the governance of health in

Africa, and will mark a transformation of the politics of health in Africa that will have global repercussions. The success of African AIDS activists in achieving the reform of international intellectual property laws to allow importation of generic AIDS drugs is so far the most salient example, but others will likely follow as the inability to deliver the drugs draws international attention to African health systems.

Understanding – and improving – governance of African health is more than a matter of prescribing mechanisms intended to increase accountability and transparency. It requires taking stock of how global policies and local politics interact, the trans-national channels through which political pressure is exercised, as well as how a broad spectrum of therapeutic alternatives is made available to, or shunned by, health-seekers. Health systems in Africa largely surpass what is accessible through the public system to encompass a patchwork of providers, whether these are biomedical entrepreneurs, churches, NGOs, or 'traditional' healers. Health systems also encompass shifting systems of social solidarity that insure against risk: there may be private health insurance for a few and some free health services here and there, but it is mainly extended social networks (which may be more or less based on varying notions of kinship) that insure against health risk. Thus, it is more apt to speak of a proliferating *therapeutic economy* where therapeutic transactions may be valued in other than monetary terms, and where affliction is not necessarily understood in a strictly biomedical idiom. The therapeutic economy is a strikingly hybridised one, where irrational use of bio-medicines coincides with the industrially produced traditional remedies, and where affliction is simultaneously understood and treated in biomedical and spiritual terms. It will be necessary to come to grips with this creolised therapeutic world, as attempts to govern health through a purely biomedical model and the illusion of its rational management are destined to run aground in the messy therapeutic politics of the real world.

Conclusion

There is recognition that accountability, transparency, and vigorous citizen participation are essential to achieving a viable society, sustainable economic growth, and equitable distribution of benefits and risk of growth. Yet African countries are characterised by persistent and in many cases worsening social, economic, gender, and health inequalities. This theme runs across the articles in this volume 'Governing the African Health System'.

Some of the key issues discussed in this volume include corruption in hospitals, transparency in Primary Health Care (PHC) delivery, citizen participation in decision-making regarding health care, and the empowerment of traditional birth attendants among others. Health sector reforms have also been widely addressed; with decentralisation, financing of health care delivery, and traditional medical practice being the key issues.

This volume on 'Governing African Health Systems' has re-focussed the debate on what makes a good health system. What makes a health system fair? And how do we know whether a health system is performing as it could?

It is our goal to clarify the uses of social science research, to provide evidence on how the health social sciences have influenced our thinking about health care issues, and to underscore some promising and relevant areas of research for the future.

II

Governance and Health
System Reforms

2

Governance and Primary Health Care Delivery in Nigeria

Omar Massoud

Introduction

The National Health Policy in Nigeria (NHP), with the main objective of 'Health for All' by the year 2000, was launched in 1988. The provision of an effective system of primary health care delivery at the local government level was one of the main goals of this policy. The central focus of the National Health Policy was a 'community-based health system in which primary, secondary and tertiary health care is organised at local, state and federal levels, with each mutually supporting the other'. Before then (in 1986), fifty-two local government areas (LGAs) had been selected as pilot project sites, with the purpose of strengthening Primary Health Care (PHC) at the grassroots. Each of these LGAs was linked with a university teaching hospital or school of health technology for the purpose of training their health officials. State governments were directed by the then federal military government to devolve all PHC responsibilities to local governments over a three-year period terminating in June 1990. The state governments were however left with the responsibilities of supervising and coordinating PHC activities, as well as playing an advocacy role. The local communities were supposed to be carried along in the programme in order to ensure its success. To this end, district and village health committees were constituted to ensure the participation of local communities. The input of these committees was to be in the form of providing information, giving suggestions for improvement, complaints, control, etc. The PHC programme as conceived then revolved around nine core functions:

- Public health education
- Nutrition improvement
- Adequate safe water and basic sanitation
- Maternal and child health care, including family planning

- Immunisation
- Prevention and control of endemic and epidemic diseases
- Provision of essential drugs and supplies
- Elderly and handicapped care
- Accident and injury care

It is almost two decades now since the NHP was launched but the ultimate goal of 'Health for all' by the year 2000 seems to be as remote as ever. Effective delivery of primary health care at the local level is almost non-existent. A study conducted in the mid 1980s and which is still relevant today shows that the spatial density of hospitals in Nigeria ranges from 415 square kilometres per hospital in Lagos State (in the South West) to 9716 square kilometres per hospital in Borno State (in the North East). The corresponding implied accessibility of hospitals ranges from 9.67 kilometres walking radius in Lagos State to 55.55 kilometres in Borno State (Idachaba: 1985:5).

Before the introduction of the NHP, it was not possible to make an accurate assessment of the health status of Nigerians. There was no system of collecting basic health statistics on births, deaths, the occurrence of major diseases, and other health indicators on a country-wide basis. There were estimates from a few centres where such data were collected from sample surveys as well as from institutional records and special studies, such as the one referred to above (National Health Policy Guidelines 1988:4). Within the framework of the NHP, Primary Health Care is defined as:

> [E]ssential health care based on practical, scientifically sound and socially acceptable methods and technology made universally accessible to individuals and families in the community and through their full participation and at a cost that the community can afford in the spirit of self reliance and self determination. It forms an integral part of the country's health system of which it is the central function and main focus, and of the overall social and economic development of the community. It is the first level of contact with individuals, the family and community with the national health system bringing health care as close as possible to where people live and work, and constitutes the first element of a continuing health care process (ibid:13).

Primary Health Care was envisaged to perform two functions under the NHP:

> To provide general health services of preventive, curative, promotional and rehabilitative nature to the population as the entry point of the health care system. The provision of care at this level is largely the responsibility of local governments with the support of state ministries of health. Private medical practitioners shall also provide health care at this level. Noting that traditional medicine is widely used, and that there is no uniform system of traditional medicine in the country but wide variations, with each variant being strongly bound to local culture and beliefs, the local health authorities shall, where applicable, seek the collaboration of the traditional practitioners in promoting their health programmes such as nutrition, environmental sanitation, personal hygiene, family planning and immunisations. Traditional health

practitioners shall be trained to improve their skills and to ensure their cooperation in making use of the referral systems in dealing with high risk patients. Governments of the federation shall seek to gain a better understanding of traditional health practices, and support research activities to evaluate them. Practices and technologies of proven value shall be adapted into the health care system and those that are harmful shall be discouraged (ibid:13).

It was envisaged that local authorities would design and implement strategies to meet the health needs of the local population, and this should be done with the guidance, support and technical supervision of the state ministries of health. In addition, the local councils should be able to elicit the support of formal and informal leaders, traditional rulers, religious and cultural organisations as well as other influential persons and groups in support of community action for health. Local health authorities were given a free hand to adopt strategies to make the programme a success. In this regard, the NHP envisaged, among other strategies, that:

- Local authorities can determine how best to provide the essential elements of primary health care;
- Provide relevant health information to the people on such matters as personal hygiene, environmental sanitation, prevention and control of communicable diseases as well as such matters where a change of lifestyle of the people can have a significant impact on their health status;
- Design and operate mechanisms for involving the communities in the critical decisions about the health services; and
- Collect relevant data about the health resources, the health status of the community and their health behaviour, including the utilisation of health services. Such data shall form the basis of the information of the local health services.

However, Primary Health Care delivery has failed almost two decades after the introduction of the NHP. Both the United Nations Children's Fund (UNICEF) and the Federal Government of Nigeria unanimously agreed recently that weak Primary Health Care Centres have largely contributed to the high level of the disease burden in the country. According to the Master Plan of Operations for 2002-2007, jointly published by the two bodies, weak PHCs have exacerbated the problem of childhood morbidity, caused largely by malaria, measles, and, in recent years, HIV/AIDS. The Action Plan noted that coverage interventions known to reduce child and maternal mortality remain very low, and only about one per cent of children under five years were reported to sleep under insecticide-treated bed nets (*New Nigerian*, 21 March, 2005). It has been estimated that Nigeria now has the unenviable record of contributing approximately ten percent of the world's maternal death and eight percent of the world's child death, and this is a trend that has been on the increase over the years. Many such deaths could have been prevented with well known cost-effective interventions if they had been available to women and children who needed them.

The Birnin Gwari Case Study

We tried to find out through an empirical study in Birnin Gwari local government some of the main causes for the failure of primary health care delivery in the country, conscious, however, that the data gathered from this local government were by no means representative, nor a fair coverage, of the operations of most local governments in the northern part of the country. What we tried to do here is to investigate empirically (which, in the end, may either validate or falsify the reasons generally given for the failure of the programme) the reasons for the failure of PHC. The data collected were based on the following broad questions we had in mind:

- Is the local government well equipped with qualified personnel and materials to ensure the success of programme implementation?
- How much, in terms of financial resources, has been spent on the programme over the past five years?
- Are the people, as stakeholders, involved in the implementation of PHC as the blueprint for the programme suggests?

Based on these broad questions, the data collected from the local government were categorised into two:

Endogenous Data: related to the internal structure and facilities available to the health services of the local government. Data collected in this regard referred to the number of health clinics, and maternity centres in the local government area. The availability of trained nurses, midwives, etc. Also considered were the financial resources available to the LGAs over a seven year period, and the materials available to the LGAs - storage facilities, drugs, etc.

Exogenous Data: material collected here enabled us to examine demographic patterns in the local government; the causes of morbidity and mortality (by age and sex); the use of health services, including maternity and child health clinics, and the degree of involvement of the people in their own health care, including the use of traditional healers.

Located in the central part of Kaduna State (in North Central Nigeria), Birnin Gwari local government has a total population of 231,617. The local government is divided into three zones – the Central zone with a population of 84, 189; the Eastern zone with a population of 76,448; and the Western zone with a population of 70,980. (Source: Birnin Gwari Local Government Council).

An examination of the statistics made available to us shows that Birnin Gwari local government has a reasonable number of facilities to cater for the health needs of the local community. The central zone has eleven clinics; the Western zone has the same number, while the Eastern zone has seventeen. In terms of storage facilities, the following are available:

- 1 Refrigerator
- 3 Deep Freezers
- 8 Cold Boxes

- 160 Vaccine carriers
- 2 Ice pack freezers
- 480 Ice packs

To ensure a constant supply of electricity, the local government has one solar energy plant and four standby generators to serve the three zones. An examination of the staff strength of the health department reveals that it is adequately staffed, with 188 personnel. This is made up of fourteen Community Health Officers, fifty-six Senior Community Health Extension Workers, seven Junior Community Health Extension Workers, three Environmental Health Officers, two Environmental Health Technicians, ten nurses and midwives, three Dental Assistants, and ninety-three Health Attendants.

The PHC unit sends out District Health Superintendents to supervise field staff from the village level to the districts. They usually assess the performance of the field staff by observing the latter performing their basic functions. Once every three months, staff planning meetings are held. This is done with the aim of identifying problems in the field. For example, some of the problems employees encounter in the clinics and with the local community include a reticence to report cases of births and deaths in the local government area, and the lack of co-operation with officials of the health department during immunisation programmes. These problems may be due to religious or traditional beliefs. During such monthly meetings the PHC staff air their views and make suggestions as to how to overcome some of the problems encountered in the field. In addition, the PHC unit also sends out staff to the field to gather health statistics. This enables the department to assess its performance and it also helps to guide them on where to concentrate their efforts. Statistics gathered usually include mortality rates, accident rates, infectious diseases, expanded programme on immunisation (EPI) activities, and control of diarrhoeal diseases (CDD).

As enumerated in the blueprint of the NHP, district and village health committees have been constituted in all the wards of the local government area. There are also the Traditional Birth Attendants (TBAs) who are recruited to supplement the efforts of the village health workers (VHWs). The minimum qualification for the TBAs is usually a certificate in adult education. While the TBAs' main focus is on child birth, the VHWs are trained in preventive health care methods, first aid etc. According to the head of the health department of the local government, the District and Village Health Committees play significant roles in primary health care delivery in the local government. They do this through the mobilisation and sensitisation of the local communities about the need for total involvement in health care programmes; supporting and maintaining the drug revolving fund; providing voluntary work (for example, there are security guards for some of the clinics who are not on the payroll of the local government); and holding frequent meetings to discuss problems such as the use of medical facilities, staff punctuality, and guarding against malpractices committed by staff of the local government.

However, the health status of the residents of Birnin Gwari leads one to question the effectiveness of the district and village health committees in performing their duties. The inhabitants of Birnin Gwari local government are still afflicted by common diseases which normally should not pose a threat to them. Presently, the causes of morbidity and mortality in the local government area are:

- Measles (in children between the ages of 1–5 years, both male and female)
- Diarrhoea
- Malaria
- Deaths related to child births
- Tetanus A – caused by injuries sustained during farming
- Tetanus B (neo-natal) in new-born babies
- Cerebro-spinal meningitis
- Malnutrition in children and pregnant women
- Road traffic accidents

Source: Health Department, Birnin Gwari Local Government.

The prevalence of these common diseases and accidents points to one basic fact: that primary health care delivery has failed in the local government. This failure, we believe, is due to two main reasons. The first reason is attributable to the lack of close and effective contact by local health officials with the local communities, consequent upon the inefficiency of the district and village health committees. Visits by the health officials to the local communities total no more than three times a year, and this is only to collect data on diseases afflicting the local communities. The organic link which is supposed to exist between policy makers and the local communities, through the district and village health committees, is non-existent. Consequently instead of being stakeholders, local communities are mere 'beneficiaries' of PHC. They thus see in the implementation of the PHC programme a similarity with all other programmes embarked on by the local government, which often end in failure, despite the enormous resources allocated to such programmes. The resultant effect is that the officials of the health department of the local government do not know their target population sufficiently well. As Tom Gabriel (1991:2) succinctly puts it:

> Development programmes, basic needs strategies, primary health care schemes etc., all share a common requirement: each has to make the most efficient use of financial and staff resources at a time when development funds are actually decreasing. Yet those responsible for planning, funding and implementing these essential activities often possess scant knowledge of how their target populations live. Insulated from food security, chronic ill health, illiteracy or powerlessness, their good intentions or occasional field visits to nearby settlements cannot adequately replace this lack of fundamental knowledge. They are usually extremely remote from the living conditions of their clients.

The second reason for the failure of the PHC programme can be traced to the lack of transparency and accountability in programme implementation. Over the past five years, from 2001 to date, the health department has witnessed its share of total budgetary spending increase significantly, as the Table below indicates.

Table 1: Figures on Local Government Finances

Year	Budget of Local Govt	Allocation to the Health Sector	Total Budget for the Health Sector %
2001	216,200,253.00	21,100,000.00	9.71%
2002	261,940,082.00	31,500,000.00	12%
2003	259,000,000.00	20,000,000.00	7.72%

For the year 2001, the health sector received 21,100,000 naira which was 9.71 percent of the total budget of the local government which stood at 216,200,253 naira. In 2002, the approved estimate for the health sector was 31,500,000, representing 12 percent of the estimates of capital expenditure of 261,940,082 for the local government. In 2003, the health sector received 20,000,000 out of a total estimate of 259,000,000 naira for the local government. This represents 7.72 percent of total spending for that year. In absolute terms, these figures represent a marked increase in budgetary allocation for health over the preceding years where for example, the health sector received in 1993, 740,000 naira, representing 4.99 percent of the total estimates of 1,950,000.

The ineffectiveness of local governments in Nigeria to provide basic services to local communities has been mainly attributed to the lack of sufficient financial resources. Financial inadequacy, we believe, is not a key constraint or obstacle to effective service delivery. This is because although local governments do not receive as much, both in terms of absolute revenues per capita and in terms of the total share of public expenditures vis-à-vis the state and federal governments, their functional responsibilities are correspondingly limited. Apart from this, the total share of fiscal revenue accruing to local authorities from federal allocations has more than quadrupled over the past four or five years. A cursory glance at the revenues which have accrued to local governments in Nigeria from the federation account, shows that their revenue base increased tremendously over a nine-year period, from 1997 to 2001 as Table 2 shows.

The increase in revenues over the past five years points to one basic fact: that poor service delivery in the local governments cannot be attributed to inadequate finances. One major problem, which contributes to the failure of local governments in meeting target goals, can be traced to the lack of transparency and accountability in governance. For example, the annual financial estimates for the health department in Birnin Gwari local government are hardly made public. They are treated as secret documents and financial reports on disbursements are hardly made available to the community, who as stakeholders have the right to know.

Table 2: Revenues Accruing to Local Governments 1993-2001

Year	Total Revenue (in billions of naira)
1993	18.31
1994	17.32
1995	22.25
1996	29.61
1997	53.06
1998	65.98
1999	116.12
2000	244.14
2001	248.63

Source: Federal Office of Statistics.

Reports of financial spending are treated as documents only for the consumption of the personnel. Even the junior nurses and community health workers have only a skeletal knowledge of how the department operates its annual budget. This problem is not peculiar to Birnin Gwari local government alone, but is widespread all over the country. According to Dr Shehu Mahdi, the executive director of the National Primary Health Care Development Agency, 'official analysis show that 60 percent of the total health spending (in the country) between 1999 and 2003 went into settling out of pocket expenses. This, in a situation where primary health care services are not available to the majority of the people and where the services are available, the quality is so bad that people prefer to go elsewhere for the services' (*The Guardian*, May 30, 2005).

Conclusion

There is no doubt that severe problems have bedevilled the Nigerian state in health care delivery. The provision of an effective system of health care delivery, as a right, and not a privilege, is but a dream in Nigeria. The failure of the Nigerian state to provide an effective, functional and sustainable health care system has led to a situation where access to heath care is not possible for the majority of the populace. Coupled with this problem is the issue of brain drain, where medical practitioners, nurses, and midwives leave the country in search of better conditions of work, often to countries in the developed world. At the heart of the economic, political and social crises bedevilling Nigeria is the lack of transparency and accountability in governance, a situation which has led to the failure of many public policies. Often, reforms of the public sector, meant to address the failure of public policies, usually focus on structural issues, relegating the behavioural to the background. Reform of public institutions is a step in the right direction, but the ultimate goal of a reform being effective and functional may not be achieved without putting in place the mechanisms which will regulate the behaviour of the individuals operating in the system. Rather than focusing on 'strong local governments' with adequate financial wherewithal, as a panacea for an ineffective service delivery, any reform, in order to be effective, should rather focus on the characteristics of the delivery system itself. To understand the failure of policy implementation, one must understand the motivations of the myriad of individuals who play major roles in the service delivery. The point made by William Dillinger (1993) cannot be clearer in this regard:

> There is no single institutional arrangement that can be universally prescribed for the delivery of urban services. What is important are not the organizational labels, but rather the relationships - the rules that govern the transactions between local political leaders, administrators and the urban dwellers. A 'good' arrangement is likely to be a very complicated one and one that is not defined merely by the designation of municipal responsibilities and revenue sources. Urban service delivery appears to be a problem that cannot be addressed by taking the organizational context as a given and attempting to change the behavior of one organization – municipal government – within it. Instead, it appears to be a problem of the public sector as a whole, and one that must be addressed by looking at the variety of factors that influence the performance of the public sector and those factors' implications for urban service delivery.

Primary Health Care Delivery has failed in Nigeria because there was no serious interaction between formal management structures and local residents. In the first place, this led to the absence of a local mechanism for ensuring public accountability and inducing greater transparency in governance. Secondly, because local communities were not seriously involved in policy making and implementation with regards to health care delivery, they did not see formal management structures in the local governments as particularly relevant to their existence. Thirdly, the local authorities, depending largely on subsidies from federally allocated revenues for their operation, saw no need to cultivate the local communities as their natural constituencies, and thus lacked the capacity to mobilise the local populace for the effective implementation of the project. This is true not only with regards to primary health care delivery, but with all other development programmes in the local governments. To enhance service delivery in the local governments therefore requires a new approach to policy making which will eliminate the prevailing dichotomy between the formal management structures and the informal sector. There is a need to put in place a unified management system injected with a strong dose of citizen participation. To achieve this, efforts must be made to ensure that:

- Local associations that have emerged to deal with particular problems in particular neighbourhoods are officially and legally recognised;
- These associations must be integrated into the normal processes of formal management;
- Efforts must be made to progressively build up the capacities of these neighbourhood associations to gradually align them with the existing modern urban management system.

These advances require the integration of traditional neighbourhood organisations into the governance of urban centres. It will be necessary, in this respect, to identify all the neighbourhood institutions in the local governments, to appreciate the nature of their leadership and their organisation, and seek to harness them for the overall administration of the locality. However, the leadership of these neighbourhood organisations must be entrusted to men and women of integrity, who have the trust and confidence of the community, and through whom information can flow from the local government council to residents of neighbourhoods and vice versa. This will have the effect of reducing the level of alienation in the local governments, because the people will know more about what is going on in the local government councils.

References

Akinkugbe, O. O., Olatubosun, D. and Esan, G. J. F. eds., 1973, *Priorities in National Health Planning*, Proceedings of an International Symposium, Ibadan, Caxton Press.

Bennett, F. J., ed., 1979, *Community Diagnosis and Health Action: A Manual for Tropical and Rural Areas*, London, Macmillan.

Carley, M., 1981, *Social Measurement and Social Indicators: Issues of Policy and Theory*, London, George Allen and Unwin.

Constitution of the Federal Republic of Nigeria, 1999, Lagos, Federal Government Press.

Dillinger, William, 1993, *Decentralization and Its Implications for Urban Service Delivery*, Washington, World Bank Urban Management Program.

Federal Government of Nigeria and UNICEF, *Master Plan of Operations: Country Programme of Cooperation, Document* 1997-2001.

Idachaba, F. S., 1985, *Rural Infrastructures in Nigeria*, Ibadan, Ibadan University Press.

Gabriel, T., 1991, *The Human Factor In Rural Development*, Belhaven Press.

Guidelines for The National Health Policy, 1988.

Marga Institute, 1984, *Intersectoral Action for Health - Sri Lanka Study*.

Report of the International Symposium on Urban Management and Urban Violence in Africa, 1994, Ibadan, IFRA.

USAID, 1994, *Governance Initiative in Nigeria: A Strategic Assessment of Primary Health Care and Local Government*, Associates in Rural Development.

3

Governing the Traditional Health Care Sector in Kenya: Strategies and Setbacks

Kibet A. Ngetich

Introduction

In Kenya, social, cultural and historical factors have led to the emergence of a plural health care system in which traditional and contemporary western medicine co-exist. The colonialists and even some westernised Africans initially regarded African traditional medicine as magic. Mission doctors described traditional health practitioners as witches and dismissed their practices as unscientific and irrational (Beck 1971, Sindiga 1995, Tinga 1998). The colonial administration outlawed witchcraft practices under which many traditional health practices were subsumed. Consequently, the colonial administration undermined traditional health practices by arraigning suspected witches in courts (Tinga 1998). These attitudes fuelled the belief that the traditional health care sector was full of fake, 'snake-oil' practitioners bent on capitalising on 'ignorant' patients and on the alleged shortcomings of modern health care.

The official recognition of traditional medicine in Kenya originated from the WHO's Alma Ata declaration of 1978 (WHO and UNICEF 1978). Since then, traditional medicine has gradually carved itself a niche in the provision of health care services in Kenya. However, this emerging sector faces a myriad of problems, of which governance features prominently.

By governance, I mean stewardship, management, leadership and guidance, which can be operationalised into organisation, supervision and control. These terms are used together in an attempt to more accurately convey the complex meaning of governance. Governance also engenders accountability and responsibility. For example, the weakening of modern health care systems in Kenya is reflected in the falling health status of the population. Over the years, the burden of disease has increased, leading to a decline in life expectancy (KDHS 1998, 2003). The decline in life expectancy is a clear indication of the modern health care system's failure or at least inability to cope with growing health care demands (KDHS 2003). This is partly due to the weakening of health system structures and governance.

It is in the context of the increasing importance of traditional medicine and the failing health care systems as indicated by the falling health standards in Kenya that the issue of governance of indigenous medicine is considered. This paper, therefore, examines governance of indigenous health care resources in Kenya with specific attention to strategies of managing and the setbacks involved.

The Quest for Governance of the Traditional Medical Sector

In Kenya, both modern and traditional medicines co-exist as parallel systems but with little coordination between them (Owour 1999). Previous efforts to coordinate the activities of traditional and modern health practitioners in Kenya have not been successful due to mutual mistrust and suspicion between ethno-medical and biomedical practitioners. In 1989 for instance, a task force committee with the objective of linking the activities of traditional health practitioners, modern doctors, scholars and researchers was launched in Nairobi but hardly took off (Kimani 1981, 1995). This effort did not take into account forms of organisation of traditional health care activities and associated operational activities.

The health provision strategies have for a long time not taken into account what the patients think about their health and where they go for treatment. As a result, there has been a mismatch between the kind of health services provided and what people actually opt for in the event of illness.

In order to make health care provision policies responsive and sensitive to the consumer (patient) preferences there is a need to understand the dynamics of the utilisation of traditional health care services. Recent research findings (Nyamwaya 1992, Ngetich 2004) indicate that there exists interaction between traditional and modern health practitioners as well as their patients in terms of cross-referrals of patients. Yet, there is no protocol governing referrals of patients between traditional and modern health practitioners.

Thus, the quest for governance of indigenous health care systems raises a number of critical issues that need to be resolved. These include: intellectual property rights and patents claims, standards of traditional medical practices and care, legal, regulatory and control issues in the traditional medicine sector, as well as organisational frameworks of traditional medical practice and utilisation.

In the light of the above, the following key questions will be addressed:

- First, what are the problems of governance facing African traditional health care sector in Kenya?
- Second, what are the strategies of governance of traditional medicine in Kenya?
- Third, what are the shortcomings or limitations of governance strategies adopted in relation to traditional medical care?

African Traditional Medicine: From 'Magic' to Medicine

A study of the utilisation of traditional medicine falls within the realm of ethno-medical research, a component of health systems research. Health System Research is 'applied research, aiming at improving the quality of health care and optimising the use of available resources in order to meet health needs in a population' (Good 1987, Nuyens 1988). According to Good (1987:17) ethno-medical systems comprise 'all the resources and responses available to a community in addressing its health problems, organised partially and changing over time'. Ethno-medical analysis therefore, focuses on the actual experiences of people and examines how they are perceived, labelled, communicated and managed in interactions with family, social network and therapists (Good 1987).

Academic research on traditional medicine and health care systems in Africa can be traced back to the works of British colonial ethnographers (Rivers 1924, Evans-Pritchard 1937). Though not particularly focussing on African medicine, these studies provided for the first time detailed descriptions of medical practices of various African peoples. However, due to the structuralist approach which was then dominant in Britain, these studies gave attention to healing only with reference to magic and rituals. The overall impact of this approach was a reduction in the study of health and illness 'to studies of witchcraft, magic and in general curative or socially re-adjustive ritual practices, with herbalists and empirical rational diagnoses, treatment and prophylaxis as residual categories' (Foster 1976: xiv-vx). As Yoder observes, 'the study of medical belief and practices became subsumed under the rubric of magic, witchcraft and religion' (1982:4).

The above works shaped subsequent in-depth studies that focussed on medical knowledge and practices of different peoples in Africa. Works along this line were done among the Batabwa and Bakongo of Congo, the Bono of Ghana, the Zulu of South Africa and the Amhara of Ethiopia (Janzen 1978, Roberts 1979, Warren 1974, Young 1975). However, these studies tended to focus almost exclusively on ethnographic descriptions of African traditional medical practices of particular ethnic groups.

In an international conference held in Alma Ata, Russia, WHO called for the use of indigenous health resources in primary health care (WHO and UNICEF 1978). This declaration inspired many researchers, who sought to determine the actual and potential role or contribution of traditional medicine in national health care (Pilsbury 1982, Young 1983) as well as identify potential areas of cooperation, conflict and integration between modern and traditional medicine (Unschuld 1976, Pearce 1982, Green and Makhubu 1984). These studies found that traditional medicine was a highly valued medical resource in many third world countries that could be promoted and tapped for primary health care.

After the recognition of the actual and potential value of traditional medicine in primary health care, attention in policy and research shifted to how to integrate traditional medicine in modern health care (Pearce 1982, Rappaport and Rappaport

1981). But efforts to integrate traditional medicine in modern health care became limited to the incorporation of traditional healers, particularly Traditional Birth Attendants (TBAs), in the national health care system. This was mainly because TBAs were viewed as being closest to biomedicine. Nonetheless, traditional medicine maintained its identity and vigour resulting in the parallel co-existence of traditional and modern health care systems.

One way of promoting traditional health care in Africa was through professionalisation. Twumasi (1984), Last (1986) and Chivundika (1994) identified areas of increased professionalisation among traditional health practitioners in Africa. These developments have seen traditional medicine achieve some measure of organisation and recognition, which is an important step towards increased governance of traditional medicine.

Governing the Traditional Health Care Sector in Kenya

It is now widely acknowledged that about eighty percent of the world's population rely on traditional medicine for primary health care (WHO 1985). Yet more than eighty percent of state resources in Kenya are allocated to modern health care delivery (Republic of Kenya 1996). This clearly demonstrates that there is a discrepancy between what the government offers in terms of health care and what the people actually accept in the event of illness occurrence. Although this scenario may be partly rooted in problems of access, there is increasing evidence that even where modern medicine is fully accessible, the people still resort to traditional medicine (Ngetich 2004).

What this suggests is that there is a need for the government to provide stewardship in the traditional health care sector with a view to harnessing indigenous health care resources by shaping and guiding its development. Thus, in the quest for a health care system that is responsive to the people's health needs and a system of health administration that is responsive to the health care practitioners and health services users, the issue of governance of the traditional health care sector needs to be addressed.

Strategies

It is evident, at least from government policy documents such as annual development plans and seasonal papers, that the Kenyan government recognises the importance of traditional medicine. But the concern is, what has it done to improve or promote this sector in the pursuit of the Millennium Development Goals for health?

First, what is needed is licensing and registration. The government, at local government level i.e., municipalities and councils, as well as at national level (ministerial), registers and licenses traditional health practitioners. This is done through the Ministry of Gender, Sports, Culture and Social Services (Department of Culture). Within the Ministry, the Department of Culture is responsible for registering the traditional health practitioners. The traditional health practitioners must also register their clinics with their local authorities as business enterprises. Through registration and licensing, the government exercises some rudimentary sense of control on the traditional medical practice.

Second, the formation of traditional healers associations is desirable. The Kenya Association of Herbalists (KAH) which has branches throughout the country, provides the individual herbal practitioners with a means to organise themselves and agitate for their interests. With swelling membership this organisation has increasingly gained some political clout and comments on issues affecting its members in various forums such as workshops, seminars and even newspapers. The KAH has increasingly moulded itself into an advocacy group seeking to promote the 'profession' and guard 'professional interests'. However, active members tend to be drawn mainly from urban areas. The bulk of rural traditional health practitioners remain relatively unorganised as they operate individually.

Third, training. The government has occasionally organised training sessions (usually seminars and workshops) for traditional health practitioners where it disseminates information on specific health issues such as the anti-HIV/AIDS campaigns. In most cases, the traditional health practitioners do not just passively receive information from the government but occasionally take the opportunity to express their concern in the training sessions.

Setbacks

Traditional medicine as a viable healthcare option faces a number of setbacks in Kenya. These setbacks, which range from policy, legal issues to attitudes, are outlined below.

First, the administrative separation of traditional and modern medicine. Traditional medicine is placed in the Department of Culture in the Ministry of Culture, Social Services, Gender and Sport, while modern medicine is placed in the Ministry of Health. This remains a major obstacle to cooperation between the two sectors, and consequently prevents the development of a coordinated and integrated health care system. What is going on between the two unrelated ministries is difficult to harmonise. This has led to major discrepancies in health policy formulation relating to the traditional health care sector. The fact that the personnel in the Ministry of Health are mainly diehard biomedics bent on seeing traditional medicine through a biomedical lens while those in the Ministry of Culture view traditional medicine through a cultural lens makes the harmonisation of issues concerning traditional medicine difficult. While traditional medicine is valued in the Ministry of Culture mainly as a cultural heritage, the Ministry of Health may want to see it from a purely medical aspect. Finding a meeting point for these two perspectives on the traditional medical sector and the formulation of appropriate health policy is primarily a governance challenge in the health care system.

Second, there is an aura of mystery and secrecy surrounding traditional health care. Also, secrecy may be understandable as a way in which traditional health practitioners guard their valuable health care knowledge on which their families depend. It has contributed to modern health practitioners finding it difficult to accept traditional medicine. As a result, many modern health practitioners have difficulties accepting religious, magical or cultural beliefs often associated with traditional medical practice. The modern health practitioners perceive these beliefs to be contrary to sound medical science, and for some, their Christian religious conscience. Thus, the association of traditional medical practice and traditional medicine in general with witchcraft and sorcery as well as the continued marginalisation of the entire sector constitutes a major setback to the utilisation of traditional medicine in Kenya.

Third, there is the lack of evidence. In spite of the acknowledgement of the continued utilisation of traditional medicine, its effectiveness in the management of various health problems is not documented. As such, the utilisation of traditional medicine continues to depend on undocumented testimonies of patients often spread through social networks.

Fourth, there is the low level of education. Most traditional health practitioners have a low level of formal education. They received their training through informal means and apprenticeship. As such, most of their knowledge is not documented, nor their practices. This poor educational level has led to poor record keeping. Furthermore, most of them have no or little formal training in basic health issues.

Fifth, the government has failed in its regulatory role. This is evidenced by the lack of adequate supervision and control of the activities of the traditional health practitioners. This has resulted in the sector being entered by quacks. This is particularly in urban areas where these healers enjoy anonymity. In this context, the clients are forced to depend on self-made claims, which may have little practical backing. Some give imagined testimonies of people whom they had previously successfully healed. This issue adds to our concern for quality care even in the context of traditional medicine. In the serious matters of health, traditional health practitioners should not be allowed to operate freely. The Association of Herbalists, which would act as a regulatory body, has no legal powers to enforce discipline among its members. As such errant members get away with malpractices.

Conclusion

The traditional health system and traditional practitioners continue to operate freely and with little control and supervision from the state. Such free operation makes traditional medical practice open to abuse by quacks bent on cashing in on the desperate patients. It is therefore clear that the state and the government in particular has failed to provide stewardship to the traditional health care sector. This has resulted in poor quality of services in the sector. Nevertheless, this paper concludes that although the traditional health care sector is peripheral in overall health care in Kenya, it is emerging as a significant alternative that requires proper governance approaches.

Policy Recommendations

The following policy recommendations are intended to improve the governance of indigenous health care systems.

Legal and Regulatory Framework

The fact that many people still use traditional medicine alongside modern medicine demonstrates the need for the promotion of traditional health care. Furthermore, as a way of reducing apprehension among traditional health practitioners that they will lose their standing, there is a need to legalise their medical knowledge and discoveries through patenting. This will encourage traditional health practitioners to share their often secretive medical knowledge for the benefit of many in the society. It is therefore necessary to incorporate and implement policies and legislation governing intellectual property rights and the sharing of rewards derived from traditional medicine. Hence, a legal framework for professional health care practice among traditional health practitioners needs to be put in place as a mechanism to guard against malpractices and enhance fair play.

Quality and Safety Control

Traditional healers need to be trained in the processing and storage of medicines to minimise the dangers to which patients are exposed through the use of traditional medicine. Quality control mechanisms would ensure the safety of the medicines. This can be attained through the acquisition of appropriate drug processing and storage facilities, which few traditional health practitioners currently enjoy.

Governance Structures

In order to promote the governance of traditional medicine there is a need for some organisational and structural changes. One problem is that traditional medicine at present falls under the Ministry of Gender, Sports, Culture and Social Services (Department of Culture), while all other aspects of health care are under the Ministry of Health. For better management of health care provision, there is a need to bring all health issues, including traditional health care, under the Ministry of Health. In addition, the finance mechanisms disadvantage traditional health practitioners in that various health care financing schemes (whether private or public) such as private health insurance and National Health Insurance Funds do not cover health services provided by traditional health practitioners. There is a need for employers to consider including traditional health practitioners in their medical schemes. This would enable their employees to obtain support from their employers or health insurance for medical costs incurred for treatments by traditional health practitioners.

The Need for Cooperation

Governance strategies should aim at promoting cooperation between traditional and modern health practitioners. Since patients consult traditional and modern health practitioners, there is a need for the practitioners of both forms of health care to cooperate for the benefit of patients and the improvement of health care in general. Such cooperation can take the form of cross referral of patients, exchange of information on illnesses, and techniques of investigation. The cross referral of patients that already exists (though on a small scale) is a step in this direction.

References

Beck, A., 1971, *Medicine, Tradition and Development in Kenya 1920-1970*, Massachusetts, Crossroads Press.

Chavundika, G. L., 1994, *Traditional Medicine in Modern Zimbabwe*, Mount Pleasant, Harare, University of Zimbabwe Publications.

Evans-Pritchard, E. E., 1937, *Witchcraft, Oracles and Magic among the Azande*, Oxford, Oxford University Press.

Foster, G. M., 1976, 'Disease Aetiologies in Non-western Medical Systems', *American Anthropologist*, 78, pp. 773-782.

Good, C. M., 1987, *Ethnomedical Systems in Africa: Patterns of Traditional Medicine in Rural and Urban Kenya*, New York, Guildford Press.

Green, E. C. and Makhubu L., 1984, 'Traditional Healers in Swaziland: Toward Improved Cooperation between the Traditional and Modern Health Sectors', *Social Science and Medicine*, (18), pp. 1071-1079.

Jansen, John, 1978, *The Quest for Therapy in Lower Zaire*, Berkeley, University of California Press.

KDHS, 1998, *Kenya Demographic Health Survey, 1998*, Nairobi, Government Printer.

KDHS, 2003, *Kenya Demographic Health Survey, 2003*, Nairobi, Government Printer.

Kimani, V. N., 1981, 'Attempts to Coordinate the Practices of Traditional and Modern Doctors in Kenya', *Social Science and Medicine*, 15B, pp. 40-45.

Kimani, V., 1995, African Traditional Health Care: The Place of Indigenous Resources in the Delivery of Primary Health Care in Four Kenyan Communities, PhD Thesis, Department of Community Health, University of Nairobi.

Last, M. and Chavundika, G. L., eds., 1986, *The Professionalisation of African Medicine*, Manchester, Manchester University Press.

Ngetich, K., 2004, 'The Utilization of Traditional and Modern Medicine in the Urban Settings: A Case Study of Nairobi City', PhD Dissertation, Kenyatta University.

Nyamwaya, D., 1992, *African Indigenous Medicine: An Anthropological Perspective for Policy Makers and Primary Health Care Managers*, Nairobi, African Medical Research Foundation.

Nuyens, Y., 1988, 'Health Systems Research in the WHO Global Strategy for Health for All', in *Methods and Experience in Planning Health: The Role of Health Research Systems*, Götenborg, Nordic School of Public Health Report, No. 4, pp. 50-70.

Owour, C., 1999, 'The Position of Traditional Medicine in Health Care Delivery: The Kenya Case', *Mila*, 4, pp. 27-36.

Pearce, T.O., 1982, 'Integrating Western Orthodox and Indigenous Medicine', *Social Science and Medicine*, 16, pp.:1611-1617.

Rappaport, H. and Rappaport M., 1981, 'The Integration of Scientific and Traditional Healing', *American Psychologist*, 36 (2), pp. 774-781.

Republic of Kenya, 1996, *National Development Plan 1997-2001*, Nairobi, Government Printer.

Rivers, W. H. R., 1924, *Medicine, Magic and Religion*, New York, Harcourt Brace Press.

Roberts, C., 1979, '*Mungu na Mitishamba*: Illness and Medicine Among the Batabwa of Zaire', Doctoral Dissertation, University of Chicago.

Sindiga, I., 1995, 'Traditional Medicine in Africa: An Introduction', in I. Sindiga, C. Nyaigoti-Chacha and M. Kanunah, eds., *Traditional Medicine in Africa*, Nairobi, East African Educational Publishers, pp. 1-15.

Tinga, K., 1998, 'Cultural Practice of the Midzichenda at Crossroads: Divination, Healing, Witchcraft and the Statutory Law', *Afrikanische Arbeitpapiere (AAP)*, 55, pp. 3-184.

Twumasi, P., 1984, *Professionalisation of Traditional Medicine in Zambia*, Nairobi, IDRC.

Unschuld, P. U., 1976, 'Western Medicine and Traditional Healing Systems: Competition, Cooperation or Integration?', *Ethic in Science and Medicine*, 3, p. 1-20.

Warren, D. M., 1974, 'Bono Traditional Healers', in Z. A. Ademunwagun, J. A. Ayoade, I. E. Harrison, eds., *African Therapeutic Systems*, Los Angels, Crossroads Press, pp. 120-124.

WHO, 1985, *Report of the Consultation on Approaches of Policy Development for Traditional Practitioners, Including Traditional Birth Attendants*, Geneva, WHO Publications.

WHO and UNICEF, 1978, Alma Ata: Primary Health Care. *Report of the International Conference on Primary Health Care*, Alma Ata, USSR, 2-6 September 1978, Geneva, WHO.

WHO, 2002, *WHO Traditional Medicine Strategy 2002-2005*, Geneva, WHO.

Yoder, P. S., 1982, 'Biomedical and Ethnomedical Practice in Rural Zaire', *Social Science and Medicine*, 16, pp. 851-1857.

Young, A., 1975, 'Magic as a Quasi-Profession: The Organization of Magic and Magical Healing Among Amhara', *Ethnology*, 14, pp. 245-265.

Young, A., 1983, 'The Relevance of Traditional Medical Culture to Modern Primary Health Care', *Social Science and Medicine*, 17 (16), pp. 1205-1211.

4

Corruption et crise des hôpitaux publics à Douala: le schémas d'une organisation tripolaire

Victor Bayemi

Introduction

Depuis la fin des années 1980, le système public de santé au Cameroun en général et à Douala en particulier, est confronté à une grave crise hospitalière qui a conduit à de profondes réformes. L'analyse des causes a conduit à la mise en relief d'une multitude de facteurs expliquant la décadence du système hospitalier par une politique sanitaire inadaptée qui, à travers la baisse de plus de 50% des salaires des personnels médical et paramédical et les mauvaises conditions de travail, a privilégié la faible productivité du travail. D'autres analyses ont mis en cause la rareté des ressources en soulignant qu'à Douala, il y a seulement: 1 médecin pour 7 023 habitants, 1 infirmier pour 1 784 habitants, 1 pharmacie pour 55 016 habitants. D'autres encore mettent l'accent sur l'iniquité du système dans la mesure ou les pauvres ont difficilement accès aux services de base et que les soins offerts sont de piètre qualité (Ministère de la Santé publique 2001).

A ces facteurs pertinents, il nous semble indispensable d'ajouter, pour une bonne compréhension de la crise des hôpitaux publics, la corruption comme une variable explicative essentielle.

En effet, depuis que le Cameroun a été classé, successivement en 1998 et 1999, au premier rang des pays les plus corrompus du monde, par l'ONG Transparency international, les dirigeants de ce pays ont pris conscience du fait que la corruption a élu domicile dans leurs administrations. Cependant, ces autorités ignorent l'organisation de la corruption qui prévaut dans ces administrations et, en particulier, dans le système public hopitalier.

À la suite de Rose-Ackerman (1978), la plupart des études [Shleifer et Vishny (1993), Cartier Bresson (1998)] soulignent que l'organisation des échanges de corruption peut être centralisée ou décentralisée. Dans le premier cas, les acteurs acceptent une règle de jeu préétablie et le corrupteur qui verse une fois le pot de vin est sûr d'être servi. Dans le second cas, pour le même service demandé, l'usager peut donner plusieurs fois le pot de vin, sans l'assurance d'être servi. L'échange peut même être anarchique et caractérisé par les marchandages permanents (les montants instables).

Ces études sont importantes car elles montrent que la corruption centralisée est moins dommageable que la corruption décentralisée. Leur limite est due au fait qu'elles ne prennent pas suffisamment en compte les liens qui existent entre les pratiques de corruption dans le secteur public et le fonctionnement non seulement du secteur privé mais aussi du secteur informel.

L'objet de ce papier est d'étudier l'organisation de la corruption dans les hôpitaux publics de Douala et son impact sur l'allocation des ressources.

Plus précisément, dans un premier temps, en s'appuyant sur les entretiens effectués auprès des personnels des hôpitaux publics de Douala et sur les apports du modèle de monopole, nous allons montrer qu'à la suite de la baisse drastique des salaires, les médecins de ces hôpitaux ont changé de comportement à travers trois phénomènes:

- la perception des pots de vin;
- le transfert des patients de l'hôpital public vers l'hôpital privé;
- le transfert des malades de l'hôpital public vers le centre informel de santé.

Ces phénomènes sont à la base d'une organisation tripolaire de la corruption.

Dans un deuxième temps, nous analyserons les effets de cette organisation sur l'offre et la demande des soins de santé.

L'organisation tripolaire de la corruption

Nous allons construire un circuit de corruption où un médecin, en situation de monopole, fait face à une multitude de malades dans trois pôles: l'hôpital public, l'hôpital privé et le centre informel de santé. Avant de décrire le comportement de ce médecin face aux patients dans chacun de ces pôles, nous allons d'abord discuter des hypothèses qui fondent cette organisation.

Les hypothèses de l'organisation

Nous distinguons trois hypothèses. Les deux premières sont relatives au comportement du médecin et la dernière concerne la stratégie des patients dans le choix de l'établissement sanitaire où ils doivent se soigner.

Dans la première hypothèse, nous supposons que nous avons à faire à un médecin en situation de monopole vis à vis des patients. Il a un pouvoir discrétionnaire qui lui permet de s'absenter de l'hôpital public et d'aller soigner les patients soit dans un hôpital privé, soit dans un centre informel de santé à des heures où contractuellement. Il devrait être présent à son poste de travail de l'hôpital public. En clair, il peut réduire l'offre de travail (Shleifer et Vishny 1993) sans être inquiété par la hiérarchie.

Cette hypothèse est restrictive dans deux cas. Premièrement, si le directeur de l'hôpital public veille au respect des lois et règlements en vigueur et, en particulier, à l'obligation de l'employé à venir à temps au lieu de service et à être présent à son poste pendant la durée officielle du travail. Cependant, elle devient réaliste, dans le cas où le directeur est laxiste ou joue de complicité avec le médecin. Deuxièmement, elle est restrictive si la pression populaire (Rijckeghem et Weder 1997) s'oppose à la corruption. Mais, à Douala, nous supposons que cette pression est faible.

La deuxième hypothèse est qu'à son poste de travail de l'hôpital public, le médecin a la possibilité de détourner les malades en les conseillant d'aller plutôt se faire soigner, soit à l'hôpital privé soit au centre informel de santé. Ce conseil est d'autant plus suivi que le médecin a un monopole informationnel sur le patient. « Dans les services médicaux, les discussions entre le patient et le médecin sont telles que ce dernier possède généralement un niveau de connaissances des problèmes immédiats (diagnostics et traitement) sensiblement plus grand. De plus, l'incitation à délivrer l'information n'est pas la même chez le médecin que chez le patient. Celui-ci veut visiblement informer le médecin, mais ce dernier n'a pas la même attitude. L'Obligation professionnelle, l'éthique et la responsabilité personnelle devraient amener le médecin à se montrer ouvert et honnête. Cependant, la simple motivation du profit peut le conduire à se comporter autrement. Pour dire les choses simplement, le médecin a la possibilité de tromper son patient et, ce faisant, de lui soutirer davantage d'argent » (Charles Phelps 1995).

Dans la troisième hypothèse, nous supposons que chaque patient part d'abord de chez lui pour se soigner à l'hôpital public. Lorsqu'il ne trouve pas la guérison dans cet hôpital, il va se faire soigner soit au privé soit à l'informel. Graphiquement, cet itinéraire thérapeutique est le suivant:

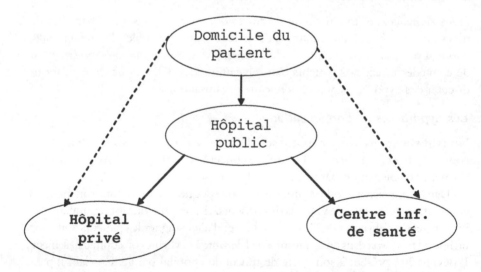

Cet itinéraire est restrictif dans la mesure où le patient peut partir de chez lui pour le centre informel de santé ou pour l'hôpital privé sans passer par l'hôpital public. Mais, en supposant que le patient cherche à bénéficier des prix moins élevés devant être pratiqués à l'hôpital public comparativement à ceux pratiqués ailleurs, il va d'abord dans celui-ci.

Une fois que ces trois hypothèses sont vérifiées, le médecin affiche un comportement que nous allons décrire à chaque pôle.

Le comportement du médecin dans les trois pôles

Nous allons décrire le comportement du médecin selon qu'il se trouve au privé, au public ou au centre informel de santé.

Le premier pôle: le médecin à l'hôpital public

La baisse drastique des salaires a poussé les médecins de Douala à adopter des attitudes relatives aux deux premières hypothèses. Le pouvoir discrétionnaire dont jouit le médecin lui permet de collecter les pots-de-vin auprès des patients en contrepartie des soins de santé offerts. À Douala, les pratiques de corruption se révèlent dans la quasi-totalité des services publics hospitaliers (Bernard Hours 1985). On peut distinguer ces pratiques selon qu'il s'agit de la radiologie, des examens de laboratoires, de la pharmacie, de la vente des médicaments et, enfin, des consultations.

Dans la radiologie et le laboratoire, la pratique la plus courante consiste à faire croire au patient que le service ne possède plus de consommables ou que les machines sont en panne. Les techniciens de la radiologie ou ceux du laboratoire lui suggèrent alors le paiement d'une certaine somme afin d'obtenir par exemple un film pour la radio ou un réactif pour le laboratoire. Les patients qui ne passent pas par ces circuits subissent des retards dans la réalisation de leurs examens de santé. Les consommables achetés pour les centres hospitaliers et auxquels les patients devaient accéder aux prix officiels, sont plutôt revendus à des prix plus élevés que ces derniers au profit des agents corrompus.

Concernant la pharmacie, la vente abusive des remèdes peut se manifester au moins de deux façons. Dans le premier cas, il y a des médecins qui vendent des échantillons médicaux. Pourtant, Il s'agit des remèdes qui leurs sont offerts, a titre publicitaire ou d'expérimentation, par des délégués médicaux et qui devraient être donnés gratuitement aux patients. Deuxièmement, suite à la consultation du patient, certains praticiens cupides (Vito Tanzi 1998) faussent souvent le diagnostic et, partant, la prescription médicale dans le but d'écouler leurs propres remèdes. À leur poste de travail, ils prescrivent des remèdes qu'ils possèdent et les vendent aux malades.

Pour ce qui est de la consultation, le principe veut que le droit d'être consulté soit payé à la caisse à un montant officiel connu de tous. Dans la réalité, on distingue au moins deux pratiques différentes de ce principe. Premièrement, certains médecins exigent que les malades leur versent une somme additionnelle en plus du paiement du droit officiel à la consultation. Deuxièmement, d'autres exigent que chaque malade leur verse une somme irrégulière et ne cherchent pas à savoir si le malade s'est acquitté du versement de la somme officielle demandée à cet effet. C'est ces deux cas de corruption que Shleifer et Vishny (1993) appellent respectivement corruption sans vol et corruption avec vol.

Par ailleurs, à partir de son poste de l'hôpital public, le médecin peut inviter certains patients à le rencontrer dans un centre informel de santé.

Le second pôle: le médecin au centre informel de santé.

Soit un centre informel de santé qui est une propriété du médecin. Un tel centre est souvent situé au domicile de son propriétaire. Les soins de santé y sont offerts en contrepartie d'un paiement fixé par le médecin. Ces soins sont donnés de manière informelle dans la mesure où le propriétaire n'a pas l'autorisation d'ouverture d'un tel centre.

Dans ce centre, le médecin travaille, souvent, à des heures où contractuellement il devrait occuper son poste au sein de l'hôpital public. En le faisant, le médecin utilise pour son propre compte une partie du temps de travail contractuel avec l'État. Le domicile du médecin devient premièrement un lieu où se donnent des soins autrefois dispensés uniquement à l'hôpital, et deuxièmement, un lieu où se rencontrent diverses personnes dont on peut déterminer les responsabilités: une infirmière embauchée par le centre informel et qui seconde le médecin, un ou plusieurs membres de la famille de la personne malade dont le rôle est d'assister cette dernière (Eric Gagnon 2001). Mais, en dehors du centre informel de santé, le détournement des patients peut se faire au profit de l'hôpital privé.

Le troisième pôle: le médecin à l'hôpital privé

Contrairement au centre informel de santé, l'hôpital privé est un établissement formel reconnu comme tel par les pouvoirs publics et en particulier par le Ministère de la Santé. Juridiquement, les soins offerts au centre informel de santé sont illégaux contrairement à ceux du privé.

Du fait du transfert des responsabilités des services publics vers les services privés, cet hôpital apparaît comme un pôle actif dans l'organisation de la corruption.

En effet, sans courir les risques de sanction, à certaines heures de la journée, le médecin de l'hôpital public peut s'absenter de son lieu de travail et aller servir les patients dans un établissement privé. Dans ce dernier, il est payé généralement au prorata du nombre de patients qu'il soigne; il a donc intérêt à soigner un nombre élevé de malades. Pour accroître la quantité de patients soignés, le médecin a intérêt à détourner un nombre important de malades de l'hôpital public vers l'hôpital privé.

Le comportement du médecin qui soigne à domicile est différent de celui du médecin qui soigne dans un hôpital privé car, à domicile, il gère tous les paiements effectués par les malades en tant que propriétaire du centre, alors qu'à l'hôpital privé, c'est des employés qui gèrent les sommes d'argent que versent les patients.

Le propriétaire de l'hôpital privé paie l'impôt à l'opposé de celui du centre informel. Le dénominateur commun à ces trois pôles est que les actes de corruption qui s'y déroulent sont effectués par le même acteur principal à savoir le médecin de l'hôpital public. En détournant les patients de l'hôpital public au profit de l'hôpital privé ou de son domicile, le médecin utilise abusivement, pour son compte propre, la charge publique qui lui est confiée. Cette organisation de la corruption qui passe par l'hôpital public, l'hôpital privé et le centre informel de santé n'affecte pas de la même façon les différents acteurs qui sont: les médecins, les patients et les hôpitaux privés et publics.

Les effets de l'organisation tripolaire de la corruption

L'organisation de la corruption que nous venons de décrire révèle, pour le patient, trois confusions: entre la caisse de l'hôpital public et celle du médecin, entre l'hôpital public et l'hôpital privé formels et enfin entre l'hôpital public et le centre informel de santé. En mettant en relief ces différentes confusions, nous analyserons en même temps leurs effets respectifs sur les acteurs du domaine de la santé.

Premier effet: Une confusion entre la caisse de l'hôpital public et celle du médecin. Au Cameroun, il est courant de distinguer le trésorier de l'hôpital public du médecin. Le premier a pour rôle d'encaisser les paiements des actes médicaux alors que le second est là pour consulter et traiter les malades. Cette distinction repose essentiellement sur la répartition professionnelle des tâches que chaque acteur doit accomplir.

Or avec les changements que nous venons de décrire au premier pôle, cette distinction devient inopérante notamment dans le cadre de la corruption avec vol. Désormais les médecins perçoivent des pots-de-vin en contrepartie des soins offerts et les patients ne versent plus rien dans les caisses de l'hôpital public. Pour le patient, il y a confusion entre la caisse de l'hôpital et celle du médecin.

Par contre, cette confusion est moindre dans le cas de la corruption sans vol car, pour un acte médical demandé, le patient paie d'abord la somme exigée par l'hôpital public et ensuite le montant demandé officieusement par le médecin. Auprès du trésorier de l'hôpital public, le versement des sommes se fait en contrepartie d'un reçu qui atteste que le patient a effectivement payé.

Dans plusieurs hôpitaux publics de Douala, à l'instar de l'hôpital Laquintinie et l'hôpital Deido, les médecins chefs ont mentionné sur les tableaux d'annonces à l'intention des usagers: « payer à la caisse ». Par cette mention, les dirigeants de ces hôpitaux demandent aux malades de ne pas verser de l'argent dans les caisses officieuses des médecins. Le patient qui verse une somme irrégulière au médecin ne reçoit pas en contrepartie un reçu de versement. La distinction entre le versement effectué auprès du trésorier de l'hôpital et celui effectué auprès du médecin repose essentiellement sur l'existence ou non de ce reçu de versement. La confusion entre la caisse de l'Etat et celle du médecin cause beaucoup de tord aux patients et quelque avantage au médecin.

Pour le médecin qui se situe du côté de l'offre de la corruption, l'opportunité de perception des pots-de-vin permet un accroissement des revenus personnels. Toutes choses étant égales par ailleurs, le pouvoir d'achat augmente et le médecin peut retrouver le niveau de vie qui était le sien avant la baisse les salaires. Lafay (1990) déclare que: « certaines formes de corruption peuvent être un moyen de contourner des règles inutilement contraignantes, d'éviter des pénuries, d'atténuer les conséquences de décisions politiques inadéquates ou même d'attirer des fonctionnaires efficaces (en leur permettant d'obtenir un complément de leur salaire officiel) ».

Si on considère que le fait de diminuer de plus de 50% les salaires au Cameroun est une décision politique inadéquate, on peut penser que les sommes irrégulières que les médecins perçoivent à Douala, en contrepartie des soins médicaux permettent d'atténuer les effets pervers de cette décision: « si le gouvernement a pris une mauvaise décision, la voie ouverte par la corruption peut bien se révéler meilleure » (Leff 1964). Cependant, les cas de corruption socialement désirables sont vraisemblablement très limités, car l'avantage précédent s'accompagne souvent des coûts encore plus importants.

En effet, pour les patients, l'accès aux soins de santé nécessite désormais plus de dépenses qu'auparavant, dans la mesure où ils doivent payer le prix officiel des soins auprès du trésorier sans oublier la somme irrégulière à verser auprès du médecin (corruption sans vol). Pour le patient, le non-versement d'un pot-de-vin au médecin peut causer l'accès tardif ou le non-accès aux soins médicaux. La hausse de prix ne permet plus à certains habitants et, en particulier, aux démunis, de se soigner. L'état de santé des plus pauvres se détériore.

Du côté du trésor public, la hausse des prix des soins médicaux entraîne la diminution des recettes dans la mesure où, du fait de la hausse des prix, certains malades évitent désormais de se soigner à l'hôpital public. Cette réduction des revenus détériore, en retour, la qualité des services publics offerts (Bearse, Glomn et Janela 2000). Les usagers évitent d'acheter les services de mauvaise qualité réduisant ainsi les recettes de l'État et l'habilité du gouvernement à offrir des services publics de qualité (Gupta, Davoodi, et Tiongson 2000).

Deuxième effet: une confusion entre le public et le privé formels
Cet effet résulte du fait que le malade qui va se soigner à l'hôpital public est détourné de celui-ci au profit du privé. Au Cameroun, comme partout ailleurs, on distingue généralement l'hôpital public de l'hôpital privé par le fait que le premier a pour objectif de favoriser l'accès de la majorité des populations aux soins de santé alors que le second a un but lucratif et vise surtout à soigner ceux des malades qui ont un pouvoir d'achat élevé. Cette distinction repose essentiellement sur une vision d'intérêt général par opposition à l'intérêt privé.

Compte tenu des changements que nous venons de décrire au troisième pôle, cette distinction n'est plus pertinente pour deux raisons au moins. Premièrement, au sein de l'hôpital public, le fait que le médecin demande aux patients d'aller se faire soigner au privé [alors qu'il aurait pu les soigner, à bas prix, dans l'hôpital public] atteste le transfert de responsabilités du public vers le privé. Deuxièmement, à partir du moment où le prix du soin médical comprend le prix officiel et le pot-de-vin, les prix pratiqués dans les hôpitaux publics peuvent égaler et même dépasser ceux des hôpitaux privés. Pour les patients, les différences de prix entre le public et le privé, qui les attiraient vers le premier tendent à disparaître. Il y a confusion entre le privé et le public.

Le secteur privé contribue à la diminution du nombre de patients devant se soigner dans le secteur public et à l'expansion de la corruption grâce au poste de travail qu'il offre au médecin de l'hôpital public et qui conduit parfois ce médecin non seulement à abandonner le public au profit du privé, mais aussi à détourner les malades du public au profit du privé. La corruption n'est plus seulement connectée au secteur public, mais aussi au secteur privé (Vito Tanzi 1998). En dehors de la confusion qu'on observe entre le public et le privé formels, le brouillage peut aussi naître entre le public et l'informel.

Troisième effet: une confusion entre le secteur public et le secteur informel
Au Cameroun, il est courant de distinguer les soins formels des soins informels de santé. Les soins formels sont offerts par les établissements officiels publics ou privés alors que les soins informels sont donnés par les établissements officieux. Les établissements d'offre de soins formels sont supposés avoir rempli les conditions réglementaires imposées par les pouvoirs publics à tous ceux qui veulent obtenir une autorisation d'ouverture d'un tel établissement. Il s'agit non seulement de disposer de moyens matériels et humains permettant de faire fonctionner un centre de santé, mais aussi de payer l'impôt.

Les usagers sont généralement sûrs de la compétence des personnels qui travaillent dans les établissements formels, car on suppose que ces établissements remplissent les conditions d'ouverture imposées par les pouvoirs publics. Au contraire, des établissements informels caractérisés par le non-respect de la réglementation en vigueur n'offrent pas de garantie aux usagers. Par conséquent, aux yeux des patients, la compétence des personnels médicaux qui travaillent dans les établissements informels est généralement douteuse. La distinction entre l'informel et le formel repose finalement sur le respect ou non de la loi et de la réglementation en vigueur et, en particulier, les conditions d'ouverture d'un établissement de santé. Cette différentiation est souvent utilisée par les chercheurs pour séparer le formel de l'informel.

À Douala, le fait que le médecin de l'hôpital public travaille à la fois à l'hôpital public et au centre informel, et le fait qu'à partir de l'hôpital public le patient est invité par le médecin à aller se soigner à l'informel rendent inopérante une distinction entre le formel et l'informel. Pour le malade, il y a confusion entre le service public et le service informel, puisqu'il peut accéder aux soins médicaux offerts par le même médecin ici ou là. Tout se passe comme si le centre informel de santé est un pavillon de l'hôpital public. Cette confusion entre l'informel et le formel affecte différemment les patients, les médecins et le trésor public.

Concernant les patients, les effets se révèlent à deux niveaux: d'abord, le médecin devient indisponible au sein de l'hôpital public puisqu'il soigne à l'informel au moment où il devait être à l'hôpital public. Dans ce dernier, les longues files d'attente de patients se constituent pour attendre l'arrivée du médecin. Cette attente réduit l'accès des patients aux soins de santé. Ensuite, les services vendus au centre informel de santé étant lucratifs, les malades reçus payent généralement plus cher comparativement aux usagers qui sont soignés dans les hôpitaux publics sans verser les pots-de-vin.

Du côté du médecin, le mode d'intervention à l'informel entraîne deux conséquences positives. *Premièrement,* les revenus des médecins s'accroissent puisque, ce que les patients versent pour payer des soins revient directement au médecin propriétaire du centre informel. De plus, ce médecin continue à percevoir le salaire auprès du Ministère de la Santé publique. *Deuxièmement,* au sein de l'hôpital public, l'absence du médecin à son poste d'emploi oblige les patients à créer une file d'attente qui devient, pour lui, une source de revenus. À son arrivée tardive à l'hôpital, le médecin a l'opportunité de collecter les pots-de-vin auprès des patients prêts à payer un surprix pour obtenir un accès privilégié (Lui 1985).

Conclusion

Dans ce papier, nous avons analysé l'organisation de la corruption et discuté des effets de cette organisation sur les principaux acteurs du fonctionnement des hôpitaux publics de Douala. Il apparaît que la corruption prospère dans ces hôpitaux à travers un circuit qui comprend l'hôpital public, l'hôpital privé et le centre informel de santé. Le fonctionnement de ce circuit crée trois confusions chez les patients: entre la caisse officieuse du médecin et la caisse du trésorier de l'hôpital public, entre ce dernier et l'hôpital privé et enfin entre l'hôpital public et le centre informel de santé. Ces confusions affectent négativement les revenus des patients et de l'hôpital public et positivement ceux de l'hôpital privé et du médecin. Cependant, on peut se demander quel est l'effet global net de ces confusions sur le bien-être des populations de la ville de Douala? Dans la mesure où la corruption suscite l'accroissement des prix des soins médicaux, elle empêche à l'hôpital public d'accomplir sa mission qui consiste à faciliter l'accès de la majorité de la population aux soins. De plus, cette corruption interfère sur la confiance des patients vis-à-vis des hôpitaux public et la crédibilité du système d'offre publique de soins. Dans le but d'améliorer la santé des populations de Douala, il est nécessaire d'engager une réflexion profonde pour combattre l'organisation hospitalière de la corruption à Douala.

Bibliographie

Banque mondiale, 1993, *Rapport sur le développement dans le monde: Investir dans la santé*, Washington DC, USA.

Bardhan, P., 1997, 'Corruption and Development: A Review of Issues', *Journal of Economic Litterature*, Vol. 35 (September), pp. 1320-46.

Bearse, P., Glomm, G. and Janeba, E., 2000, 'Why Poor Countries Rely Mostly On Redistribution In-Kind', *Journal of Public Economics*, Vol. 75 (March), pp. 463-81.

Cartier B. J., 1998, « Les Analyses économiques des causes et des conséquences pour les PED », *Mondes en Développement*, tome 25, pp. 102-25.

Ehrlich, I., and Lui, F. T., 1999, 'Bureaucratic corruption and Endogenous Growth', *Journal of Political Economy*, Vol. 107 (December), pp. 270-93.

Gabah, I., 2001, « Les médecins acteurs dans les systèmes de santé. Une étude de cas au Burkina Faso », in *Systèmes et politiques de santé*, sous la direction de Bernard Hours. Paris, Éditions Karthala.

Gagnon, E., 2001, « Soins domestiques et services publics: une transformation de l'espace des soins au Quebec », in *Systèmes et politiques de santé*, sous la direction de Bernard Hours, Paris, Éditions Karthala.

Gruénais, M., 2001, « Communauté et État dans les systèmes de santé en Afrique, in *Systèmes et politiques de santé*, sous la direction de Bernard Hours, Paris, Éditions Karthala.

Gupta, S., Davoodi and H. Tiongson E., 2000, 'Corruption and the Provision of Health Care and Education Services', IMF Working Paper WP/00/16.

Hours, B., 1985, *L'État sorcier: santé publique et société au Cameroun*, Paris, l'Harmattan.

Huntington, S. P., 1968, *Political Order in Changing Societies*, New Haven, Yale University Press.

Jones, C. and Roemer, M. (eds), 1989, 'Modeling and Measuring Parallel Markets in Developing Countries', *World Development*, Vol. 17, 12.

Lafay, 1990, « L'économie de la Corruption », *Les Analyses de la SEDEI S.* 74, pp. 62-66.

Leff, N. H., 1964, 'Economic Development through Bureaucratic Corruption', *The American Behavioural Scientist*.

Lui, F. T., 1985, 'An Economic Queing Model of Bribery', *Journal of Political Economy*, 93, (4), August.

Medtoul, M., 2001, « Les acteurs sociaux face à la santé publique: médecins, État et usagers (Algérie) », in *Systèmes et politiques de santé*, sous la direction de Bernard Hours, Paris, Éditions Karthala.

Ministère de la Santé publique, 2001, *Stratégie sectorielle de la Santé. République du Cameroun*.

Phelps, C. E., 1995, *Les fondements de l'économie de la santé*. Nouveaux horizons.

Rose-Ackerman, S., 1978, « Une Stratégie de Réforme anti-corruption », *Mondes en Développement*, tome 26, pp. 102-41.

Rose-Ackerman, S., 1978, *Corruption: A Study in Political Economy*, New York, Academic Press.

Sam, P., 1995, *Evaluating Public Services: A Case Study on Bangadore*, India, New Directions for Evaluation, 67 (Autumn).

Schleifer, A. and Vishny, R. W., 1993, 'Corruption', *Quaterly Journal of Economics*, (August) 108 (3), pp. 599-617.

Tanzi, 1998, 'Corruption Around the World: Causes, Consequences Scope and Cures', IMF Working Paper, WP/98/63.

5

Health Sector Reforms in Kenya: User Fees

Alfred Anangwe

Introduction

Health sector reforms were introduced under the umbrella of Structural Adjustment Programmes (SAPs) implemented in the 1980s, necessitated by the debt crisis. The economic crisis was evident in the diminishing financial abilities of government to provide social services such as health and education. With or without Structural Adjustment Programmes, African governments were faced with the challenge of sourcing funds in order to continue financing social service provisioning. One of the ways of sourcing funds was located in the potential to pay by users, hence the introduction of cost sharing.

Cost sharing is variously called by such terms as user fees, co-financing, and cost-recovery. In Kenya, the introduction of user fees was the first reform in the health sector. As part of health sector reforms, cost sharing in public health facilities was meant to improve the provision of quality health care services. Funds generated from user fees would supplement government's diminishing expenditure allocated to health care services and, therefore, would ensure continued provision of health care services through supply of drugs and medical equipment, as well as in maintaining and expanding health facilities.

Health sector reforms in Kenya were tailored to meet Kenya's health sector policy goal of providing accessible, affordable and efficient health care services to all Kenyans. Before their implementation, it was feared that health reforms would marginalise the poor and vulnerable in accessing health care. However, the government of Kenya took care of this concern by introducing the system of waivers and exemptions. Under exemptions, certain categories of patients were automatically exempted from user fees. These included those seeking family planning, children under five years, sexually transmitted disease patients, and those suffering from HIV/AIDS. Exempting children under five years was in realisation of the fact that such children have a low immunity development, which predisposes them to sickness. Indeed, statistics on malaria morbidity attests to this fact, as children under five years are the most affected both in terms of morbidity and mortality.

On the other hand, waivers were supposed to take care of those who could not afford to pay for health services because of their inabilities. Waivers and exemptions were put under the care of medical staff and social workers at the hospitals who were charged with the responsibilities of assessing the financial position of patients and waiving part or all of their bills. This paper discusses the impact of health sector reforms, especially users fees, on Kenya's health policy objective of "Health for All".

Meeting Kenya's Health Policy Objectives

Over the years, Kenya's health policy was designed to achieve the following objectives:

- Increase coverage and accessibility of preventive and promotive curative health services especially in rural areas.

- Consolidate urban and rural curative and preventive/promotive health services, i.e. rural-urban referral system.

- Increase emphasis on Maternal-Child Health (MCH) and Family Planning (FP) in order to reduce morbidity, mortality and fertility through related public health education programmes.

- Strengthen the Ministry of Health's Health management capabilities, with emphasis being placed at the district level in order to take care of management problems such as facility management, drug supply, and transport and equipment maintenance.

- Increase inter-sectoral coordination between the Ministry of Health and other ministries such as agriculture, water, education, social ser-vices, information and NGOs.

- Increase alternative mechanisms for financing health care programmes.

- Improve and expand the National Health Insurance.

In pursuing the above health care objectives, the Government of Kenya targeted achievement of its long-term goal of Health for All by the year 2000 (Owino 1997). The government realised that this objective would be achieved if citizens lived within a radius of ten kilometres of the nearest health facility, and if primary and preventive health care services were extended countrywide. As a result the Government of Kenya pursued various initiatives: It constructed new health facilities in 'under-served' areas and upgraded existing ones. Grants were provided to church or mission hospitals to complement the government in providing health care services. The government made efforts aimed at ensuring that essential medical supplies and equipment were made available through the construction of depots in strategic locations. It encouraged and promoted community and NGO participation through grants for capital development. Training opportunities and career development for health personnel were expanded through the government's continuing education and on-the-job refresher and residential training programmes.

Kenya's health policy, at independence, was shaped by both historical and global factors, and was designed to achieve both political and health objectives. Many independent African countries began their lives as populist regimes (Walt 1994), and came up with populist policies. In the case of Kenya, health services were made 'free' in order to meet health needs of all Kenyans while at the same time making the government popular among the masses. In fact the introduction of 'free' medical care in government facilities was done in line with the guidelines of the Kenya African National Union's (KANU) manifesto (Odada and Ayako 1989). By then KANU was the political party, which had won elections at independence and formed government. Providing 'free' public health care services served two very important functions. One function of 'free' health care was to discontinue African experiences of the colonial past. Africans were not accorded the best health care services, as was the case with members of the European descent in the period of African colonisation. The second function was to make the government popular among the people. 'Free' health care delivery was part of the government's scheme of centralising its functions and having control and discipline over its population. The Government of Kenya designed a health care delivery system that would serve its entire population both in the rural and urban areas. The Cold War that underlined global politics at the time contributed to this situation because supplementary financing for health care could be easily obtained from foreign debts and aid depending on a country's political leaning.

Kenya's health care delivery system, which is charged with meeting health policy objectives, is organised around the Ministry of Health (MoH). The Ministry of Health headed by the Minister is charged with the responsibility of setting policies, coordinating the activities of Non-Governmental Organisations (NGOs), and managing, monitoring and evaluating policy implementation (Owino 1997). Kenya's Ministry of Health is the largest provider of health care (curative, preventive and promotive) and undertakes environmental protection and pollution surveillance (Odada and Odhiambo 1989). In general, the Ministry of Health is involved in six-health related programmes, namely promotional and preventive health care, family planning and population control, environmental protection and programme supervision, special programmes (such as disease control projects), and research. The Government of Kenya has also encouraged the plural system of health service delivery. Other providers of health care services include local authorities which, by law, are required to undertake public health activities, supported by public finance. They provide curative in-patient and out-patient care. In addition, there is a for-profit private sector, which comprises private hospitals and nursing homes and concentrates on curative services. Missions and religious groups charge fees for their curative services but much below the prices charged by the for-profit private sector. Parastatals and private companies provide curative services for their staff within their own facilities. Finally, the traditional medicine sector is often a resort of those in ill-health.

Kenya, in pursuit of its health policy, was able to achieve much in the field of health care provisioning especially in the 1960s through to the late 1980s. This was demonstrated over the years through increasing the number of, and expanding, health facilities and training medical personnel. The government dominated the provision of health care services and by 1996 'it provided 43 percent of the total sector funding and 70 percent of hospital beds of which the Ministry of Health (MOH) provided 62 percent. As a result, the government realized a decline in crude death rate from 20 per 1000 persons in 1963 to 13 in 1987, and 12 in 1991; life expectancy increased from 40 years in 1960 to 58 years in 1994; infant mortality declined from 126 per 1000 in 1962 to 60 per 1000 in 1994; and the immunization coverage rose to 70 percent in 1994 from less than 40 percent at independence in 1963' (Kenya Development Plan, 1997/2001). According to Rae et al. (1989), measles immunisation coverage increased from about 55 percent in 1982 to about 60 percent in 1987 as a result of the Kenya Expanded Programme on Immunisation (KEPI).

Declining mortality rates are some of the indicators of improvement in the health status of society (Rae et al. 1989). As the table below shows, Kenya made remarkable reductions in infant mortality rates since 1948.

Table 1: Mortality and Life Expectancy, Kenya, 1948-1987

Year	Crude death rate per 1000 population	Infant mortality rates per 1000 live births	Life expectancy at birth
1948	25	184	35
1962	20	120	44
1969	17	119	49
1979	14	104	54
1987	13	84	58

Source: Kenya Contraceptive Prevalence Survey 1984 – First Report.

In 1979 'Kenya had one doctor per 10,107 population, and this had risen to about one doctor per 7,542 in 1987 despite population growth' (Rae et al. 1989:54).

Table 2: Estimated Personnel/Population Ratio 1979-1987

Type of personnel	1979 (ratio)	1980 (ratio)	1981 (ratio)	1982 (ratio)	1983 (ratio)	1984 (ratio)	1985 (ratio)	1986 (ratio)	1987 (ratio)
Doctors	10,107	10,408	8,898	8,850	8,368	7,482	7,535	7,473	7,542
Nurses	1,144	1,142	1,138	1,107	1,058	1,039	1,038	1,009	1,004
Clinical officers	11082	10,889	10,623	10,506	10,306	10,290	10,163	10,013	9,834

Source: Rae *et al.* (1989:55).

However, constraints resulting from the debt crisis, which was evident in many developing countries in the late 1980s, curtailed government's ability to continue with its expansion of the health sector. Challenges occasioned by new diseases such as AIDS notwithstanding, the success story of the pre- SAPs began to diminish resulting from government's diminishing per capita expenditure on health. According to Owino (1997:4) the increases in nominal funding notwithstanding, Kenya's Ministry of Health's 'total and recurrent spending as a percentage of the GDP and treasury budget allocations were on the decline, which coincided with the implementation of adjustment in the early 1980s'. The story in other countries is the same. For example, in Zimbabwe it has been noted that 'child mortality figures have began to rise reversing the gains made in the previous decade as a result of declining per capita expenditure on health and the declining quality of health services' (Bijlmakers et al. 1996:14).

Faced with financial constraints, inefficiency and inequities, poor management and inappropriate pricing of services, there was a need to rethink a proper method of improving quality health care delivery. These formed the background of health sector reforms, especially cost sharing.

Rationale of Health Sector Reforms

Cassels (1995) asserts that reforms are triggered by crisis, which may be economic or political. The economic crisis of the late 1980s formed the background for Structural Adjustment Programmes (SAPs). Health sector reforms were an outcome of SAPs. Health reforms try to correct system-wide problems that hinder the delivery of priority health services (Dmytraczenko et al. 2003). Kenya introduced health sector reforms in line with its health sector policy objectives of providing affordable, accessible and efficient health services for all (Kenya Development Plan 1997/2001). The rationale of introducing health reforms was predicated on the realities of the 1980s - the debt crisis - in which the government found itself unable to continue financing health services yet at the same time was committed to achieving health for all. As a result, the government introduced cost-sharing or user fees. The user fees were intended to enable individual health facilities to meet their financial demands that would in turn make possible the provision of drugs and medical equipment. The same funds generated would also cater for those who could not afford health care. Aware that there was a poor section of the population that could not afford to meet the user fees, the government introduced a system of waivers and exemptions in order to ensure that health care was accessible to all. In general, therefore, reform policy in the health sector was in line with the general health policy as it was geared towards improving accessibility, affordability and efficiency of health services for all.

The World Bank (1992) admits that 'implementation of macro-economic adjustment policies causes various groups to become vulnerable and these include the poorest in society, the relatively scattered rural communities who have not benefited greatly from public expenditure and are facing discontinued subsidies during SAPs, and the urban dwellers who, prior to reforms, have disproportionately benefited from quality public services and subsidies like the civil servants and other middle income groups and the poorest groups'. Several scholars debated the side effects of SAPs on vulnerable and poor groups in society as early as 1989. According to Rae et al. (1989) the various components of SAPs, which fall under six broad categories, were considered to have a direct and indirect impact (positively or otherwise) on the health sector. The six SAP components were the devaluation of the Kenyan currency; cuts in government spending on social services, especially in health and education; additional taxation on mass consumption goods; the removal of price controls; the removal of subsidies on food, etc.; and improvements in public sector planning and execution.

Scholars projected possible impacts of various SAP measures outlined above on the delivery of health care services and health status of vulnerable groups. Rae et al. (1989:60-61) outlined some of them as in Table 3.

Even though SAPs entailed negative impacts on the health sector, the need to institute health reforms rested on the positive side of SAPs because waivers and exemptions, which the government would provide to the poor and vulnerable, would contain the negative effects of SAPs. As a result health sector reforms were instituted.

Health Sector Reforms in Kenya

The cost sharing programme was mooted in the 1984/88 Development Plan (MoH 1984, Owino 1997). The most forceful policy statements on user fees are contained in the Ministry of Health 1984-88 Development Plan, Seasonal Paper No. 1 of 1986, and the Ministry of Health Concept Paper of 1989 on cost-sharing. Details about overall health sector reforms are contained in the Health Policy Framework Paper (MoH 1994). These health reforms, which were to be implemented over fifteen years, included mobilising additional resources; enhancing the role and participation of the private/NGO sector in health care delivery; redefining the role of MoH in health care delivery; organisational and management adjustments; and resource reallocation.

Table 3: Possible Impacts of Various SAP Measures on the Delivery of Health Care Services and Health Status of the Vulnerable

SAP measure	Negative effect	Positive effect
Devaluation	*Rise in domestic prices of imported goods such as drugs, vehicles and medical equipment *Increase in cost of health inputs *Rise in the cost of availing safe and clean water *Fuel inflation further causing rises in prices of commodities *Placing of more burden on vulnerable groups	*Stimulation of exports hence raising incomes and employment. When poverty declines, health improves *Protective effect on domestic industries as import prices rise
Cuts in public spending	*Reduction of funds for buying drugs, vaccines and other medical supplies *Reduction in available training funds, reduced number of trained manpower and reduced access to trained health personnel *Limitation of the ability of MoH to employ more health manpower, thereby inhibiting further improvements of ratios of health manpower to population *Reduction of funds for preventive and promotional health interventions	*Reduction of government deficits and debt *Fall of rate of inflation and rise of purchasing power *Improvement of health status *Release of resources for development expenditure and capital formation for further economic growth *Benefit to vulnerable groups
Additional taxation on mass consumption goods	*Further training of the already trained will be slowed down *Welfare of poor households will be reduced	*Fall of Central government *Improvement of health status
Removal of subsidies on basic foodstuffs and other basic needs	*Reduction of access to food and increase of malnutrition *Poor Housing	*Reduction in government deficits and debt. Fall of inflation and benefit to vulnerable groups as purchasing power rises
Removal of price controls	*Cause of additional burden on vulnerable groups because of the tendency of prices to go up	*Creation of incentives for more production and employment in the medium and long term vulnerable groups benefit
Improvements in public sector planning and execution		*Increase of efficiency of health care delivery resulting in savings on resource inputs and enhancing the quality of health care services

Source: Rae *et al.* (1989:60-61).

Of all of these, health financing was identified as the key constraint to increasing the efficiency and quality of health services in the public health sector. For the same reason, reforms in the health sector were mainly focussed on developing alternative financing mechanisms to those provided by government. On the list are strategies such as increased cost recovery, social insurance, maintaining health facilities through communal fundraising efforts (the 'harambee' spirit) and community-based health care. A priority area became the introduction of user charges. The main objectives of cost-sharing were to encourage increased cost-recovery from users of public health facilities as one of the ways of mobilising additional revenue to augment the financing of the under-funded non-wage recurrent expenditure items, minimise on excessive use of services, promote functioning of the referral system, and improve access by the poor to health services by charging those who make most use of the curative care and who are most able to pay, and channelling the subsidies to those least able to pay (Owino 1997).

In August 1989, the results of the discussion on cost-sharing, which took place between the Government of Kenya and its development partners (mainly donors), were put before the Kenyan cabinet, which basically endorsed the proposed system of health financing for the public sector. The Ministry of Health expressed its fears about the introduction of user fees and complained to the World Bank that the proposed fees to be charged were high. The introduction of user fees also coincided with the introduction of multi-party politics in Kenya and this threatened the popularity of the ruling party KANU among the masses. The opposition political parties took advantage of the introduction of user fees to challenge the government's inability to provide 'free' health care services to its citizens. Generally, the government was not willing to introduce user fees and even after their introduction, revisions were continuously announced, mostly at public rallies, in order to rally the support of the masses. User fees charged on patients was deemed as low in the first instance, but the statistics regarding hospital attendance began to take a downward trend, prompting the president to intervene. The president called for a reduction from 100 to 20 Kenyan shillings per day at Kenyatta National Hospital for in-patients (Dahlgren 1990). This was done after it was realised that the utilisation of the hospital service had fallen drastically due to reasons related to affordability, and subsequently bringing to the fore the issue of accessibility. But despite all this, Ake (1996) asserts that 'Africa still lost out as it continued complaining while implementing SAPs, imposed on these societies by the World Bank and the IMF as a condition for additional extension of credit'.

A system of waivers and exemptions was provided in the new policy to address the concern that the policy could not be affordable to the vulnerable who would in turn be denied access to modern health services. Initial beneficiaries of this system included children under five years, prisoners, the destitute and the mentally handicapped, patients attending family planning, antenatal and post natal care, child welfare, sexually transmitted diseases, psychiatric illnesses, tuberculosis, leprosy, AIDS, and patients referred 'downward' or 'upward' within the Ministry of Health system.

Exemptions were also extended to civil servants including spouses and children under 22 years old. The responsibility of adjudicating the system rested with the individual facilities. Those entrusted to grant waivers included clinical officers and community nurses at the health centres, and clinical or medical officers in the case of hospitals. After the first consultation, patients were referred to the area chief or sub-chief with an exemption form for endorsement to certify the person's hardship. After this, the authorised officer issued an exemption certificate valid for a period of one year. The whole system of cost sharing with its attendant waivers and exemptions was not able to work efficiently enough to guarantee every Kenyan adequate heath care. This is based on a number of reasons as stated below.

Firstly, several changes have been made to the system of exemptions such as a rise in the exemption ages to 10 and later to 15, excluding civil servants and omitting certain diseases and categories of patients originally included. Secondly, there was limited consultation between government and stakeholders in the design of the programme, and the modalities of its implementation. Thirdly, the six-week period given for the implementation was too short to build acceptance of the policy (Mbugua 1993). Fourthly, the management and administrative structures for implementation were either not in place or inappropriate. Fifthly, funds raised during the initial period of the programme were tied up in bureaucratic obstacles or lay idle in bank deposits, instead of being used to improve the quality of health services (Owino 1993).

As a result of the above reasons the cost-sharing programme was suspended in 1990 in order to put in place institutions that would solve the administrative and management problems. The first institution was the Health Care Financing Division (HCFD), which was set up in 1991 to improve revenue generation and the utilisation of such funds. The second institution to be set up was the District Health Management Board (DHMB), in May 1992, to oversee the operations of the cost-sharing programme at the district level. Thereafter, there were fee adjustments and then the re-introduction of the cost-sharing programme in early 1992.

The management of financial resources deriving from user fees was entrusted to the Health Care Financing Division (HCFD), centrally placed under Ministry of Health headquarters. This division was in charge of controlling revenue generated from the cost-sharing programme and authorising expenditure by public health facilities (MoH 1994). HCFD was inadequately prepared to handle this immense task. In 1993, HCFD was overburdened by the additional responsibilities of strengthening the National Hospital Insurance Fund (NHIF) and rehabilitating major equipment in the health facilities, comprising eight provincial hospitals, ninety-four district hospitals, and four hundred health centres (Owino 1997a).

HCFD could not afford to carry out these responsibilities given its lean technical staff of six at the secretariat. Its performance was inadequate and this translated into deteriorating health standards in health facilities, bringing into debate the issue of quality and efficiency of health services. This time again, the 'free' media highlighted the problem. Deterioration in health services was evident in the lack of curative patient care items like drugs and laboratory reagents, poorly maintained medical equipment and buildings, and congestion (Owino 1997). It was against this background that a proposal was mooted to transfer financial management to lower levels in the health care hierarchy to strengthen and empower districts and individual health facilities in order for them to develop and build capacities in modern management and planning. The rationale was to improve organisation and decision making abilities at the local level, greater community involvement in health programmes, closer integration of the activities of the government, the NGO sector and the private sector, and reductions in red tape.

This did not, however, mean that the DHMBs were fully authorised to determine their user fees and implement them. They were required only to propose budgets and forward them to the HCFD for approval. The result was that it took too long for the HCFD to respond to individual proposals and this resulted in individual facilities implementing their proposed, but yet to be approved, changes. This translated into increases in fees beyond the reach of the poor. Corruption led to further deteriorating conditions of the health facilities because the money raised from user fees for improving the quality of health services ended up in the pockets of individuals, thereby impacting on efficiency. This further put Kenya's health policy objective into question as well as the rationale of health sector reforms. Studies on user fees have provided empirical evidence for the negative impact of user fees on the poor and vulnerable.

Impact of Health Reforms on the Poor and Vulnerable

Bijlmakers (2003:104) asserts that 'the effects of user fees on clinic attendance in low-income countries have been documented extensively in the international literature'. Studies undertaken during the early years of the introduction of user fees give different results of the impact of user fees on hospital attendance. There are studies which have documented major and long-lasting declines in the use of health services as a result of users fees (Waddington and Enyimayew 1989, Moses et al. 1992). Others have claimed that after an initial period of decline, utilisation gradually reverted to 'normal levels' after some time (Nyonator and Kutzin 1999), or even that there was no significant decline at all (Chawla and Ellis 2000).

It has been noted that there is no universally accepted definition of the quality of health (Campbell et al. 2000). Definition is subject to perceptions of the different stakeholders – users, health care providers, health care managers – who have different perspectives of quality of care based on different dimensions in their definitions, such as availability of physical structures, adequacy of staff, technical quality of clinical care, the nature of interpersonal interaction between the provider and the user, the efficacy outcome of treatment and user satisfaction. These varying perceptions also impact on the conceptualisation of the impact of users fees on access to quality health care.

Health sector reforms are aimed at correcting system-wide problems (Dmytracsenko 2003). In the case of Kenya, 'Cost-sharing aimed at making people more responsible for their own health care by sharing in the cost of the services they received' (Quick and Musau 1994). Ngugi (1995), Mwabu (1992) highlight the rationale for the introduction of cost sharing which was to relieve the government of the financial burden of providing public health services. Cost sharing mobilises resources to supplement government contributions so as to improve the quality of services provided.

Decentralisation regarding the determination of the level of user fees has led to health institutions putting their fees so high as to be beyond the ability of poor people to pay (Owino 1998, Sauer et al. 1994). The latest case of arbitrary increases in user charges took place at Kenyatta National Hospital in January 2004, in which the daily bed charges for in-patients rose from 300 to 450 Kenya Shillings, while clinic consultation charges shot up from 200 to 350 Kenya Shillings. The registration fee also went up from 150 to 200 Kenya Shillings. The question of raising fees notwithstanding, there is evidence that funds generated through user fees were diverted through corruption. According to recent internal audit reports (Nos. KNH/1A/57/51 and KNH/FIN/35) at Kenyatta National Hospital, senior management officers have defrauded the hospital of 51 million Kenya Shillings.

This sum of money was enough to buy anti-retroviral drugs for 17,000 people living with AIDS, or for building two well-equipped operation theatres to boost the already strained hospital theatres. The systems of waivers and exemptions put in place to cushion the poor are continually collapsing (Owino 1998). Since its inception, several changes have been made to the system, which have included raising the exemption ages to 10 and later to 15, excluding civil servants, and omitting certain diseases and categories of patients originally included. The collapse in the system of exemptions and waivers has had the greatest impact on the vulnerable population, especially children under five years whose immunity to common diseases like malaria is very low. For example, Kenyatta National Hospital introduced user fees for children under five in January, 2004. Children who had previously been exempted from user fees now have to pay the mandatory 200 Kenya shillings as a registration fee besides their parents meeting the costs of any further medical investigations or treatment (*Daily Nation* 2004). According to Doctor Fred Were, chairman of Kenya Paediatricians' Association, the new policy will worsen the already poor child survival rate.

The consequences of de-exempting children are already emerging at the Kenyatta National Hospital where the number of children under five years attending the hospital has gone down. Statistics indicate that there has been a drop in seeing between 300 and 500 children a day to less than 200 (*Daily Nation* 2004:25). Several studies have revealed a declining demand for public health services with the introduction of fees (Ngugi 1995, Mwabu et al. 1995, Quick et al. 1994, Kirinjia et al. 1989). Findings from these studies reveal that the introduction of user fees where none existed before may create the perception of a high percentage increase and also that the demand for health services is highly sensitive to price levels. According to Rae et al. (1988:61), 'cost-sharing through charging fees for health services at public institutions worsened the plight of the vulnerable groups'.

Experience in Zimbabwe is also telling. Bijlmakers et al. (1996:13-14) have observed that during the 1980s, infant mortality especially among children under one year of age in Zimbabwe declined from pre-independence levels of 120 to 150 per 1000 live-births, to 61 by 1990. In addition, they observed that child mortality among children one to four years also declined from 40 per 1000 in 1980, to 22 in 1990. However, there is accumulating sad evidence that mortality figures have started to rise in the 1990s, and that 'the gains made in the previous decade are being reversed'. They have attributed this to several reinforcing factors, namely: the declining per capita expenditure on health and the declining quality of health services, the drought, the HIV/AIDS epidemic and the general deterioration in the living conditions of large segments of the population. Turshen (1999) is among the outspoken opponents of user fees in Zimbabwe and has observed that Structural Adjustment Policies were, in general, designed to reduce the demand for public health services, and user fees, in particular, were a mechanism of rationing care. This assertion has been reinforced by studies conducted in Chitungwiza and Murewa Districts in Zimbabwe, which have added evidence to the existing literature on user fees and service utilisation, and bring in the dimension of quality of care to help explain the relationship between user fees, quality of care, and clinic attendance. Creese (1997) makes a very important observation, arguing that user fees have detrimental effects on health seeking by the poor and the vulnerable. He adds that user fees are a political strategy for shifting health care costs from the better off to the poor and sick and that this method of raising revenue and maintaining access to care is based on need rather than ability to pay.

The concept of stewardship as it relates to the issue of good governance demands that government should try to overcome its inadequacies in terms of enhancing responsiveness, improving and maintaining health, and assuring fairness of financial contribution (Sama 2004). According to Sama (2004), the poor emerge as receiving the worst level of responsiveness as they are treated with less respect, given less choice of service provision, and offered lower quality amenities.

Governments have failed to address the question of corruption (black market) in the health sector and this has further worsened the situation because the few funds generated from user fees end up in private pockets. Through involvement, governments can achieve good stewardship through receiving information that would help improve and correct system-wide problems in the health sector. Stewardship 'encompasses the tasks of defining the vision and direction of health policy and collecting and using information' (Sama 2004).

Conclusion and Recommendations

Studies on user fees in Kenya have shown that cost-sharing is having a negative impact on attendance at health facilities. User fees have denied access and created inequity in health care seeking. This study proposes two ways that will promote access to health by the poor and the vulnerable, namely advocacy and the expansion of the Kenya National Insurance Fund (NHIF).

The first recommendation is advocacy. Health is a human right (Committee on Economic, Social and Cultural Rights 2000) and the 'core element of the right is prevention of ill-health' (Packer 2002). The state is duty-bound to respect and protect the human rights of its people, otherwise, under the International Law, the state is held responsible for its omissions (Packer 2002). It is therefore, the recommendation of this paper that advocacy groups engage the health agenda in their activities. Advocacy in the area of health has worked under certain circumstances such as in women's reproductive health. Advocacy groups have questioned the usefulness of certain cultural practices, which have posed risks to women's health and thereby contributed to the violations of the right to health, such as female circumcision, early pregnancy, and incisions in pregnancy, some traditional birth practices and delivery taboos. Advocacy groups have opposed these practices and made some progress. Advocacy in conjunction with the media can bring desired ends in the field of health care access. An example is the Kenyan government's legislation against female circumcision, and this has gone a long way in improving women's reproductive health. In order for advocacy to be effective, those advocating must come up with a scheme that can work to ensure that all Kenyans have access to health as a basic right. One such scheme is social health insurance.

The second recommendation, therefore, is the expansion of the Kenya Health Insurance Fund (NHIF). This Fund was established in Kenya in 1968 as a social insurance fund. In its initial years it was meant to assist Government employees to gain access to higher quality private hospitals, thereby relieving congestion in the 'free' public hospitals. NHIF provided a cover for the contributors, including their families, for in-patient care in NHIF-approved hospitals. Contributions, benefits and reimbursement rates remained static until mid-1990, after which they were reviewed upwards. The importance of such a scheme has been indicated by Owino (1997) and Kraushaar and Akumu (1993), who have observed that the NHIF's potential reimbursements to public health facilities alone could increase the state's vote for preventive and primary health care funds by about 25 percent. Together with the mandatory enrolment requirement and long experience in handling third party payments for health care, the future impact of the

NHIF on financing, coverage and access to health services could be very signifi-cant. Other than the government, and despite its low population coverage, the NHIF remains the largest financier of health services, apart from direct govern-ment funding, providing approximately 50 percent of actual revenue generated from the cost-sharing programme.

All that the NHIF requires, therefore, are necessary reforms, which include broadening its functions and coverage, promoting competition, and providing an enabling environment for its operation and expansion (GoK 1995). Reforms should be targeted to solve current problems and inadequacies of the NHIF, which include provision of low benefits for in-patient care, weak administrative mechanisms, lower than expected returns on investments, poor incentive for health care providers to meet high standards of quality health, low claims at public health facilities, accumulated huge surpluses that bear no relation to the claims volume, lack of transparency in the management and accountability of funds, among others. Only a small population of Kenyans has coverage from commercial health insurance and, in its present form and structure, the NHIF covers between about 20-35 percent of the total population (that is the contributors and their dependents). The rest of the population cannot qualify for the more traditional insurance, and need to be enrolled in some flexible risk-pooling schemes. A state health insurance scheme is the only feasible insurance cover for the poor and vulnerable who cannot meet the insurance costs of private insurance companies from their pockets.

References

Ake, C., 1996, *Democracy and Development in Africa*, Washington DC, Brookings Institution.

Alam, M. M., Huque, A. S. and Westergaard, K., 1994, *Development Through Decentralization in Bangladesh: Evidence and Perspective*, Dhaka, University Press Ltd.

Anderson, J., 1975, *Public Policy Making*, London, Nelson.

Bijlmakers, L. A., Basset, M. T. and Sanders, D. M., 1996, 'Health and Structural Adjust-ments in Rural and Urban Zimbabwe', Research Report No. 101, Nordic African Institute.

Chawla, M. and Ellis, R. P., 2000, 'The Impact of Financing and Quality Changes on Health Care Demand in Niger', *Health Policy and Planning*, 15 (1), 76-84.

Creese, A., 1997, 'User Fees – They Don't Reduce Costs, and They Increase Inequity', *British Medical Journal*, 315, 202-203.

Collins, D. H., Quick, J. D., Musau, S. N. and Kraushaar, D. L. 1996, *Health Financing Reform in Kenya: The Fall and Rise of Cost Sharing, 1989-94*, Management Sciences for Health and U.S. Agency for International Development, Stubbs Monograph Series No. 1, Boston.

Dahlgren, G., 1990, 'Strategies for Health Financing in Kenya - The Difficult Birth of a New Policy', *Scandinavian Journal of Social Medicine*, Supplement 46, pp. 67-81.

Deolalikar, A. N., 1997, 'Cost and Utilization of Health Services in Kenya', Mimeo, August.

Dmytraczenko, et al., 2003, 'Health Sector Reform: How it Affects Reproductive Health', Population Research Bureau, Policy Brief.

Dunn, K., 2000, 'Tales from the Dark Side: Africa's Challenge to International Relations Theory', *Journal of Third World Studies*, Vol. XVII, No. 1, Spring 2000.

Government of Kenya (GoK), 1965, Sessional Paper No. 1 of 1965, *African Socialism and Its Application to Planning in Kenya*, Nairobi, Government Printer.

Government of Kenya (GoK), 1979, *Development Plan 1979-83*, Nairobi, Government Printer.

Government of Kenya (GoK), 1986, Sessional Paper No. 1 of 1986, *Economic Management for Renewed Growth*, Nairobi, Government Printer.

Government of Kenya (GoK), 1993, *Strategic Action Plan for Financing Health Care in Kenya*, Nairobi, Government Printer.

Government of Kenya (GoK), 1995a, *Kenya Health Policy Framework Paper*, Nairobi, Government Printer.

Government of Kenya (GoK), 1995b, *Guidelines for District Health Management Boards*, Nairobi, Government Printer.

Government of Kenya (GoK), 1996, 'Health Sector Reform Programme: Annual Summary Report', Nairobi, Health Sector Reform Secretariat (HEROS).

Gros, J., ed., 1998, *Democratization in Late Twentieth-Century Africa: Coping with Uncertainty*, Westport, CT., Greenwood Press.

Kenyatta National Hospital, Audit Reports Nos. KNH/1A/57/51 and KNH/FIN/35 2003.

Mbiti, D., Mworia, F. and Hussein, I., 1993, 'Cost Recovery in Kenya', [Letter] *Lancet*, 341, 376.

Mills, A.V., Smith, J.P., et al., 1990, *Health System Decentralization: Concepts, Issues and Country Experiences*, Geneva, World Health Organisation.

Moley, D. and Lovel, H., 1986, *My Name is Today*, London, Macmillan.

Moses, S., Manji, F., Bradley, J. E., Nagelkerke, N. J., Malisa, M. A. and Plummer, P. A., 1992, 'Impact of User Fees on Attendance at a Referral Centre for Sexually Transmitted Diseases in Kenya', *Lancet*, 340, pp. 463-466.

Mwabu, G. M., 1992, 'A Framework for Analyzing Health effects of Structural Adjustment Policies', Paper presented for Social Science and Medicine Africa Network (SOMA-NET) Nairobi, 10-14 August.

Mwabu, G. M., 1993, 'Health Sector Reform in Kenya 1963-93: Lessons for Policy Research', Paper Presented at the Conference on Health Sector Reform in Developing Counties, 10-13 September, New Hampshire, USA.

Mwabu, G. M., 1993, 'Quality of Medical and Choice of Medical Treatment in Kenya; An Empirical Analysis', Working Paper No. 9, African Technical Department, Washington DC, The World Bank.

Mwabu, G. M., 1995, 'Health Care Reform in Kenya: A Review of the Process', *Health Policy*, 32.

Mwabu, G. M. and Wang'ombe, J., 1995, 'User Charges in Kenya Health Service Pricing Reform: 1989-93', *International Health Policy Program*, Working Paper.

Mwanzia, J., Omeri, I. and Ong'ayo, 1993, 'Decentralization and Health Systems in Kenya: A Case Study', Nairobi.

Nyonator, F. and Kutzin, J., 1999, 'Health for Some? The Effects of User Fees in the Volta Region of Ghana', *Health Policy and Planning*, 14 (4), pp. 329-341.

Odada, J. E. O. and Ayako A. B., eds., 1989, Report of the Proceedings of the Workshop on 'The Impact of Structural Adjustment Policies on the Well-being of the Vulnerable Groups in Kenya', November 3-5, 1988.

Odada, J. E. O. and Odhiambo, L. O., 1989, Report of the Proceedings of the Workshop on 'Cost-sharing in Kenya', 29 March-2 April 1989.

Okwemba, A., 2004, 'KNH Raises Fees Amid Graft Claims', *Daily Nation*, 4 March 2004, pp. 23-25.

Owino, P. S. W., 1993, 'The Impact of Structural Adjustment on the Production and Availability of Pharmaceutical Products in Kenya', PhD Thesis, University of Sussex.

Owino, P. S. W., 1997, 'Public Health Sector Efficiency in Kenya: Estimation and Policy Implications', IPAR Discussion Papers.

Owino, P. S. W., 1998, 'Public Health Care Pricing Practices: The Question of Fee Adjustment', IPAR Discussion Papers.

Owino, P. S. W., 1998, 'Enhancing Health Care Among the Vulnerable Groups: The System of Waivers and Exemptions', IPAR Discussion Paper.

Owino, P. S. W. and Munga, S., 1997, 'Decentralization of Financial Management System: Its Implementation and Impact on Kenya's Health Care Delivery', IPAR Discussion Papers.

Packer, C. A. A., 2002, 'Using Human Rights to Change Tradition: Traditional Practices Harmful to Women's Reproductive Health in Sub-Saharan Africa', Utrecht University, Institute for Legal Studies.

Quick, J. D. and Musau, N. S., 1993, 'Impact of Cost-sharing in Kenya – 1989/93, Kenya Health Care Financing Project', Nairobi, Ministry of Health, Kenya.

Rae, G. O., Manandu, M., and Mondi, F. V., 1988, 'Health Care Delivery', in A. B., Ayako, and J. E. O., Odada eds., Report of Proceedings of the Workshop on the Impact of Structural Adjustment Policies on the Well-being of the Vulnerable Group in Kenya, Nairobi 3-5 November.

Rondinelli, D. A., Nellis, J. R., and Cheema, G. S., 1983, 'Decentralization in Developing Countries: A Review of Recent Experiences', World Bank Staff Working paper No. 581, Washington DC, The World Bank.

Sama, M., 2004, 'Malaria Intervention in Central Africa: A Health Systems Challenge', Paper presented at the CODESRIA's Governing African Health Systems Institute, 8 March-2 April.

Stover et al., 1996, *Report on Status and Observations on Cost-sharing: Issues in Supervision and Decentralization*, Nairobi, Ministry of Health.

Turshen, M., 1999, *Privatizing Health Services in Africa*, New Brunswick, New Jersey and London, Rutgers University Press.

Waddington, C. and Enyimayew, K. A., 1989, 'A Price to Pay: The Impact of User Charges in the Volta Region of Ghana', *International Journal of Health Planning and Management*, 5 (4), 287-312.

Walt, G., 1994, *Health Policy: An Introduction to Process and Power*, Johannesburg, Witwatersrand University Press.

World Bank, 1997, *The State in a Changing World - World Development Report*, Oxford, Oxford University Press.

6

Decentralisation of Health Care Spending and HIV/AIDS in Cameroon

Christopher Sama Molem

Background Information

As Claude Ake pointed out in 1981, 'productive forces (comprising labour power, objects of labour and means of labour) express the overall capacities of a society. They tend to develop over time. When one talks of the development of productive forces, one may be thinking of the quantitative and qualitative improvements in labour power, for instance when people acquire more scientific education and technical skills. One could be thinking of the improvement of natural assets such as the irrigation of arid land to make it arable. One could also be thinking of the development of the technology with which man produces. The importance of the development of productive forces to society cannot be overemphasized. The state of the development of productive forces decisively influences social organizations, culture, the level of welfare and even consciousness'.

Labour power comprising the physical, psychological and intellectual capabilities of people constitutes the subject matter of productive forces. Good health is a major determinant of labour power and consequently, the health sector is generally one of the most sensitive of any in the economy and usually attracts a lot of attention from governments and institutions. Improved health contributes enormously to economic growth and development in four ways: it reduces production losses caused by worker illness; it permits the use of resources that can be totally or nearly inaccessible because of disease; it increases the enrolment of children in schools and makes them better able to learn; and it frees resources for alternative use that would otherwise have to be spent on treating diseases or illnesses. This implies that good health leads to productivity gains and therefore improves the efficiency in the use of our scarce and depleting resources. Economic gains are relatively greater for poor people who are typically most handicapped by ill health and who stand to gain the most from the development of underutilised resources. Throughout Africa, the privatisation of health care has reduced access to necessary services. The introduction of market principles into health care delivery has transformed health care from a public service to a private commodity. The outcome has been the denial of access to the poor, who cannot afford to pay for private care.

The relation between economic change and health has been of interest to both social and medical scientists. Empirical studies have generally focussed on mortality or its opposite, survival, expressed as life expectancy at birth, probably because of the difficulties of collecting sound morbidity data, particularly in developing countries. Although a long-run general relation between economic and health conditions is evident in both cross-sectional and longitudinal analyses, the debate has centred on the relative importance to mortality reduction of income gains and of improvements in public health or medical technology. Most studies suggest that there is a very strong relationship between per capita income and life expectancy in the long-term (Wagstaff 2000). Historical records also show that mortality rates do respond to short-term economic fluctuations, particularly in poor and agricultural settings. The usage of health care facilities depends on the availability and accessibility of these facilities to users. The government, in most countries, plays a leading role in this regard. Existing literature also shows that the usage of health care facilities is sensitive not only to availability and accessibility alone but also to the quality of health care provided by each facility (Collier et al. 2002).

Over the past fifty years, life expectancy has improved more than during the entire previous span of human history, although the last twenty years have been ravaged by the HIV/AIDS pandemic. In 1950, life expectancy in developing countries was forty years; by 1990, it had increased to sixty-three years before dropping to below fifty-five by 2002 due to the HIV/AIDS pandemic. In 1950, twenty-eight of every one hundred children died before their fifth birthday; by 1990, this had fallen to ten (World Bank 1993). Despite these remarkable improvements, enormous health problems still remain. New fatal diseases like HIV/AIDS and to a lesser extent SARS, have surfaced; whereas old ones that were already under control like tuberculosis are reappearing. Absolute levels of mortality in developing countries remain unacceptably high. Child mortality rates are about ten times higher than those in developed countries. In addition, every year, seven million adults die of conditions that could be inexpensively prevented or cured. Surprisingly, remarkably few attempts have been made to estimate total national financing or expenditures from all sources and relate them to their various uses by all the health providers within the context of national health priorities. This study therefore is structured to answer the following questions that are essential

in evaluating the success of the decentralisation of health care spending in
Cameroon:

- Who finances health care, how much and for what?
- Are expenditures consistent with health priorities (including the fight against
  HIV/AIDS)?
- How can resources be mobilised by the health providers and are the generated
  resources used more efficiently to reduce the spread of the HIV pandemic?

Objective of the Study

The main objective of this study is to examine the effectiveness of the decentralisation of health care spending in Cameroon. Specifically the study is structured to
achieve the following minor objectives:

- Identify the respective sources of finances and the health care providers;
- Examine the changing trends in public and private health spending;
- Assess the trend and socio-economic impact of the HIV/AIDS pandemic;
- Make policy recommendation on the way forward.

Methodology

The main sources of data for this study are secondary. The data are extracted
from reports of ministries involved in health related issues. Principally, the Ministry of Public Health provides the bulk of information, and to a lesser extent, the
Ministries of Planning and Regional Development, Finance, Armed Forces, National Education, Higher Education and Social Affairs. Other relevant data, particularly on the external financing of health, are collected from the World Bank
and World Health Organisation documents.

Basic analytical tools include descriptive statistics. These are complemented by
the National Health Accounts Framework (NHA) technique. Peter Berman
developed this technique in 1997. The choice of the above methodologies is aimed
at ensuring simplicity in the analysis such that results should be more policy oriented.

Theoretical Considerations

When economic functions are shared among the various tiers of government
with each tier handling its own activities, efficiency is enhanced. Efficiency, which
is concerned with the need to finance or provide services in a way that maximises
the well-being of the people, can be divided into two, namely, allocation and
internal efficiency (World Bank 1997). Allocation efficiency, with respect to health
care, for instance, involves the pursuit of health care programmes or services
whose benefits are maximised. To be worthwhile; they must be expanded up to
the point where marginal benefit equals marginal cost. Internal efficiency, on the
other hand, deals with the avoidance of waste, which may be an aftermath of
deficient administrative or managerial resources within the production process.

Both forms of efficiency manifest themselves in the health sector in various ways. Examples of allocation inefficiency include under-funding of health services, misallocation of resources among the primary, secondary and tertiary subsectors etc., while over-centralisation of financial decision making and under-funding of specific complementary inputs like drugs, fuel, working vehicles etc., are examples of internal inefficiency (World Bank 1987). Efficiency, whether allocation or internal, covertly or overtly relates to equity. Equity deals with access to health care services, especially for the poor in society. It looks at distribution rather than the processes through which distribution is achieved. More so, it does not necessarily emphasise an equal degree of health care for everyone, rather, its emphasis is on accessibility in physical and financial terms.

The efficiency and equity arguments tend to show why decentralisation is appropriate primarily for services provided directly to people in dispersed facilities, where there are user charges for drugs and curative care. This agrees with the argument that access to improved quality of health care through effective sharing of health care functions enhances, to some degree, the performance profile of labour, which, in turn, will increase productivity for the betterment of health care delivery.

Health Problems in Developing Countries

The characteristics and performance of the health sector vary tremendously among developing countries. However, in most cases the sector faces three main problems. It is argued here that each of these problems is due in part to the efforts of the government to cover the full cost of health care for everyone from general public revenues.

The first problem concerns the allocation of insufficient spending on cost-effective health activities. Current government spending alone, even if it were better allocated, would not be sufficient to fully finance for everyone a minimum package of cost-effective health activities, including both the truly 'public' health programmes noted above and the basic curative care and referral services on health. Not enough funding goes towards basic cost-effective health services. As a result, the growth of important health activities is slowed despite the great needs of fast expanding populations to pay at least some of the costs of health care.

The second problem concerns the internal inefficiency of public programmes. Non-salary recurrent expenditures for drugs, fuel, and maintenance are chronically under-funded, a situation that often dramatically reduces the effectiveness of health staff. Many physicians cannot accommodate their patient loads, while other trained staff are not productively employed. Lower level facilities are underused while central out-patient clinics and hospitals are overcrowded. Logistical problems are pervasive in the distribution of services, equipment and drugs. The quality of government health services is often poor; clients face unconcerned or harried personnel, shortages of drugs, and deteriorating buildings and equipment.

The third problem refers to the inequity in the distribution of benefits from health services. Investment in expensive modern technologies to serve the few continues to grow while simple low cost interventions for the masses are under-funded. The better off in most countries have better access to non-governmental services, because they live in urban areas and know how to use the system. The rural poor benefit little from tax-funded subsidies to urban hospitals, yet often pay high prices for drugs and traditional care in the non-government care sector.

Decentralisation of the Health Sector in Cameroon

The decentralisation of the health sector in Cameroon has generated a lot of controversy, especially because of the concern for effective and rapid provision of health services nation-wide, given the threats of HIV/AIDS in the country.

The movement from colonial to independent state in the 1960s paved the way for Health Sector Reform in Cameroon. The colonial master, as was the case in other African countries, established health services in towns where the poor had little or no access. More so, the model of health care was purely colonial, intended to serve the needs of colonial administrators and expatriates, with separate or secondary provision made for Africans. It was characterised by the irrational distribution of health infrastructure, as hospitals were concentrated in the urban areas to the detriment of rural areas. It was also more curative than preventive oriented. Critical in the colonial period was the mobile medical team initiated by Dr Eugen Jamot to treat sleeping sickness and malaria with the aid of community members. Patients were treated on the spot and through preventive strategies. The post-independent period saw Cameroon in an experimental stage.

The DASP zone was introduced to replace the mobile team for the fight against endemic diseases with vertical programmes. Extension workers were trained and new institutions were created like the University Teaching Hospital (CHU). Although the DASP zone proved that communities were ready, to a certain de-gree, to finance health care and organise them to create village hospitals, it lacked inter-sectoral collaboration and was cost-ineffective, hence subject to revision.

For effective implementation of the decentralisation policy, the Cameroon health system adapted a pluralistic system because it was characterised by multiple sources of financing and health care providers. The main financing sources nowa-days are the government, public enterprises, and foreign aid donors. Private en-terprises, households, religious missions, NGOs, government health facilities, public enterprise health clinics, private clinics, pharmacies and drug retailers, and tradi-tional doctors are the providers of health care. It is also a vertical system in the sense that financing sources deal directly with the providers without going through intermediaries or financing agents.

The Declaration of Health Sector Policy organised health services at three levels. The Cameroonian government clearly defined the roles and functions to be performed by each tier of government in its 1990 circular letter.

The constitution stipulates that the central government should support in a coordinated manner, three sub-systems of health care. The Ministry of Health

(MOH) prepared the schedule of responsibilities assigned to the different levels in such a way as to provide effective health services at all levels. These levels are:

a) Local health centres, usually staffed by certified nurses and providing preventive and basic curative care to the surrounding population;

b) Provincial and central level hospitals providing specialised medical services;

c) District and Departmental hospitals usually staffed by at least one physician and providing first referral health services.

Co-management of the health system, linked to both decentralisation and cost recovery measures, has been promoted since June 1990 when the minister of public health signed a 'lettre circulaire' authorising the creation of community health and management committees at the village, health centre and sub-divisional levels. Health Committees (called COSA) are being established for each catchment area and will have responsibilities for planning activities and expending resources made available to the community health facilities. A subcommittee of COSA (called COGE) will be responsible for managing the funds obtained through cost recovery. At the district level, COSADI are being established with similar responsibilities.

Financing the Health System

Cameroon's public health care system is financed by the national budget, revenues from the authorities to retain the proceeds from cost recovery at the local level, and external aid.

Government Financing

The government finances health care service delivery through the use of buildings and land ceded to the Ministry of Public Works; from civil servant medical and para-medical staff salaries paid by the Ministry of Finance; and from investment and operating support provided by the Ministry of Public Health.

Overall government spending on health has never substantially exceeded five percent of the national budget (compared with the ten percent recommended by WHO) but did attain approximately US$12 per capita (35.58 billion CFAF, or eight percent of the national budget) in 1985-86. The economic crisis forced deep budget cuts in 1986-87 and 1987-88. Since 1988-89 the budget has remained selectively stable both as a percentage of the national budget and in absolute terms, while obviously declining in real terms.

Community Financing

Since 1964 all health facilities have been authorised to charge fees for services, which, except for a percentage retained by consulting physicians as incentive payments, were retained by the treasury. Laws passed in 1990 and 1992 are designed to significantly increase financial resources available to meet operating expenses.

The drug financing law of 1990 authorises public health care facilities to establish community-managed drug revolving funds through which drug sale revenues can be retained locally. The Hospital Financing Law of 1992 authorised selected tertiary-level hospitals to retain fifty percent of fee-generated revenues.

The existing system of cost recovery in Cameroon (confessional health centres, bilaterally funded projects, and private non-profit health facilities) exhibits a wide variation in the kinds and amounts of managing revenues. The fundamental issues affecting the viability of cost recovery include the availability of essential drugs, an equitable pricing policy, and common approaches for dealing with chronic under-utilisation of health services.

External Financing

The principal sources of external support for Cameroon's health sector include the traditional multilateral donors (WHO, UNFPA, UNICEF, EU) etc.; a wide range of bilateral donors, several with many years of experience in the country (Germany, USA, Belgium, and France); and a significant non-profit sector comprising both international NGOs and local confessional groups. Germany (GTZ) is involved in the development of the decentralised health districts in the South West and North West Provinces. USAID financed maternal and childcare programmes in the Adamoua and South provinces. France for its part is providing assistance in hospital management in the North and Littoral provinces.

Discussion of Results

Sources of Funds to Providers of Health Care

A matrix of the sources of funds to providers in the Cameroon NHA for the 2000/2001 fiscal year is presented in Table 1. This Table illustrates the decentralised health care spending in the country. It portrays not only the allocation inefficiency but also the internal inefficiency in the utilisation of resources at the disposal of public health care providers. Sources of financing are presented at the top, and providers on the left, of the matrix. The country's total health expenditure for that year was estimated at CFA francs 2,225,103 million - equivalent to about US $347 million. Total GDP that year stood at CFA Francs 6,320 billion (US $8.262 million). National health expenditures represented 3.3 percent of GDP, equivalent to an annual per capita expenditure of CFA francs 13,332 (US $26.7). Total public spending on health (government plus state-owned enterprises plus foreign aid) was CFA francs 665,539 million, equivalent to US $6 per capita or 0.9 percent of GDP; while private spending (households, private enterprises, and religious missions/NGOs) totalled CFA francs 1,013,820 million, equivalent to US $20.6 per capita or 2.42 percent of GDP.

Table 1: Financial Sources to Providers Matrix (in millions of CFA francs)

Providers	Ministry of Economy & Finance	State Owned Enterprises	Foreign Aid	Private Owned Enterprises	House-holds	Private Non Profit	TOTAL
Ministry of Public Health	56.3,148		38.285			55.2,172	149.8,17
Other Ministry Facilities	4.1,292				27		31.1,292
State owned Enterprise Facilities		6.0,853			1,472.5		1,478.5853
Non Profit Facilities					90.1,542	5.58	95.7,342
Pharmacies & Drug Retailers		13.3,796		12.7,255	206.5,034		232.6,085
Private - Profit Clinics		3.3,511		7.6,353	9.1,388		20.1,252
Traditional Healers					27.1,033		27.1,033
TOTAL	60.4,440	22.816	38.285	20,360.8	2,022.4	60.797.2	2,225.103

Source: Data for this core matrix was obtained from numerous sources

The Providers of Health Care

In Table 1 we observed the allocation of health spending among the various categories of providers. The most important single use of expenditure in the Cameroon health system is for drugs, which came to CFA francs 232,608 million or 88.9 percent of total household health expenditure. This Table includes the actual cost of drugs in public and private health facilities, private pharmacies, drug retail stores, as well as sales by roadside vendors. It does not include profits on drugs in public and private health facilities. Unfortunately, no information is available permitting a breakdown by facility. The amount reflects the high cost of drugs in the country, due partly to the fact that virtually all drugs are imported, and partly to major inefficiencies in the drug procurement system. These are due to the long and cumbersome administrative procedures as well as the lack of transparency in the authorisation of drug imports.

In terms of the allocation of health spending between public and private facilities, CFA francs 1.478.585 million went to government facilities. Private not-for-profit and private for-profit providers received, respectively, 95.7,342 million and 3.3511 million, while 27.103.3 million was estimated to have gone to traditional healers.

There has been a long-standing debate in Cameroon concerning the relative importance of the public and private sectors in the provision of health care. On the basis of the frequency distribution of patient consultations by category of health provider, information from the 1995 household budget-consumption survey suggests that 14.8 percent of these consultations were with traditional healers. As far as consultations in modern health centres are concerned 43.8 percent took place in public facilities and 56.2 percent in private facilities, even though services in the latter are 50 percent more expensive, and the former outnumber the latter by a ratio of 3:1.

These percentages are also confirmed in the North West province where excellent records of monthly consultations at health centres during the period 1989-1995 show that in 1995 there were 173,450 consultations in religious mission facilities and 129,569 at government facilities (Ghogomu et al. 1996). This is testimony to the superior quality of private sector health services. The household budget-consumption survey did not, however, provide any indication of the relative importance of public and private inpatient care (such as the total number of inpatient days for the two categories of facilities). But the records of monthly hospital consultations in the North West province show the domination of the government sector with 154,396 consultations in 1995 as opposed to 92,274 for the missions and 16,327 for the private for-profit sector. The evidence from the North West province during the past several years also suggests a steady decline in health care provision by the government sector: the share of the government sector in both health centre and hospital consultations fell from 72.9 percent in 1989 to 50.1 percent in 1995, while the share of mission and private sectors increased from 25.5 percent to 47 percent, and 1.6 percent to 2.9 percent respectively (Ntangsi 1996). The main reason cited for the declining role of the public sector was the economic crisis, which has drastically reduced resources for the maintenance of facilities and led to the demoralisation of health staff following the more than 60 percent cut in civil servant salaries in January 1991. Owing to a rapid deterioration of facilities the bed occupation ratio at the General Hospital in Yaoundé fell from 45 percent in 1985 to 23 percent in 2001, and since then this has been reported to be a generalised phenomenon throughout the country. These figures strongly demonstrate the ineffectiveness of the decentralised health care system in Cameroon. Also it explain the raison d'être for the increase of out-of-pocket expenditures by respective households.

High Transaction Costs in Government Spending

The low levels of government health spending and the advent of the economic crisis in 1985, combined with shrewd political expediency, ushered a new and harsh reality into the Cameroon budgetary system, which has had far-reaching consequences for health care. Year after year, and in an apparent attempt to satisfy the demands of various political constituencies, government budgets approved by the National Assembly (Parliament) and allocated to ministries in the form of treasury vouchers (with the exception of salaries which are paid directly to staff by the Ministry of Economy and Finance) have largely failed to reflect the severe and steady decline in government revenues. The approved budget exceeded actual government revenues by 42 percent in the fiscal year 2000/2001. The total value of treasury vouchers issued in any one year for the purchase of goods and services has far exceeded government revenue, and a substantial number of vouchers have remained unpaid for several years. Treasury offices have been besieged by long queues of suppliers and other contractors waiting to be paid, but without any pre-established order of priority for payment. The end result has been that treasury officials at various levels of the bureaucracy have capitalised on the situation by extorting 'commissions' or bribes of up to 60 percent of the value of a voucher as a condition for payment.

Since the non-salary health expenditures by government involve substantial transaction costs, one must distinguish between expenditures for health and expenditures for health care. Expenditures for health are the resources that have actually been mobilised for the health sector. In the 2001 fiscal year they amounted to CFA francs 60.4434 billion of which 19.2 billion was in the form of salaries (for government health personnel). The expenditure balance of 41.24 billion in the form of treasury vouchers would have involved transaction costs evaluated at 20.62 billion (assumed to be approximately 50 percent of nominal value). This means that actual expenditures on health care were therefore only 20.62 billion. In NHA, transaction costs are counted as health expenditures even though they are not spent on health care; they are viewed as a penalty or a toll that must be paid in order to have access to the 20.62 billion. This is a demonstration of the internal inefficiency inherent in the health care system in Cameroon.

In a recent analysis of the Cameroon budgetary system undertaken for the European Union by AEDES, consultants Jean Benoit Burrion and Philippe Vinard made the following assessment:

> Whatever the level in the health pyramid, the testimony is unequivocal: the delegated credits [approved budgets to the regions] are utilized at no more than half their nominal value for the purpose for which they were intended. Some speak of 30% but it is difficult to evaluate. At any rate this is not rumor or widespread prejudice but a reality lived and experienced by everyone.

For about ten years the Treasury has experienced an acute shortage of liquidity. At first this shortage induces a 'waiting line' of suppliers for the settlement of their claims at the counters of the treasury. Delays of payment can be long (sometimes a couple of years). In the long-run an informal system of management of the waiting line installed itself based on the law of supply and demand. Given the limited resources of the treasury, these are sold to the most intransigent suppliers.

Progressively the informal system becomes a near institutionalised system in which everyone follows their interests. The system transforms itself into a network of complicity.

The system has two consequences. The first is some sort of natural selection of suppliers who are capable of negotiating their claims or who are financially solid. The second is the regulation of the market, which results in 'the law of 50 percent'. However, according to the authors, it is not that the authorities are ignorant of what is going on. At least one cabinet minister attempted unsuccessfully to fight the system. Indeed, as the authors have implied, far stronger action is needed at the highest political level to change the system. 'The system is known to everyone and the authorities at the central level are fully conscious about what is going on. Given the interests in play, it is very unlikely that an improvement of the liquidity situation or that a few exemplary "sanctions" will be sufficient to change the "system"'.

Equity Considerations

Given the low level of per capita incomes in sub-Saharan Africa, large segments of the population may not even have access to the basic package of health care. An important policy by its stewards should therefore be to improve equity of access through an appropriate distribution of health expenditures, either across geographical regions or across income groups. This is because stewards of the health system are entrusted to provide an optimal control and intervention package to reduce the prevalence of HIV/AIDS and to minimise the unfair financial burden.

The NHA sources regarding geographical regions and prevalence of AIDS matrix and the distribution of household per capita health expenditures by population deciles (which is a partial source to income group matrix) are presented in Tables 3 and 4. They are used to discuss equity as concerns of the spending in health care, given the challenges of HIV/AIDS.

The NHA geographical distribution analysis demonstrates that some regions are disproportionately penalised over the others in the allocation of public funds. Table 3 reveals more dramatic inequalities. Cameroon's political strategy, like in any sub-Saharan country where universal coverage has not been achieved, was to ensure that the limited public resources benefited the rural poor. A careful review, using national health accounts data revealed that, contrary to policy intentions in Cameroon, the allocation of resources for the rural poor disfavour the regions with greater epidemiological challenges such as HIV prevalence. The sources to regions matrix shows considerable inequalities in the distribution of health expenditures between urban and rural areas (and also to a lesser extent among rural areas).

Table 2: Sources to Geographical Regions and Prevalence of AIDS Matrix (in $ per capita)

Regions	Government	Public Enterprises	Foreign Aid	Private Enterprises	Households	Religious Missions	Total by region	HIV prevalence rate by region%
Yaounde	13.1	4.5	4.3	4.0	77.9	-	103.8	2.023
Douala	6.5	5.4	4.3	2.9	82.9	-	102.0	27.9
Other towns	5.4	6.3	4.3	-	29.5	-	45.5	31
Rural Forest	5.4	6.4	4.3	-	32.4	-	48	34.1
Rural Plateau	4.5	-	4.3	-	33.8	-	42.6	32.054
Rural Savana	4.0	-	4.3	-	43.6		51.9	52.545
All Regions	6.8	2.4	4.3	2.2	43.6	68.1	127.6	34.1

Source: Computed by the author, 2004.

Following the presentation in the household surveys, Douala (the country's largest town), Yaoundé (the capital) and 'other towns' are treated as regions (they held some 40 percent of the country's population in 2000/2001) and there are also three rural regions: the forest area (covering the Centre, South and East provinces), the plateau area (covering the North West, West, South West, and Littoral provinces) and the savannah (covering the Far-North, North, and Adamaoua provinces).

As can be seen, per capita health expenditures were respectively $102.0 and $103.8 in Douala and Yaoundé compared with $42.6 and $51.9 in the rural plateau and rural savannah respectively. The high expenditures in Douala and Yaoundé are explained by the combination of high household expenditures (due to high incomes), high government spending, and a concentration of public-owned and private-owned enterprises. In other words government expenditures have helped to aggravate, rather than attenuate, existing regional inequalities in health spending by the other sources.

A cursory look at the distribution of health expenditures across income groups reveals more dramatic inequalities. Per capita household expenditure for health by the poorest ten percent of the population was only $11.4 while for the richest ten percent it was $191.2.

Table 3: Household Per Capita Health Expenditures
by Decile of the Populations

Deciles of Population	Total Per Cap. Expenditure (C F A Francs)	Per Capita Health Exp. (CFA)	Per Capita Health Exp. (in dollars)	Total Population	Percentage of Total Population
1	87.2	8.3	11.4	1,894,784	12.47
2	132.7	12.7	17.3	2,097,108	13.8
3	161.5	15.5	21.1	2,048,879	13.48
4	200.7	19.2	26.2	1,815,854	11.95
5	236.2	22.6	30.9	1,661,053	10.93
6	291.5	27.9	38.1	1,379,780	9.08
7	373.1	358.1	48.8	1,362,861	8.97
8	489.6	470.0	64.1	1,107,016	7.28
9	679.5	652.3	89.0	921,984	6.07
10	145.9	140.1	191.2	907,868	5.97
Entire Pop	324.7	311.7	42.5	15,197,500	100

Computed by the author, 2004.

As noted earlier, the World Bank has evaluated the cost of a basic package of health care delivered to ninety percent of the population in a low-income country like Cameroon per capita to be approximately $50 (World Bank 2003). On the basis of our estimate the actualised cost in 2000/2001 was $42.2 per capita. This means that the sixth deciles of the population (with a per capita household expenditure of $38.1) all by themselves could not have been able to afford the totality of the basic health package. However, if it were assumed that the government expenditure of CFA francs 41.24 billion (after transaction costs) were to be distributed equally to the population (15 million in 2000/2001), this would have resulted in an extra per capita expenditure of $2.6. If foreign aid expenditures of $5.8 per capita were also added the extra expenditure would increase to $8.4. Expenditures for the sixth deciles would now be $46.5 (38.1 + 8.4) and the basic health package would become accessible. However, for the first five deciles of the population corresponding to a population of approximately five million (about forty percent of the total population) the health package would still not be accessible. At any rate, as we have seen, government expenditures are not distributed equitably, and therefore far more than five million would not have had full access to the health package. This is partly responsible for the high prevalence of HIV in the poorer segment of the society as demonstrated in Table 3 above. Also it is an indication of the allocation inefficiency, internal inefficiency and inequity in health care spending in Cameroon.

The Prevalence of HIV/AIDS

The low levels of government health spending coupled with gross mismanagement and misappropriation of funds in the health sector, usher in a new and harsh reality in fighting the spread of the HIV/AIDS in Cameroon. It is evident that the problems of budgetary allocation inefficiency, management inefficiency and inequitable distribution of revenue associated with decentralisation of the health system in Cameroon has resulted in poor maintenance of health care facilities, low incentives for health personnel, lack of essential infrastructure and in most cases insufficient hospital beds for patients. All these have culminated in an increase in the HIV/AIDS pandemic. According to the analyses of the Ministry of Public Health, the incidence of HIV/AIDS in the sexually active population of Cameroon was eleven percent in 2000, which is twenty-two times greater than its incidence in 1987 when it was only 0.5 percent. The World Health Report (2003) reported that the number of persons living with HIV was estimated at more than 937,000: one person out of nine in the sexually active population.

The prevalence rate in Yaoundé and Douala stood respectively at 10.33 percent and 9.0 percent, the rural forest and savannah stood at 16 and 11 percent respectively. It is worthwhile to note that the HIV prevalence rate in pregnant women in rural areas stood at 18 percent compared to 13.59 percent of pregnant women in urban areas.

Prevalence among ante-natal clinic attendees in twenty-eight sites was 10.8 percent; HIV prevalence in Yaoundé was 11.2 percent, and median HIV prevalence in Douala was 11.6 percent. In areas outside the major urban centres, the HIV prevalence among ante-natal attendees increased from less than one percent in 1989 to eight percent in 1996 and has continued to rise. In 2000, median HIV prevalence in 25 sites outside the major urban areas ranged from six percent to thirteen percent. HIV prevalence in 2000 among the 20-24 years old was 12.2 percent. HIV prevalence among sex workers tested in Yaoundé increased from 5.6 percent in 1990 to 45.3 percent in 1993.

In 1994, 21 percent of sex workers tested in both Yaoundé and Douala were HIV positive; in 1995 the rate was 17 percent. A couple of studies among truck drivers, conducted between 1993 and 1994, found that between 9 to 17 percent of those tested were HIV positive. In 1996, 15 percent of military personnel tested were HIV positive. HIV prevalence increased among male STI clinic patients tested from 5.6 percent in 1992 to 16 percent in 1996. Outside of the major urban areas, HIV prevalence among STI clinic patients tested in six sites had reached 8 percent in 1992. In 1994, 9 percent of patients tested in Banka, Central province were HIV positive (UNAIDS 2002).

Although HIV/AIDS-related issues affect everybody, they affect the vulnerable, the poor and women more. Details are contained in Table 4.

Table 4: Country HIV and AIDS Estimates, End 2003

Adult (15–49) HIV prevalence rate	6.9% (range: 4.8%–11.8%)
Adults (15–49) living with HIV	520,000 (range: 360,000–740,000)
Adults and children (0–49) living with HIV	560,000 (range: 390,000–810,000)
Women (15–49) living with HIV	290,000 (range: 200,000–420,000)
AIDS deaths (adults and children) in 2003	49,000 (range: 32,000–74,000)

Source: 2004 Report on the global AIDS epidemic

In response to this growing social and economic threat of the HIV/AIDS epidemic for the population, the Prime Minister launched a strategic plan in September 2000. This document, entitled 'A Strategic Document for the National Plan for the Fight against AIDS in Cameroon 2000–2005', better known by its French acronym 'Comité National pour la Lutte contre le SIDA (CNLS)', sets out the basis for collaboration between the state, national actors and bilateral and multilateral partners in countering the epidemic. The Minister of Public Health chairs this committee. The Committee's Central Technical Group coordinates the implementation of activities throughout the country, with the assistance of ten provincial technical groups run by ten provincial coordinators.

The CNLS is made up of thirteen representatives of the public sector, including the offices of the President of the Republic and the Prime Minister, representatives of the private sector (an employers' organization and a trade union), national and international NGOs, the representatives of the two networks of associations of people living with HIV, the representatives of donors, and in particular la Coopération Française, GTZ, the European Union, the members of the Theme Group, including the UNAIDS country coordinator and representatives of parliament. The CNLS holds two statutory meetings per year, convened by its chair.

Its joint monitoring Committee supervises the action of the CNLS. This is an audit and control body, which also serves as an advisory body to the CNLS. The Ministry of Territorial Administration and Decentralisation meets it four times a year. It approves the annual and quarterly plans of action and the annual activities report. The Theme Group takes part in its work.

The Country Coordinating Mechanism has just taken its place in this organisation, specifically in connection with the follow-up of activities funded by the Global Fund. The Country Coordinating Mechanism has thirty members and is chaired by the Chairman of the CNLS.

National initiatives such as agreements signed between the government and the private sector are subject to a further level of coordination, determined by their specifications and at the proposal of the private sector.

The main objectives of the plan are to preserve the health of children, women, and men at home, or at work, at leisure and in hospital. This is to be achieved through a series of measures: minimising the risk of contamination with HIV/AIDS among children aged five to fourteen by promoting a healthy lifestyle and the development of responsible sexual behaviour, developing information mechanisms aimed at bringing about changes in the behaviour of the sexually active population, reducing the risk of transmission of HIV from mother to child, minimising the risk of infection through blood transfusion, and developing a national mechanism for solidarity with persons living with HIV/AIDS.

The strategic plan adopted a decentralised sectoral approach aimed at reducing the spread of the virus and involving among others the educational, agricultural, transport and military sectors. A summit bringing together several African First Ladies, international experts and other delegations was held in Yaoundé in November 2002 with the theme 'African Synergy against HIV/AIDS and its Sufferings'. In order to ensure adequate financing for the implementation of the National Plan for the Struggle against AIDS, the government of Cameroon committed itself to setting up mechanisms to mobilise resources for the campaign from internal and external sources and to ensure rigorous and effective management of the resources.

UNAIDS Support to the National Response

Given the inherent limitations of the decentralisation of the health sector, in 2004 the government of Cameroon embraced the activities of the United Nations HIV/AIDS. The activities focused on the following points.

For the first time ever the country team organised a retreat to draw up the United Nations plan in support of the national response to HIV/AIDS (2004-2005). This retreat was divided into two phases: first of all, the heads of agencies defined priorities, after which the technicians translated the priorities into operational terms; the outcome was the plan referred to above.

The country team held three meetings with the Chairman of the National Committee to draw his attention to the following needs: the organisation of a forum among partners involved in the HIV/AIDS control effort, follow-up for major interventions (prevention of mother-to-child transmission, access to antiretroviral therapy, and the private sector), documentation of best practices, assessment of the impact of HIV and AIDS on the national economy and on the main sectors of activity (private sector, agriculture, and education), an increase in the national budget allocated to the other ministerial departments for AIDS control and the urgent need to introduce efficient management mechanisms for activities funded by the Global Fund. Also planned was the production and dissemination of a liaison bulletin highlighting actions by the United Nations system in the field of HIV and AIDS. Technical and financial support for activities was linked to DHS (funding) through UNFPA and the World Bank. In addition, there was input for activities linked to the Global Campaign and to World AIDS Day by helping to draft the appeal made by the First Lady. Finally, implementation was planned together with the government and with synergies from Africans of the NO SIDA (AIDS) Caravan in all of Cameroon's provinces.

The Socio-economic Impact of HIV/AIDS

HIV/AIDS follows a different pattern in each locality. Geographical and ethnic factors, agro-ecological conditions, religion, gender, age and marital status play a role in the pattern and impact of HIV/AIDS and in people's perceptions of the disease. Urban and rural disparities in infection rates have also been observed. Initially, the prevalence was more in townships in Cameroon but is gradually engulfing rural areas at a more rapid rate. This has critical implications for the design of HIV/AIDS interventions.

HIV/AIDS is disproportionately affecting poor households, and particularly people in the most productive age groups. Women are more exposed to infection than males. There are far more AIDS widows than widowers. Young widows with dependent children tend to become entrenched in poverty as a result of socio-economic pressures related to HIV/AIDS. The HIV/AIDS stigma, for instance, which largely results from the prevailing stereotype that it is the women who are responsible for transmitting HIV, is undermining traditional coping mechanisms accessible to young widowed women and changing the socio-economic fabric of the extended family.

The socio-economic impact of HIV/AIDS is beginning to have an effect on the value system of the family in Cameroon as traditional norms and customs are breaking down under the pressures triggered by the HIV/AIDS epidemic. The result is that the social fabric of the extended family is showing signs of erosion and the close bonds that hold family members together are disappearing. To give but some examples:

The stigma attached to those infected with HIV/AIDS is as discussed above, in some cases, breaking up families and distancing widows from their children. Parents are forced to either send their children to work or to take them out of school. In both cases, youths are being deprived of family life education, which is instrumental in establishing a code of conduct between men and women and husbands and wives. Family life education is critical in the social development of young men and women, ensuring the transmission of family values, mores and norms, establishing a social and sexual code of conduct and setting limits in sexual conduct. Many parents attribute early sexual activity and multiple or casual partners to the disappearance of family life education.

In some areas in the country, families are being forced to adjust burial rites and ceremonies to cope with economic pressures resulting from HIV/AIDS. Firstly, the mourning time is being shortened to only two to three days. Secondly, less money is being spent. And thirdly, the drinking and socialisation taking place during burials is changing to discourage substance abuse and casual sex. Traditions such as ritual cleansing and wife inheritance are threatening the well being of the extended family as a result of HIV/AIDS but no acceptable alternative mechanisms have been developed.

Apart from affecting the value system of the family, HIV/AIDS has the potential to create severe economic impacts in Cameroon. It is different from most other diseases because it strikes people in the most productive age groups and is essentially 100 percent fatal. The effects will vary according to the severity of the AIDS epidemic and the structure of the national economies. The two major remarkable economic effects are a reduction in the labour supply and increased costs.

On the labour supply side the loss of young adults in their most productive years affects the overall economic output. If AIDS is more prevalent among the economic elite, then the impact may be much larger than the absolute number of AIDS deaths indicates.

On the costs side, the direct costs of AIDS include expenditures for medical care, drugs and funeral expenses. Indirect costs include lost time due to illness, recruitment and training costs to replace workers, and care of orphans. If costs are financed out of savings, then the reduction in investment could lead to a significant reduction in economic growth.

The economic effects of AIDS are felt first by individuals and their families then ripple outwards to firms, businesses and the macro-economy. The household impacts begin as soon as a member of the household starts to suffer from HIV-related illnesses. There is a loss of income of the patient (who is frequently the main breadwinner). Household expenditures for medical expenses increase substantially. Other members of the household, usually daughters and wives, miss school or work less in order to care for the sick person.

Death results in a permanent loss of income from less labour on the farm or from lower remittances; from funeral and mourning costs; and the removal of children from school in order to save on educational expenses and increase household labour, resulting in a severe loss of future earning potential.

Conclusion and Recommendations

Developing countries such as Cameroon that achieved a remarkable reduction in morbidity and mortality in twenty years are now confronted with the HIV/AIDS pandemic. An unfortunate collateral effect of the disease is the resurgence of certain almost eradicated infectious diseases like tuberculosis. This has increased the demand for the conventional services of hospitals and physicians. In Cameroon where managerial resources are scarce, communication is difficult, transportation is slow, and many people are isolated, decentralisation of the government service system should be considered as one possible way to improve effectiveness in the fight against this deadly disease.

Decentralisation is appropriate primarily for HIV/AIDS intervention services, provided directly to people in rural households. These programmes are more effective if they are contracted out to local health providers. These health providers could easily create awareness of the existence of HIV/AIDS and knowledge on how the rural people can protect themselves. Myths, misconceptions, superstitions, stereotypes and stigmatisation are widely prevalent in poor, illiterate households. The less people know about the disease, the more negative they tend to be about HIV/AIDS-afflicted and affected families and the stronger the stigmatisation. What is particularly significant is that individuals tend to blame their partners for transmitting the HIV virus, not themselves for engaging in high-risk sexual behaviour.

Decentralisation of financial planning should include the general principle that revenue collected in the form of user charges should be retained as close as possible to the point at which they were collected. This improves the incentive for collection, increases accountability of local staff within limits that ensure that the choice of expenditures reflects local needs, and fosters the development of managerial talent at the community level.

To encourage community-run and private sources of health services that could enhance the fight against HIV/AIDS in the country, there is the need to reverse past tendencies toward unnecessary restrictions, hostility and neglect. Other positive steps in this direction include helping community-based non-governmental organisations. Government could start by increasing public funding for training and backup support, including technical supervision and assistance in procurement of the anti-retroviral drugs. The provision of technical and financial assistance to private voluntary organisations for training (especially such areas as management) and the coordination of activities are very desirable.

Other steps include making credit accessible (especially where markets are restricted) to private ventures that want to expand or upgrade services and facilities for major interventions.

One possibility is transferring the operation of government facilities to non-governmental health providers (through sales, lease or contract). Such a step is appropriate for preventive facilities where the benefits of care and support accrue directly to those served.

It is necessary to mobilise support for people with AIDS or people who are vulnerable to HIV/AIDS. Young widows/widowers whose families have been affected by AIDS could be involved in HIV/AIDS education and related activities and possibly given some incentives. They can also be assisted with information on how to live positively with AIDS within the community, and instructed how to make wills.

The promotion of condom use should include extensive sensitisation, covering issues such as how to raise the subject with their partners, when to use condoms, how to use them properly, how to dispose of them properly, underscoring the importance of consistent use, especially under the influence of alcohol.

Perhaps the most important role for the government in the fight against HIV/AIDS is to ensure an open and supportive environment for effective programmes. Governments need to make HIV/AIDs a national priority, not a problem to be avoided. By stimulating and supporting a broad multi-sectoral approach that includes all segments of society, governments can create the conditions in which prevention, care and mitigation programmes can succeed and protect the country's future development prospects.

References

ADE, 1996, République du Cameroun, *Revues des Dépenses Publiques*; Volet Santé, Rapport Final, Yaoundé, Ministry of Public Health.

Ake, C., 1981, *A Political Economy of Africa*, Longman Inc., New York.

Akin, J., Birdsall, N. and de Ferranti, D., 1987, *Financing Health Services in Developing Countries: An Agenda for Reform*, Washington DC, World Bank.

Alesina, A., Bagir, R. and W. Easterly, 1993, 'Public Goods and Ethnic Divisions', *Quarterly Journal of Economics*, 114 (4):1243-84 November.

Amin, A. A., 1995, 'The Problem of Decreasing Incomes and Increasing Cost of Health Care in Cameroon', *Les Camers d'OCISCA*, no. 23, Yaoundé.

Arndt, C., and Lewis, 2000, 'The Macroeconomic Implications of HIV/AIDS in South Africa: A Preliminary Assessment', *South African Journal of Economics*, Volume 68:5, pp. 856 - 87.

Bardhai, P., and Mookherjee,D., 2000, 'Capture and Governance at Local and National Levels', *American Economic Review*, 90 (2): 135-39, May.

Bergstrom, T. C., and Goodman, R. P., 1973, 'Private Demands for Public Goods', *American Economic Review*, 63 (3), pp. 280-96, June.

Berman, P. A., 1997, 'National Health Accounts in Developing Countries: Appropriate Methods and Applications', *Health Economics*, Vol. 6, pp. 11-30.

Besley, T. and Coate, S., 1999, 'Centralized versus Decentralized Provision of Local Public Goods: A Political Economy Analysis', NBER Working Paper No. W7084.

Besley, T. and Burgess, R., 2002, 'The Political Economy of Government Responsiveness: Theory and Evidence from India', *Quarterly Journal of Economics*, 117 (4): 1415-51, November.

Betancourt, R., and Gleason, S., 2001, 'The Allocation of Publicly-provided Goods to Rural Households in India: On some Consequences of Caste, Religion and Democracy', *World Development*, 28 (12): 2169-82, December.

Bonnel, R., 2000, 'HIV/AIDS and Economic Growth: A Global Perspective', *South African Journal of Economics*, Volume 68: 5, pp. 820-55.

Carria, G. and Politi, C., 1996, 'Exploring the Health Impact of Economic Growth, Poverty Reduction and Public Health Expenditure', Macroeconomics, Health and Development series, *WHO Technical paper*, No. 18.

Collier P., Dercon, S., and Mackinnson, J., 2002, 'Density versus Quality in Health Care Provision: Using Household Data to Make Budgetary Choices in Ethiopia', *The World Bank Economic Review*, Vol. 3.

Cuddington, J., 1993, 'Modelling the Macro-Economic Effect of AIDS with an Application to Tanzania', *The World Bank Economic Review*, Vol. 7, No. 2.

Cuddington, J., Hancock, T. and Rogers, A., 1994, 'A Dynamic Aggregative Model of the AIDS Epidemic with Possible Policy Interventions', *Journal of Policy Modelling*, Vol. 16: 5, pp. 473-96.

Direction de la Statistique et de la Comptabilité Nationale, 1998, *Enquête Budget Camerounaise Auprès des Ménages: Synthèse Méthodologique, Opérations sur le Terrain et Exploitations des Données,* Yaoundé, Ministry of Planning and Regional Development.

Dixon, S., McDonald, S. and Roberts, 2001a, 'HIV/AIDS and Development in Africa', *Journal of International Development*, Vol. 13, No. 4, pp. 391-409.

Dixon, S., McDonald, S., and Roberts, 2001b, 'AIDS and Economic Growth in Africa: A Panel Data Analysis', *Journal of International Development*, Vol. 13, No. 4, pp. 411-25.

Foster, A. D. and Rosenweig, M. R., 2001, 'Democratisation, Decentralization and the Distribution of Local Public Goods in a Poor Rural Economy', Research Paper.

Griffin, C. C., 1989, *Strengthening Health Services in Developing Countries Through the Private Sector,* Washington, International Finance Corporation Discussion Paper 4.

Korte, R., Richter H., Merkle F. and Gorgen H., 1992, 'Financing Health Services in Sub-Saharan Africa: Options for Decision Makers During Adjustment', *Soc. Sci. Med.* Vol. 34, No. 1, pp. 1-9.

Miguel E. and Gugerty, M. K., 2002, 'Ethnic Diversity, Social Sanctions and Public Goods in Kenya', mimeo, Berkeley, University of California.

Ministry of Public Health, 1997, 'National Health Management Information System', Annual Activity Report, Yaoundé.

Ministry of Economy and Finances, 1996, *Conditions de Vie des Ménages au Cameroun en 1996: Enquête Camerounaise Auprès de Ménages (ECAM),* Yaoundé.

Ntangsi, J. V., 1996, 'An Analysis of Health Sector Expenditure in Cameroon Using a National Accounts Framework,

Oates, W., 1972, *Fiscal Federalism,* New York, Harcourt Brace Jovanovich.

Tanzi, V., 1995, 'Fiscal Federalism and Decentralization: A Review of Some Efficiency and Macroeconomic Aspects in Development Economics', Annual World Bank Conference Washington DC, World Bank.

Wagstaff, A. and van Doorslaer, 2002, 'Overall vs Socio-economic Health Inequalities: A Measurement Framework and Two Empirical Illustrations from Canada and Vietnam'.

World Bank, 1987, *World Development Report,* New York, Oxford University Press.

World Bank, 1990, *World Demographic and Health Survey,* Washington DC, World Bank.

World Bank, 1993, *World Development Report,* New York, Oxford University Press.

World Bank, 1994, *Better Health in African Experience and Lessons Learned*, Washington DC, World Bank.

World Bank, 1994, 'Cameroon: Diversity, Growth and Poverty Reduction', Working draft, Human Resources and Poverty Division, African Region.

World Health Organisation, 2000, *The World Health Report 2000, Health Systems Improving Performance*, Geneva.

7

Another Look at Community-Directed Treatment (ComDT) in Cameroon: A Quality Challenge to Health System Development

Martyn T. Sama and Richard Penn

Introduction

Onchocerciasis is the world's second leading infectious cause of blindness with an estimated 123 million people under risk, and about 18 million people in the world suffering a grave burden imposed by the disease (WHO 1997a). In Africa, some 17.5 million people are infected with *Onchocerca volvulus* (WHO Technical Report Series no.852). It is estimated that more than 6 million people are suffering from Onchocerca skin lesions and severe itching (Remme, Murray, and Lopez 1990).

The vector *Onchocerca volvulus* produces millions of microfilariae worms which migrate to the skin and the eyes of the human host, causing severe itching and pigmentation. The most severe manifestations of onchocerciasis are irreversible: ocular lesions of both the anterior and posterior segments of the eye, resulting in impaired vision and ultimately total blindness. In Africa, it is one of the leading causes of visual impairment and blindness. Rarely life threatening, but causing chronic suffering and severe disability, onchocerciasis constitutes a serious obstacle to socio-economic development (WHO 1996).

Mass-treatment of onchocerciasis is carried out in meso- and hyper-endemic areas once a year, and in hypo-endemic areas, treatment is clinic-based. The target population is persons of five years and above, with the exception of seriously sick persons, pregnant women, nursing mothers whose babies are aged below eight days, and very old persons.

The process of Community-Directed Treatment (ComDT) with Ivermectin (CDTI), has been adopted for onchocerciasis control in some places of Africa. A multi-country study (WHO 2002) conducted in some of the endemic countries has demonstrated that Community-Directed Treatment (ComDT) is an effective strategy for drug distribution. Those communities are deeply involved in their own health care on a large scale. An assessment by the African Programme for Onchocerciasis Control (APOC 2000) showed that ComDT is effective also for other health and development activities like distribution of Vitamin A, Malaria control, Guinea worm control, and Sanitation. Despite the success, several questions remain unanswered about community and health system interaction for sustained coverage of Ivermectin distribution (WHO 2002a).

Ivermectin distributors, the Community Directed Distributors (CDD), are supposed to be members of their community chosen by the community through a democratic process, trained to distribute Ivermectin and supervised by health services staff. Ivermectin is considered safe enough to be administered by non-health personnel.

Treatment coverage varies between contexts where ComDT has been tried. The mean reported coverage over different ongoing projects is 70 percent. Problems in the selection of CDDs, inadequate supervision by health staff and limited community participation in decision making are common obstacles. The following problems are common to all project sites, these range from poor selection of CDDs, inadequate supervision by health staff to limited community participation in decision making (APOC Technical Report 2002). The urgency of research on ComDT is underscored by the fact that advocates of ComDT want to also use it for other community-based interventions.

This paper reports on a study of ComDT Ivermectin treatment in Cameroon. More specifically we give results on coverage and the views of the CDDs, the health personnel and the community on the ComDT of Ivermectin. The study is an exploratory single case-embedded design, seeking to understand the factors influencing the effectiveness of community-based approaches to drug distribution, in this case ComDT Ivermectin treatment.

Methods

The study was conducted in the south western part of Cameroon where the NGO Sight Savers International (SSI) currently has a Community-Directed Ivermectin Treatment (CDTI) programme. The South West Province lies between 5°20 and 4° N and 8°45 and 9°45 E. The study area includes the health districts of Muyuka, Kumba, and Konye. The areas were purposely selected for this study because they were among the meso- and hyper-endemic communities. Two of them are hyper- and one meso-endemic, thus meeting the criteria for mass treatment with Ivermectin. The study area has a very rich network of drainage systems, most of which flow from high altitude and are interrupted by numerous cascades, rapids, and waterfalls. These streams provide sites for *Simulium* vectors, which can be found at high altitude in the area.

A traditional chief heads each community, and links the communities and the administration. However, the influence of the chieftaincies over the communities varies from one ethnic group to the other. In some communities the people are better organised around the administrative authorities.

Several channels of communication are used. Each community has a town crier whose role is to transmit messages in the local languages to the community. Churches and 'Njangi houses' are also commonly used for disseminating information. Other traditional channels include the talking drum, and flute.

For this study information was obtained from the study population which consisted of different actors involved in the process of ComDT with Ivermectin at the community level. These include the CDDs, the health facility staff, and the community members and their leaders. At the Local Government Area/District level, the heads of the other health and developmental activities operating within the study communities were also studied. The team that conducted the study comprised of a social epidemiologist, a medical doctor, an anthropologist, a communicator, a bio-statistician (part-time) and six interviewers.

The interviewers were under-graduate students of the Department of Sociology and Anthropology at the University of Buea. Training was carried out for two weeks on the techniques of using quantitative and qualitative instruments for data collection. Confidentiality protection was guaranteed by demanding and receiving oral reports from all CDDs, households, community leaders and health workers to insure data quality before interviews.

Quantitative Data Collection

Forty communities within which at least two CDDs were found were randomly selected for data collection. In each community, two CDDs who covered a minimum of fifteen households were selected for surveys - hence a total of eighty CDDs, seventy-five male and five female, who met these criteria, were interviewed. A semi-structured questionnaire was administered to each CDD to collect information on the different health and development activities in which he/she was involved, how and when they got involved, their motivation, the number of days spent on each activity, similarities to the other activities in their work as CDDs, and how their involvement in the other H&D activities affect their work as CDDs.

A total of 1200 households in which the eighty CDDs worked were surveyed to estimate for household treatment coverage, using a pre-tested standard household survey form. Fifteen households per CDD were used to collect information on sex, age, treatment coverage, period of treatment, treatment effect and side-effects. Information on actual coverage was obtained from 1185 households with 5812 individuals, consisting of 2919 (50.2 percent) males and 2893 (49.8 percent) females.

Qualitative Data Collection

Forty focus group discussions (FGDs), one per community were conducted; twenty male FGDs and twenty female FGDs. Each FGDs ranged from eight to twelve persons. A FGD guide was used to direct the moderator, note-taker and observer during the discussions.

Forty in-depth interviews were conducted with each community leader using an in-depth interview guide. In-depth interviews were conducted with all nine people (eight nurses and one DMO) from health facility staffs that supervise the CDDs in the study communities. An in-depth interview guide for health staff was used to guide the interviewers.

Quantitative Data Analysis

EPI-info was used for entering data from the household surveys and CDD surveys and for the questionnaire's descriptive analysis. For more detailed analysis, SPSS was used to examine variation and correlations.

Qualitative Data Analysis

Data were transcribed from tapes to records. MSWord was used for entry and transfer to text files. Textbase-Beta was used for content analysis.

Results

Quantitative Results

Two questions in the household survey give estimates of the proportion of persons that report they received tablets and those that report they swallowed the tablets. The overall estimates for persons five years and older were 73.5 percent and 72.6 percent (14 percent of the persons in the household survey were under five). Among those that reported tablets swallowed, 46.3 percent reported side effects and 3.5 percent reported having taken any health care action. Table 1 shows the detailed estimates by age and sex. Both sexes report lower coverage in the age groups 15–34 years. Children and older people have higher frequencies of persons that received and swallowed tablets. Women have generally lower coverage. The proportion having swallowed tablets was about one percent lower than the proportion that received tablets quite systematically. Women more often reported side effects than men and also sought health care more. Both these proportions were larger for the older groups.

There is a large variation between CDD areas and between households within these areas. The coverage estimated from reported numbers in the CDDs questionnaire is considerably lower, less than 50 percent. No correlations were found between the coverage estimated from the household survey and the information from the CDDs. We did not find any correlation between CDD age, sex and educational level, time spent on CDTI, involvement in other activities and motivation. An attempt to use a multiple regression model gave the result that the CDD variables only explained 1.9 percent of the variation in coverage between the areas where CDDs operated. The model was not statistically significant, i.e. all correlations were fully explainable by chance variation.

There were five female CDDs among the eighty that filled in the questionnaire. The ages ran from 22 to 59 years. Ten reported having attended secondary school. Seventy percent reported having been selected by the village leaders and most of them were appointed during 1999. As many as 77 reported that they had spent two weeks or more in a year on CDTI.

Some opinions expressed in the questionnaire answers are summarised in Table 2. There are some doubts about CDTI working well. The question on support from the health sector was mainly answered positively but a reasonable number of CDDs did not share that opinion. The views on CDDs' improvement, community involvement and the feasibility of taking on other tasks were quite uniform. Generally, the last four questions point to the negative view regarding other tasks. Table 2 provides data on the responses from the CDDs.

Table 1: Estimated Coverage, Proportions of Persons that Received and Swallowed Tablets, Frequencies of Side Effects and Health Care Seeking Actions by Age and Sex in the Household Survey

	Male				Female			
Age	Receive tablets	Swallow tablets	Side effects	Health care seeking	Receive tablets	Swallow tablets	Side effects	Health care seeking
5-14	77.1	76.8	36.1	2.4	77.6	76.8	42.3	1.8
15-24	68.7	67.2	40.7	3.0	62.7	61.5	46.6	5.3
25-34	73.6	72.6	48.4	2.5	66.7	66.2	56.8	8.6
35-44	77.7	77.4	48.9	1.3	76.8	76.2	54.2	6.2
45-54	78.9	77.8	46.5	1.9	77.8	76.5	56.4	3.3
55-	80.4	78.8	56.2	3.4	74.3	74.3	55.5	2.7
Total	75.4	74.5	43.4	2.5	71.7	70.9	49.4	4.5

Table 2: Frequencies of Responses to CDTI Given by CDDs in Questionnaire

Question	Do not at all agree				Agree fully
CDTI works satisfactory	21	41	1	15	2
The support received is enough	6	31	2	22	19
The CDDs are capable for the job	3	12	5	44	16
CDDs have improved during work	21	48	7	2	2
Community is involved in process	13	49	3	12	3
CDD should not do other acts.	1	3	3	47	26
Other acts would be helpful	41	37	0	1	1
CDD will have to do other acts.	20	45	3	11	1
CDD will enhance health	31	47	1	1	0
Better monitor. With other acts.	19	48	10	3	0

Most CDDs reported that community members selected them during gatherings or general meetings but some reported that the procedures did not follow CDTI guidelines. A CDD could be selected by the village chief alone or with his cabinet or by a health worker. The village head could also appoint himself, by village head alone, or by a health worker and village chief together.

Various problems in carrying out activities were identified in the process of preparing for and implementing the distribution of Ivermectin. Transportation was a major concern. Several CDDs complained because they received no provision to cover the transportation cost needed to collect Ivermectin. Some complained that they spent their own money. Shortages of Ivermectin were noted creating tension between CDDs and community members. Poor storage facilities existed. Batches of supplies were often known to have expired because of bureaucratic delays in the system.

The issue of the fear of side effects and the impact on compliance concerned several CDDs. They noted that the issue is complicated by the lack of drugs that relieve side effects, for example itching. CDDs reported low morale due to the lack of incentives and compensation for time spent on distribution. CDDs observed that people were often absent during distribution, and this required the CDD to make repeated additional home visits. The CDDs often complained that 'I have no time of my own. People can come to me any time of the day'.

Several CDDs said they faced difficulties in reporting and documenting their activities. The problems were said to be caused by the short time for training and by community members not providing towards buying or recording supplies like notebooks and pens.

The overwhelming majority of CDDs reported they received no assistance from the health facility. Only a few reported receiving assistance, which took the form of the mobilisation of community members and making announcements about the availability of drugs. Training on implementation, reporting and management of side effects was not sufficient. Supervision and monitoring of CDD activities from the health sector was not at an acceptable level.

In a similar manner, CDDs often reported that community members did not play an active role in the distribution of Ivermectin. One response that summed up a common reason for low community involvement was: 'Nobody assisted. They did not know about the procedure. They did not receive any information about it'.

Views and Experiences of Health Workers

Selection and training of CDDs were reported to present problems. It was difficult to find literate candidates; even semi-literate CDDs find it difficult to cope with the task and the training. The health staff, as well as the CDDs, face transportation problems in getting to the training venue. Health workers also noted the lack of response and support from health authorities: 'We have written a proposal on how to train CDDs but we have not received any response yet'.

Most front-line health workers were not involved in CDD or programme supervision. This was actually left in the hands of the onchocerciasis coordinator of the District Health Service. The need for reinforced supervision was clearly recognised.

Management of side-effects was another important task discussed by health workers. They noted that 'Some people fear side-effects so they don't want to take the drug. They complain of itching, swelling of body, dizziness, and stomach-ache'.

A finding from the in-depth interviews with health personnel was that supervision of CDDs was a major problem:

'CDTI is a very difficult programme. I am the chief nurse, mid-wife, consultant, leprosy inspector and in charge of delivery and outreach activities. The CDTI programme is a burden to me. It adds too much work on me'.

The DMO for Muyuka noted: 'Some nurses are not competent enough to manage and handle records, especially financial reporting. The programme lacks a good information management system. More so, issues of onchocerciasis endemicity are not yet clear to the community members. They do not understand why some people are supposed to be treated in the hospital and some through mass treatment in the communities'.

The perceived roles of the health worker were captured in the following statement. 'Delivery has been regular for the past three years. The health worker spends about one hour to discuss health issues but they rarely talk about onchocerciasis'.

Views and experiences of community members

In a female FGD it was noted that CDD selection criteria were not always observed. 'We do not know who chose them. We only saw them with the nurse moving from house to house taking our names, after which they came with Mectizan. They said we should take it to treat our filaria'. Some community members were of the opinion that the CDDs were chosen by the health personnel. 'To me, I know that he was chosen by the mid-wife to help to distribute Mectizan. We were not asked to choose them'. In an in-depth interview, a community leader admitted having appointed all the CDDs in his village after he 'received a letter from the chief of post, to select four people and send to him for training. I called three of my councillors and my daughter and sent them for the training course'.

A major issue raised in FGDs, in-depth, and key informant interviews with community members was that of ownership of the programme. The majority of respondents said that CDTI belonged to the community. On why they thought that the programme belonged to the community, they gave responses such as: 'we are the beneficiaries', 'we plan the distribution', 'we do the distribution', 'we select the distributors', 'the distributors is ours', and 'because we are told so'.

Those who thought that the programme does not belong to the community stated that it belonged to the government or the ministry of health. 'It is the government that brought this programme to us but we have been told that in the near future, it will be our own.' Most community members saw their role in CDTI as mainly passive.

Community members also identified other problems with the programme. These included non-involvement of certain segments of the population (especially men). On the subject of absenteeism, one woman said, 'Our men are sometimes not present when distribution takes place'. Others observed poor compliance, including both low turnout and refusal to take the drug. Others noted that there was a lack of awareness of the importance of the drug. This problem is compounded by the wrong messages which are sometimes passed to community members. Community members also pointed out organisational problems. The major complaint of communities with no health facility is that they do not have an opportunity to discuss their health needs with health workers.

Discussion

The study provides an overall estimate of Ivermectin treatment coverage as about 73 percent - not much lower than the long term sustained 75 percent stipulated as necessary to effectively interrupt transmission. The results from this study show that the overall treatment coverage (68.2 percent) is low in the study area.

In order to interrupt transmission, APOC sets a minimum coverage rate of 75 percent sustained for a long period (APOC 2002). However, there are large variations in coverage between districts as well as between households within districts. No single factor can conclusively be identified as responsible for coverage variations. Some suggestions are that overall low treatment coverage may be attributed to: poor selection and training of CDDs, poor supervision of CDDs, management of severe side effects, and the distribution process. The quantitative analysis fails at this point. Different mechanisms might be the reason for low coverage in different districts. The qualitative analysis reveals some of these.

In the CDTI approach the community, as an administrative, geographical and social construct, plans their own distribution system. They make decisions on who should distribute the drug, the mode (house to house, central location) and place (chief's compound, school, or church) of the distribution system. Communities collect Ivermectin from the collection point if it is not located far from them and decide when to distribute. The CDTI approach is an evolution from other community-based delivery strategies. It is supposed to promote active community participation as an integral part of Ivermectin distribution, to improve access to the drug and give a sense of community ownership of the process.

The information obtained in interviews reveals that the guidelines for selection and training of CDDs were sometimes ignored by some health personnel and community leaders. In addition, the health system generally did not provide adequate training skills to the health personnel. CDDs to some extent lacked the skills to conduct a household census, keep good records, maintain treatment registers, observe and identify side-effects, report severe side-effects and give information to the community about side-effects. The lack of management skills of side-effects provided a major barrier to high treatment coverage of Ivermectin. The programme for side-effect management did not train nurses. When severe side effects occurred, nurses were not available for management. The referral and counter referral system was not working.

A lack of adequate supervision during distribution was reported, and can be one reason for low coverage. Enormous supervision problems existed at the level of the health system. There was a gross lack of transportation for the local health staff to supervise CDDs during distribution. Many of the health facilities are under-staffed and the health personnel are not properly trained to conduct supervision. No incentives were provided for supervision; therefore no health personnel were motivated to supervise the CDDs.

The Ivermectin distribution process appears to be flawed with various systemic problems. There were no drug distribution plans for CDDs, communities were given responsibility to take decisions on the mode, time, and place of distribution, but were not empowered in the decision-making process. Although the entire community should decide the selection of distributors, the decision-making process that may exist in a given community prior to the commencement of the control programme led to village leaders in some communities selecting themselves or relatives as distributors (Amazigo 2001).

A TDR Report identifies constraints influencing the task of Ivermectin distributors as: delays in the delivery of Ivermectin from the port to the country; follow up and treatment of the members of the community who are absent during the period of mass treatment (absentees); refusals; the house to house mode of distribution; and the complex record keeping demands. The schedule and work load of distributors resulted in some instances in a high attrition rate among distributors.

The success of Community-Directed Treatment with Ivermectin (CDTI) using Community-Directed Distributors (CDDs) in Onchocerciasis control has drawn attention from other disease control programmes (Walsh 1979). However, the health system is faced with quality challenges regarding their selection, training, supervision, management of severe side effects, and the distribution process. There are systemic issues that need to be addressed before ComDT can take on its role as an entry point to community-based healthcare interventions at a time when there is a need to critically examine determinants of treatment coverage of Ivermectin distribution. The main purpose here is to propose some basic conceptual elements that may help establish a consistent basis for policy, action, and research before CDDs can take on additional health care activities.

There have been various attempts in Cameroon to use a Community-Directed Treatment System and Community-Directed Distributors for other health interventions but the implications of this development for the treatment coverage of CDTI are not clear. It is expected that the integration of additional community level heath care activities into CDTI would enhance treatment coverage. However, treatment coverage may be at risk if the health system starts using CDDs for other activities without ensuring sustained high coverage. Overloading CDDs without sustained treatment coverage can erode the health system. Opinions have been expressed, rather strongly, as to the negative effects of the ultimate consequence of overloading CDDs with programmes built essentially on top-down approaches on the effective implementation of CDTI. (Brieger 2000; Zekus and Lysack 1998; Schwap 1997, Walsh and Waren 1979). What this means is that more evidence on the nature of the effect of involving CDDs in other health and development programmes on CDTI implementation is needed. This study points to some major weaknesses.

Conclusions

Community-Directed Distributors find it difficult to achieve high coverage and sustain it due to programmatic obstacles in their selection, training, supervision, and management of severe side effects and non-empowerment of the communities in decision-making.

Although coverage is not extremely low overall, there are large variations and pockets of the population are left without treatment.

At the organisational level, the issue of the quality of the distribution process has not been addressed, and because of this, the programme suffers from technical inefficiency.

Serious systemic problems still exist, and need to be rectified before community-directed distributors can take up additional health and development activities.

The communities are not involved in decision-making regarding selection of distributors, mode, place, and time of Ivermectin distribution, hence ownership and sustainability of the programme seems to be eroded.

The support from the health sector in terms of training, supervision and assistance is not sufficient everywhere since health facilities are under-staffed, poorly equipped, and poorly paid.

It is necessary, therefore, for health systems to address systemic programmatic and organisational issues before undertaking large-scale implementation programmes like community-directed treatment with Ivermectin.

To obtain high and homogenous coverage there is a need to use better routines for the selection of CDDs and select only persons that can be effectively trained. CDDs must be given better training for strengthening the health system involvement. It is necessary to give the CDDs information and knowledge about the management of severe treatment side effects including the capacity to report adequately and inform the community. Communities must be empowered to take decisions. The linkage between research-to-policy-to-action-to-practice should be clear.

References

Amazigo, U., et al., 1998, 'Delivery Systems and Cost Recovery in Mectizan Treatment for Onchocerciasis', *Ann. Trop. Med. & Parasitol.*

APOC Partners Meeting, 2000, DIR/APOC, Meeting May-June.

APOC Technical Report, 2002, 'Community Directed Treatment with Ivermectin', SW1 Project July.

Blas, E., and Limbambala, 2001, 'The Challenge of Hospitals in Health Sector Reform: The Case of Zambia', *Health Policy and Planning*, 16 suppl. 2.

Brieger, W. R., 1996, 'Health Education to Promote Community Involvement in the Control of Tropical Diseases', *Acta Tropica*, 61: 93-106.

Frenk, J., 1993, 'Dimensions of Health System Reform', *Health Policy*, 27.

Godin, 1998, 'Cameroon Chad: Cost Recovery', *Annals of Tropical Medicine & Parasitology*, vol. 92, supplement no.1.

Paphassarang, C., Philvong, K., Boupha, B. and Blas, E., 2002, 'Equity, Privatization and Cost Recovery in Urban Health Care: The Case of Lao PDR', *Health Policy and Planning*, 17, suppl.1.

Remme, J. H. F., 1990, 'Onchocerciasis', in C.J.L., Murray and A.D. Lopez , *The Burden of Diseases: Global and Regional Estimates for 1990*, World Health Organisation.

Schwab, M., and Syne, S. L., 1997, 'On Paradigms, Community Participation and the Future of Public Health', *American Journal of Public Health*, 87 (12):2049-2051.

Walsh, J. A., and Warren, K. S., 1979, 'Selective Primary Health Care - An Interim Strategy for Disease Control in Developing Countries', *New England Journal of Medicine*, 301: 967-976.

Wealth Health Organisation, Technical Report, Series no. 852.

World Health Organisation, 1996, 'Community-Directed Treatment with Ivermectin: Report of the multi-country study', Document TDR/AFR/RP/96.1.

World Health Organisation, 1997, 'Twenty Years of Onchocerciasis Control Review of the work on Onchocerciasis in West Africa from 1974-1994', Geneva, WHO.

World Health Report, 2000a, *Health Systems: Improving Performance.*

World Health Organisation, 2000b, 'Implementation and Sustainability of Community-directed Treatment of Onchocerciasis with Ivermectin: Report of the Multi-Country Study', Document. TDR/IDE/RP/CDTI/00.1.

World Health Report, 2002, WHO/WHR/02.1.

Zakus, J. D. L. and Lysack, C. L., 1998, 'Revisiting Community Participation', *Health Policy and Planning*, 1998, 13 (1):1.

III

Les systèmes de santé
et le VIH au Maghreb

8

Le Système de santé au Maghreb

Sofiane Bouhdiba

Introduction générale

Le concept de santé

Mais qu'entendons-nous par *Santé*? La santé est une notion ambiguë, relative et fluctuante selon les époques et les régions géographiques, qui déterminent toutes deux un environnement socioculturel, élément lui-même primordial dans la définition de la santé.

Si l'on se réfère aux textes officiels, la santé est définie par l'OMS comme étant: « …un état optimal de bien-être physique, mental et social, et pas seulement l'absence de maladie et d'infirmité ».[1]
Le terme *optimal* signifie qu'il y a une comparaison permanente entre un état de santé observé dans une population, et un état considéré comme souhaitable. Nous retrouvons ici le concept d'*Iitidal* (équilibre), cher à Ibn Sina (Avicenne), pour qui:

> La maladie est avant tout perçue comme une rupture par rapport à une norme psychique, physiologique, somatique ou physique, laquelle norme n'a rien d'absolu puisque d'une région du monde à l'autre, d'une ethnie à l'autre elle peut varier considérablement.[2]

Et il est vrai que, dans les populations musulmanes, la santé est perçue comme un état d'équilibre interne; la maladie est de ce fait profondément ressentie comme une situation de déséquilibre.

Dans la suite de notre exposé, nous considérerons la santé prise comme le bien-être physique, et nous retiendrons également la définition négative « *absence de maladie* ».

L'autre aspect qui nous semble extrêmement important dans la définition de la santé, c'est justement le fait qu'elle s'inscrit dans la durabilité. On peut reprendre la définition globalisante de K. Schaapveled, pour qui: « La santé est un état durable qui suppose un mode de vie durable dans un environnement durable ».[3]

Cette approche intègre la notion de qualité de l'environnement dans la problématique de santé. On pourra ainsi considérer la pollution de l'air et du littoral, la congestion urbaine, la pollution sonore ou même l'épuisement des ressources naturelles comme des questions de santé publique.

Si à présent on part du principe que la santé constitue un bien durable, au même titre que d'autres produits, cela signifierait qu'il existe un véritable « *marché* » de la santé, soumis à une loi de l'offre et de la demande. Nous essaierons de voir au travers de cette série de cours s'il existe un principe régulateur sur ce marché, dans lequel la santé est alors considérée comme un output émanant d'un processus de production complexe.

Le temps limité de ces cours ne permettra pas bien entendu de répondre à l'ensemble des questions et de traiter tous les aspects de la santé. Il s'agira tout au plus d'avancer un certain nombre d'éléments permettant de mieux cerner les problématiques spécifiques de l'Afrique du Nord, ce qui nous permettra d'avancer autant que possible dans la formulation de la problématique régionale de l'Afrique.

Mon objectif sera, au-delà de l'observation et l'analyse, l'ouverture de quelques pistes de recherche, et éventuellement de partager les leçons de l'expérience maghrébine en matière de santé.

L'Afrique du Nord

Pour la clarté de l'exposé, nous considérerons que l'Afrique du Nord regroupe les trois pays suivants: Algérie, Maroc et Tunisie, c'est-à-dire les pays du Maghreb. Commençons donc par présenter brièvement ces trois pays:

Tableau 1: L'Afrique du Nord

Pays	Superficie (km²)	Population (millions)	ISF	Tx de croissance	Part de la population de moins de 15 ans	Part de la population de plus de 64 ans	Tx d'urbanisation	PNB/ hab	Densité
Algérie	2 384 000	31	3,1	+2,4%	39%	4%	49%	1 500 $	13 hab/km²
Maroc	447 000	29,2	3,4	+1,7%	33%	5%	54%	1 260 $	65 hab/km²
Tunisie	164 000	9,7	2,03	+1,6%	31%	6%	63%	2 110 $	59 hab/km²

Source: Nations Unies.

Le Système de santé au Maghreb

Introduction

Dans les années soixante, les trois pays d'Afrique du Nord nouvellement indépendants se sont engagés dans la modernisation et le développement de leur économie, afin d'assurer la satisfaction des besoins d'une population qui allait augmenter très rapidement. Si l'on peut parler de similarité, en ce qui concerne les objectifs globaux et à long terme, il n'en est pas de même pour les options et les stratégies retenues par chacun de ces pays. Celles-ci diffèrent en fonction de nombreux éléments géographiques, historiques, sociologiques, économiques,...

Ces différences étaient également surdéterminées par les idéologies qui s'affrontaient à l'époque et qui divisaient le monde en deux blocs, si bien que les choix et les options stratégiques de développement pouvaient être différents d'un pays à l'autre dans une région pourtant relativement homogène à plus d'un titre.

Cependant, quel que soit le modèle choisi, il accordait une large place à l'édification d'un système de santé moderne, capable de prendre en charge les immenses besoins d'une population dont l'état sanitaire, hérité des autorités coloniales, était médiocre.

Or, à l'époque, des données démographiques et épidémiologiques suffisamment détaillées, qui permettraient d'évaluer les besoins de la population dans le domaine de la santé et serviraient d'éléments fondamentaux dans la fixation des priorités, étaient quasiment inexistantes.

Les trois jeunes pays Nord-africains n'avaient donc pas la possibilité d'étudier ces besoins de façon scientifique et de mettre en place les stratégies les plus adaptées à l'état sanitaire et les mieux ajustées aux réalités économiques, démographiques et sociales. La planification sanitaire étant donc impossible dans ces conditions, des programmes d'investissement plus ou moins importants ont été lancés.

Ce n'est que longtemps après, dans les années 80, sous la contrainte de la crise économique que se sont posées les questions suivantes:

- De quelle façon, en l'absence d'une politique sanitaire explicite, d'une planification cohérente et d'objectifs précis, s'est édifié le système de santé?
- Dans quelle mesure un tel système permet-il de répondre effectivement aux besoins réels de la population?
- Quel a été son impact précis sur le profil démographique et sur le profil épidémiologique des populations?

Plus que dans les autres, il faut prendre en compte dans le secteur sanitaire, l'influence de différents intervenants, des groupes de pression qui sont impliqués et qui représentent des intérêts différents, voire conflictuels.

Ce sont en fait les décisions de ces différents groupes de pression le plus souvent professionnels, qui ont été déterminants dans les choix technologiques et les choix stratégiques, choix qui n'ont pas toujours été les plus judicieux.

Beaucoup de ces groupes étaient moins préoccupés par les vrais besoins des populations que par l'acquisition de moyens parfois sophistiqués. Longtemps, on a cru que l'accumulation de moyens entraînerait automatiquement une amélioration des résultats sanitaires. Cela était particulièrement vrai pour l'Algérie, qui bénéficiait alors d'une manne pétrolière, et qui s'était lancée dans des programmes sanitaires démesurés.

On s'aperçut très vite alors que la croissance des moyens et des dépenses était nettement plus rapide que l'amélioration des indicateurs sanitaires. Après les premiers instants d'euphorie, les difficultés financières ont fait découvrir que la disponibilité des ressources est, certes importante, mais que les techniques de gestion de ces ressources et leur adaptation aux problèmes l'étaient davantage.

Ces difficultés qui se sont posées d'une manière particulièrement vive en Afrique du Nord, ont suscité des préoccupations nouvelles et ont permis de focaliser l'attention sur de nouvelles problématiques débouchant parfois sur une véritable remise en cause du système de santé et sur son impact réel sur les populations.

On peut affirmer aujourd'hui, avec le recul, que la santé de la population ne dépend pas que du système de soins, et que la réponse médicale n'est que l'une des réponses possibles aux besoins de la population. Il existe en effet des facteurs tels que la nutrition, l'hygiène, l'assainissement, l'adduction en eau potable, l'éducation, l'émancipation de la femme qui se situent, certes hors du champ sanitaire, mais qui n'en ont pas moins un impact déterminant sur la santé.

Sur un autre plan, les comparaisons établies entre les trois pays d'Afrique du Nord ont montré qu'à niveau de développement égal et en mobilisant les mêmes ressources, on n'obtenait pas les mêmes résultats.

Ainsi, certains pays utilisent plus de ressources matérielles, humaines et financières qu'il n'est nécessaire pour atteindre un état de santé donné. C'est le cas par exemple de l'Algérie, où on relève un décalage important entre les indicateurs de santé, tels que le taux de mortalité ou le taux de mortalité infantile, et les indicateurs de développement économique, comme le Produit national brut (PNB).

La question centrale qui se pose alors, et à laquelle il est très difficile de répondre, est donc la suivante: quels sont les facteurs qui sont réellement déterminants sur les profils épidémiologiques et démographiques?

Beaucoup de chercheurs ont essayé d'y répondre. Parmi ces tentatives, il nous a semblé intéressant d'exposer celles de John Caldwell qui, à partir d'une série de comparaisons entre pays de même niveau de développement économique, a abouti à des hypothèses et des explications intéressantes même si elles peuvent paraître contestables pour certains.

Nous allons, à travers ce cours, tenter de comparer les systèmes de santé dans les trois pays d'Afrique du Nord et essayer de comprendre pourquoi, à partir d'une situation de départ relativement similaire, les choses ont évolué de manière différente.

Le Maroc, la Tunisie et l'Algérie présentent des structures politiques, des modes de légitimation du pouvoir et des choix de développement différents. L'organisation sanitaire de ces trois pays, malgré un profil épidémiologique assez semblable, est relativement différente, tant au plan du financement des soins médicaux que des modalités de leur production et de leur distribution.

Dans cette première partie, nous tenterons de situer le système de santé maghrébin par rapport au reste du monde.

Les modèles de systèmes de santé

Nous avons pu recenser dans la littérature quatre principaux modèles de système sanitaire, qui varient selon leur degré d'intégration horizontale et verticale.[4] Ces schémas simplifiés distinguent trois étapes dans un système sanitaire.

Le premier niveau représente la collecte des contributions, c'est-à-dire les paiements directs des ménages, les participations des caisses sociales et la redistribution des impôts et taxes.

Au deuxième niveau intervient le processus d'achat au travers duquel les contributions collectées sont allouées à des prestataires institutionnels ou individuels pour la construction d'établissements hospitaliers ou l'acquisition de produits consommables.

Enfin, le dernier niveau du modèle comprend la phase de prestation de soins proprement dite.

On peut alors représenter graphiquement les quatre modèles de la manière suivante:

- modèle 1: intégration complète: une seule institution gère les 3 phases du processus (cas exceptionnel de la Grande-Bretagne avant les réformes Thatcher);
- modèle 2: intégration verticale: différents organismes, chacun assurant les trois phases du processus, gèrent les soins de chaque sous-population (cas des pays latino-américains);
- modèle 3: intégration horizontale: a chaque fonction correspond une seule institution qui gère les soins de l'ensemble de la population (modèle le plus fréquent dans le monde, et vers lequel tendent la majorité des pays en développement);
- modèle 4: système mixte: chaque institution gère une seule phase du processus de santé et, à chaque phase, agissent différents intervenants, chacun gérant une tranche spécifique de la population.

Les pays du Maghreb semblent plutôt s'aligner sur le *modèle n°4*, puisqu'à chaque étape du processus sanitaire correspondent plusieurs institutions spécialisées, chacune assurant la couverture sanitaire d'une tranche particulière de la population.

En effet, la collecte des fonds est assurée par les ménages, les patrons des employés ou les caisses sociales.

L'achat est ensuite assuré par les différentes institutions (Pharmacie centrale, Ministère de la Santé Publique,...) ou directement par les ménages.

Enfin, au niveau de la phase de prestation, interviennent de nombreux établissements sanitaires publics et privés, ainsi que des professionnels privés.

Comme nous aurons l'occasion de le voir tout à l'heure et à l'instar de nombreux autres pays en développement, c'est vers le *modèle n°3* que tend à s'orienter la politique maghrébine de santé publique. En effet, il semblerait que nous allons actuellement vers une intégration horizontale, c'est à dire la mise en place de super-structures qui assureraient d'une manière autonome chacune des trois fonctions du modèle.

Figure 1: Modèles de soins de santé selon le degré d'intégration horizontale et verticale

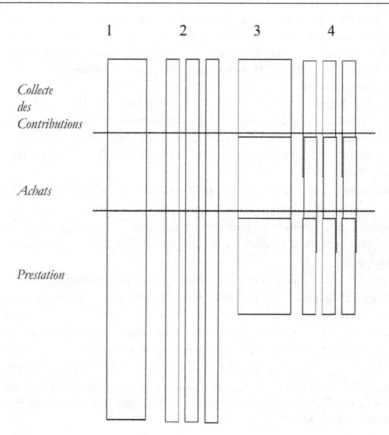

Source: OMS

Essayons à présent de décrire brièvement et successivement les principales stratégies de développement sanitaire en Afrique du Nord.

Les stratégies sanitaires en Afrique du Nord

L'Algérie

L'Algérie est, parmi les trois pays du Maghreb, celui qui a connu la plus profonde et la plus longue colonisation. La légitimité du Front de Libération nationale (FLN) et de l'armée, principale force politique, a été acquise au cours de la lutte pour l'indépendance. Cette légitimité n'a pu être prolongée et maintenue en temps de paix qu'en s'appuyant sur des structures s'identifiant à l'état providence pourvoyant à la quasi totalité des besoins du citoyen.

Finalement, et grâce à des ressources en hydrocarbures importantes, c'est un modèle de développement volontariste qui est retenu, avec une concentration des efforts sur l'industrie lourde, au détriment de l'agriculture, des industries manufacturières et de l'habitat.

Le décès du Président Boumédienne en 1979 et la recomposition du paysage politique se traduisent dans les années 1980 par des changements au niveau des choix économiques. Ainsi, une nouvelle stratégie de « *conservation des ressources naturelles* », l'abandon des investissements onéreux pour la valorisation des richesses du sous-sol (Plan Valhid) est au programme du plan quinquennal 1980-1984.

Par ce biais, l'Algérie s'efforce d'échapper au « *tout pétrole* » et s'oriente vers un développement intégré. De nouvelles priorités sont alors dégagées et une place plus large est accordée à l'habitat, l'agriculture, l'hydraulique, les industries manufacturières afin, selon les auteurs du plan quinquennal, de préparer « *l'après-pétrole* ». À cette modification de la structure des investissements va s'ajouter à partir des années 1980, une diminution de leur volume, sous l'effet de l'effondrement des prix pétroliers et du poids de la dette extérieure (44% du PNB).

Le volontarisme des premières années de l'indépendance marquera fortement l'édification du système de santé. Le droit à la santé est un devoir de l'état providence qui décidera officiellement de la gratuité des soins pour tous en 1974.

En pratique, et malgré la mise en place de ressources considérables en infrastructures, en équipements et en personnels, l'Algérie a beaucoup de difficultés à assurer une offre de soins publics généralisée et efficace. Malgré les options proclamées, le secteur privé se développe timidement jusqu'aux années 1980, puis très rapidement après cette date. Mais c'est surtout le secteur parapublic qui a connu une expansion considérable grâce aux investissements de la caisse de sécurité sociale et à ceux des entreprises publiques.

Au fur et à mesure de l'aggravation de la crise économique, c'est précisément la caisse de sécurité sociale qui finance de fait le système de soins, la part de l'État diminuant régulièrement d'année en année.

La crise a très vite révélé et amplifié les insuffisances et les dysfonctionnements d'un tel système et sa quasi-totale dépendance de l'extérieur pour tous les intrants nécessaires à son fonctionnement. Le système de santé se caractérise en effet par une très forte extraversion et importe environ 80% de ses besoins en médicaments et la quasi-totalité des équipements, instruments et réactifs.

Le Maroc

Au Maroc, le système politique et la légitimité du pouvoir royal et de l'État reposent sur une tradition historique nationale et un fondement religieux (le roi commandeur des croyants).

Le modèle de développement marocain témoigne de la volonté d'éviter des mutations trop profondes et trop rapides susceptibles de remettre en cause les structures traditionnelles sur lesquelles s'appuie le pouvoir royal.

La priorité est ainsi donnée au développement de l'agriculture. L'industrie reste peu développée et à forte participation de capital public. Des progrès certains ont pu néanmoins être observés grâce à la mise en valeur du sous-sol et à l'appel précoce et massif aux investissements extérieurs.

Sur le plan sanitaire, le système de soins marocain a connu peu de bouleversements reproduisant à peu de choses près l'organisation et les méthodes de l'époque coloniale. Les effectifs médicaux, malgré une sensible augmentation, restent toutefois en deçà des efforts de formation des deux autres pays maghrébins.

L'intervention de l'État est cantonnée aux domaines conventionnels de la formation du personnel médical et paramédical, de la réglementation des activités médicales et de la gestion de quelques institutions et établissements de soins.

Une importante infrastructure sanitaire privée et parapublique se concentre aujourd'hui dans les zones urbaines (60% des médecins privés exercent dans les deux villes principales du Maroc).

La couverture collective des soins est assurée par des organismes de prévoyance sociale et la caisse de sécurité sociale, mais elle reste peu étendue. Ainsi, les petits paysans, les chômeurs et une grande masse de salariés précaires ne bénéficient d'aucune protection sociale effective.

En théorie, la gratuité des soins dans les établissements sous tutelle du Ministère de la Santé permet aux indigents d'accéder aux soins médicaux, mais l'éloignement et l'encombrement limitent considérablement leur accès et leur efficacité.

La Tunisie

En Tunisie, dès l'acquisition de l'indépendance en 1956, s'est posé le problème du choix d'une politique économique nationale. La première option retenue fut celle du socialisme étatique et d'une économie centralement planifiée. Malheureusement, la collectivisation progressive de la plupart des terres agricoles et d'une partie du commerce à un système coopératif mal conçu et mal organisé provoque dès 1969 un mécontentement général.

Face à l'inefficacité de la gestion bureaucratique, un changement s'opère et un retour rapide au libéralisme économique s'effectue sans toutefois remettre en cause le rôle du parti unique et de son principal dirigeant de l'époque.

Concrètement, dans les années 1960, la Tunisie accorde la priorité aux investissements tournés vers l'exportation, notamment dans le secteur des textiles. L'agriculture est reléguée au second plan et sa part dans les exportations décroît régulièrement. À côté d'une industrie extractive prospère dans les années 1970, s'est développée une industrie manufacturière (textile, agro-alimentaire, produits chimiques). Malgré des progrès certains, la situation reste difficile. La production agricole largement déficitaire, les importations massives de biens, le recours aux crédits, et surtout une baisse de l'activité touristique ont entraîné une inflation préoccupante.

La politique sanitaire tunisienne a bien évidemment largement subi les fluctuations des choix économiques. Jusqu'en 1970, le système de soins se développe dans un cadre étatique avec des résultats impressionnants: construction massive d'hôpitaux et de dispensaires, programme élargi de vaccination et large protection maternelle et infantile.

L'abandon d'une économie centralement planifiée se traduit sur le plan sanitaire par la mise en place d'un système mixte où le secteur privé se développe rapidement à côté d'un secteur public relativement important. On observe alors une augmentation du nombre de médecins exerçant à titre privé.

La couverture du « *risque maladie* » est financée par de multiples régimes d'assurances maladies, les prestations associent l'octroi de soins directs dans les formations relevant du Ministère de la Santé publique, le remboursement des soins en cas de « *longue maladie* » et une compensation des pertes de salaires éventuelles. Plus de 45% des assurés sociaux sont affiliés à des régimes de base, aux prix de cotisations supplémentaires. La gratuité des soins reste assurée pour les plus pauvres dans les établissements publics.

Le développement de ce système est cependant remis en cause à partir des années 1980, où s'accentuent les insuffisances et des dysfonctionnements posant ainsi la question centrale du financement et des dépenses de santé.

On constate donc l'existence de trois systèmes économiques et trois systèmes de santé assez différents en Afrique du Nord.

À l'immobilisme marocain s'oppose le pragmatisme tunisien et le volontarisme algérien. Cependant, à quelques nuances près, les niveaux de développement atteints dans les systèmes de santé restent comparables, malgré la variété des options retenues. Cette observation est surtout vraie en ce qui concerne les premières décennies de l'indépendance, elle reste cependant à nuancer depuis quelques années, chaque pays en effet réagissant différemment à l'impact des chocs extérieurs et à la difficile conjoncture mondiale actuelle, sans oublier la situation politique particulière qui prévaut en Algérie.

Nous allons donc dans cette deuxième partie observer l'évolution des états de santé des populations à partir de quelques indicateurs de base.

Évaluation des systèmes de santé

Les outils de mesure du système de santé

La santé, définie par l'OMS comme un *état de complet bien-être physique, mental et social*, n'est pas une entité aisément quantifiable.

D'une manière générale, les relations entre le niveau de santé et le système de santé sont très complexes à établir, la santé procédant d'un enchevêtrement d'activités où la détermination des moyens, de leurs coûts, et l'évolution de leurs conséquences et de leurs résultats sont très difficiles à isoler.

En réalité, la santé de la population ne dépend pas que du système de soins, et les causes des écarts entre les pays ne sont pas liées essentiellement aux dépenses consenties pour le système de soins.

Comme ailleurs, les pays maghrébins ont défini différentes étapes à court et moyen terme censées leur permettre d'atteindre l'objectif fixé par Alma-Ata en 1978 (*La santé pour tous en l'an 2000*). Ils ont lancé de grandes actions de santé publique, telles que la vaccination de tous les enfants contre les principales maladies infectieuses, l'hygiène du milieu, l'assainissement, l'alimentation en eau potable ou l'éducation.

Il semble cependant qu'il y ait eu un décalage entre les déclarations de principe, les objectifs généraux fixés par les différents plans et la réalité. C'est le cas en particulier de l'Algérie où la mise en œuvre concrète des plans a souffert des déficiences voire de l'absence d'une stratégie de réalisation et où les liens entre planifications et programmations ne sont pas formulés de manière explicite.

Ce décalage est cependant difficile à apprécier faute d'instruments méthodologiques, capables de mesurer le degré de mise en œuvre et les progrès effectivement réalisés par rapport aux objectifs fixés. Il est vrai cependant que chacun des trois pays a tenté d'intégrer à sa stratégie un processus de contrôle et d'évaluation. Ce processus s'appuie en général sur les indicateurs de l'OMS.

En 1981, l'OMS proposait dans le cadre de la *stratégie mondiale de la santé pour tous*, trois catégories d'indicateurs permettant d'évaluer un système de santé:

* *des indicateurs de la politique de santé* mesurant l'engagement des pays vis-à-vis de la santé, l'affectation des ressources et leur répartition;

* *des indicateurs sociaux et économiques* en rapport avec la santé concernant les mutations démographiques, l'éducation, le logement, le travail;

* *des indicateurs de l'état de santé* abordant les résultats de développement en matière de santé.

Pour l'OMS, ces indicateurs devraient être considérés comme des instruments à utiliser dans un processus national bien défini de contrôle et d'évaluation des stratégies adoptées. On voit donc que « *La santé pour tous en l'an 2000* », que certains ont qualifié « *d'utopie mobilisatrice* »,[5] a permis d'élargir la portée et la signification des indicateurs. Jusque-là en effet l'accent était surtout mis sur les mesures de morbidité et de mortalité.

Il faut relever d'ailleurs que malgré ces progrès, l'état de santé tel que mesuré par les indicateurs de mortalité et de morbidité continue à être la mesure la plus opérationnelle dont on dispose.

Pour prendre la mesure des problèmes de santé, on continue à se fonder sur la mortalité, mais cet indicateur ne rend évidemment pas compte des autres conséquences de la morbidité (souffrances, handicaps, incapacités). C'est cette constatation qui a poussé l'OMS et la Banque mondiale a définir d'autres indicateurs prenant en compte ces aspects, et en particulier les concepts d'incapacité, vie sans incapacité, EVSI,...

Quoi qu'il en soit et concernant les pays du Maghreb, ce sont les indicateurs classiques qui sont utilisés et pour lesquels on dispose d'informations relativement fiables. Ceci est particulièrement vrai pour la mortalité infantile qui, traditionnellement, a toujours été un indicateur de grande signification pour la santé publique. Un taux élevé de mortalité infantile reflète en général des déficiences au niveau de l'environnement physique et socio-économique, de la nutrition, de l'éducation et des soins.

On le voit donc, à la complexité des problèmes s'ajoute la grossièreté des instruments méthodologiques disponibles, pour pouvoir effectuer des comparaisons valables entre pays. Cette imprécision est parfois elle-même aggravée par l'absence ou l'insuffisance des données nécessaires à l'élaboration des indicateurs. Voyons ce qu'il en est en Afrique du Nord.

Évaluation du système de santé en Afrique du Nord

Pour les trois pays du Maghreb, dans le domaine sanitaire le legs de la période coloniale reste aujourd'hui encore très difficile à apprécier, même s'il est possible d'affirmer qu'il a été globalement négatif, malgré la mise en place d'une infrastructure plus ou moins importante selon les pays.

Au moment de l'indépendance, chacun des pays se caractérisait par des niveaux de santé extrêmement bas, aggravés par la désorganisation liée au départ des personnels médicaux et paramédicaux français. En 1962, l'Algérie comptait environ 300 médecins pour une population de douze millions d'habitants.

Voyons ce qu'il en est aujourd'hui, à travers l'observation des quelques indicateurs de santé suivants:

Tableau 2: Indicateurs de santé au Maghreb (2003)

Pays	TMI	TM	Années			Rapport de mortalité maternelle	Part d'enfants vaccinés contre la rougeole	Part du PIB consacrée aux dépenses de santé
			Hommes	Femmes	Total			
Algérie	55 ‰	6 ‰	68	70	69	150 ‰	74%	3.3%
Maroc	53 ‰	6 ‰	67	71	69	390 ‰	92%	1.6%
Tunisie	28 ‰	6 ‰	70	74	72	69 ‰	92%	3%

Source: Nations Unies.

Dans les années 50, les taux de mortalité infantile étaient supérieurs à 200 ‰ dans les pays du Maghreb. C'est en Tunisie qu'elle commencera à baisser sensiblement, dès 1969-1970, parallèlement au taux de fécondité. En Algérie et au Maroc, même si elle diminue un peu dès 1965, elle demeurera forte jusqu'en 1977. Le Maroc connaît une évolution moins rapide jusqu'en 1983. Il faut y voir probablement le démarrage plus tardif des campagnes de vaccinations dans ce pays.

Les Taux de mortalité infantile

Aujourd'hui, le taux de mortalité est élevé en Algérie et au Maroc, mais relativement faible en Tunisie. La Tunisie se démarque donc encore aujourd'hui, mais il faut y voir en partie les effets de la baisse plus rapide de la fécondité.

Les pays du Maghreb ont suivi le schéma classique des déclins de mortalité des pays en développement: c'est entre 0 et 1 an que les progrès sont les plus rapides, et c'est là que se creusent les inégalités entre pays ou entre classes sociales dans un pays. La première année de vie est un âge où frappent essentiellement des maladies infectieuses et parasitaires, où les facteurs culturels jouent pleinement, parfois même plus que les facteurs sociaux et économiques.

Les Taux de mortalité

Le mouvement de déclin des taux de mortalité est enclenché dès le début des années 60. Dans les trois pays, le taux de mortalité se situe entre 15 et 17 ‰ jusque vers 1970. Il s'accélérera ensuite dès 1971 pour la Tunisie, vers 1975 et 1977 pour le Maroc et l'Algérie.

Dans les années 70, les écarts entre les trois pays se creusent: la Tunisie se distingue rapidement avec un taux de mortalité de 8.8 ‰ dès 1976, tandis que l'Algérie traîne (16 ‰ à la même date). La situation évolue ensuite rapidement: le Maroc poursuit régulièrement son déclin alors que l'Algérie en plus mauvaise position jusqu'alors récupère rapidement son retard: son taux de mortalité diminue de moitié en 1978 (13.4 ‰) à 1988 (6.6 ‰).

Aujourd'hui, les taux de mortalité oscillent autour de 6 ‰ dans les trois pays.

L'espérance de vie

Depuis 1960, l'évolution des espérances de vie confirme ces déclins sensibles de la mortalité dans la région: très basse jusque vers 1970, 49 ans environ, elles vont rapidement décoller. Dès 1975, elles sont déjà à près de 60 ans en Tunisie, dans les 55 à 56 ans ailleurs. En 1980, la Tunisie est à près de 65 ans, les deux autres pays toujours groupés dans les 58 à 59 ans. L'Algérie et le Maroc accélèrent alors le rythme pour atteindre en 1989 une même espérance de vie de 65 ans. Aujourd'hui, les espérances de vie ont des valeurs proches de 70 ans dans les trois pays, et on note que la Tunisie a fait les plus grands progrès.

Ainsi, entre 1960 et aujourd'hui, la Tunisie a gagné 23 ans d'espérance de vie, l'Algérie et le Maroc 20 ans. On peut juger de l'effort accompli en matière de santé en considérant qu'il a fallu près de trois fois plus de temps aux pays industrialisés comme la France pour atteindre la même espérance de vie. Le passage d'une espérance de vie de 40 à 60 ans s'est réalisée en 10 ans au Maghreb contre 30 ans en France.

Enfin, il est significatif de noter que les différences d'espérance de vie entre les deux sexes sont faibles dans les trois pays.

Pour résumer tous ces éléments, on peut dire qu'il existe une similitude d'évolution en Algérie, en Tunisie et au Maroc puisque ces trois pays ont considérablement fait reculer leurs taux de mortalité et leurs taux de mortalité infantile, et augmenter l'espérance de vie depuis le début des années 1960. Il existe cependant des différences dans la « vitesse » de réalisation de ces progrès qui font que la Tunisie semble en avance, alors que le Maroc enregistre un retard par rapport à ces deux voisins.

On note donc beaucoup plus de concordances dans l'évolution des trois pays que de discordances. Pourtant, ce sont précisément les causes de ces discordances et de ces différences qu'il est le plus intéressant d'analyser. En effet, pourquoi à partir d'une situation épidémiologique et démographique assez semblable, ces différences existent-elles aujourd'hui?

Ces différences peuvent-elles s'expliquer uniquement par le système de santé? Dans ce cas, pourquoi le pays qui a investi le plus dans son système de soins et qui dispose du PNB le plus élevé, en l'occurrence l'Algérie, ne se situe-t-elle pas en tête?

Quels sont les autres facteurs les plus déterminants sur l'état de santé, quels sont les autres mécanismes qui améliorent effectivement les indicateurs de santé?

Pourquoi les mêmes causes ne produisent-elles pas les mêmes effets dans les différents pays, même si à long terme les tendances lourdes sont les mêmes?

Les réponses à ces questions sont loin d'être simples. Elles ne se retrouvent en effet ni totalement dans le système de santé, ni dans des facteurs hors champs.

Les ressources sanitaires et les équipements collectifs

Infrastructure et densité médicale

Dans les trois pays du Maghreb, la densité du personnel médical s'est améliorée. Les effectifs de médecins et de personnels paramédicaux ont augmenté régulièrement, mais l'on remarque un certain contraste des niveaux atteints dans les trois pays.

Tableau 3: Infrastructures médicales au Maghreb (2003)

Pays	Médecins		Hôpitaux		Pharmacies	
	nombre	1 pour x habitants	nombre	1 pour x habitants	nombre	1 pour x habitants
Algérie	19 487	1 591	447	70 000	1 752	17 800
Maroc	5 100	5 725	186	160 000	1 351	22 000
Tunisie	7 700	1 260	148	64 000	1 264	7 500

Source: Ministères de la Santé publique.

En Algérie et en Tunisie, la densité de médecins a fortement augmenté. C'est en Algérie que la démographie médicale a été la plus forte: 342 médecins en 1962, 1425 médecins en 1974, et 19 487 médecins aujourd'hui, soit près de quatre fois l'effectif du Maroc pour une population quasiment équivalente.

Lors de l'élaboration du plan de développement 1981-1985, les autorités marocaines visiblement déjà préoccupées par cette situation, s'étaient fixé deux objectifs: le premier pour 1985, visant un médecin pour 6000 habitants a été jugé à la portée des possibilités du système interne de formation dégageant en moyenne 500 nouveaux diplômes tous les ans. Le second objectif, pour l'horizon 2000, visant un médecin pour 1500 habitants s'est révélé irréalisable sans un doublement de la capacité de formation des facultés de médecine.

Le retard accumulé par le Maroc entre 1965 et 1980 s'avère donc, de l'avis même des autorités, difficile à combler aujourd'hui.

En matière d'infrastructures sanitaires, les trois pays se sont efforcés d'augmenter le nombre d'hôpitaux, de multiplier les centres de santé et d'ouvrir des dispensaires. Si on s'en tient au nombre de lits d'hôpitaux, les efforts sont très nets en Algérie où l'effectif total a augmenté de plus de 70% en vingt ans.

En Algérie, en Tunisie et au Maroc surtout, la situation se dégrade: la croissance démographique prend de vitesse la croissance des infrastructures.

Ici encore, les autorités ont pleinement conscience des insuffisances et ont réagi différemment. En Algérie, le gouvernement a retenu de privilégier l'amélioration du fonctionnement des équipements existants, l'augmentation du taux d'occupation des lits hôpitaux et les actions de prévention.

Au Maroc, face aux coûts très élevés des infrastructures, les autorités ont conclu que l'objectif était irréalisable et ont opté pour un développement privilégié de la médecine préventive.

En Tunisie, les mêmes conclusions ont conduit à mettre l'accent sur la conservation et la rentabilisation de l'infrastructure existante et sur une réorientation des efforts vers la médecine de base.

L'industrie pharmaceutique

Un système de santé ne saurait se concevoir sans une industrie pharmaceutique qui permettrait de mieux asseoir la stratégie sanitaire du pays, mettant à sa disposition les produits consommables sans pour autant dépendre des aléas économiques et politiques des marchés extérieurs. C'est pourquoi les nouvelles approches des systèmes de santé intègrent la composante pharmaceutique.

C'est ce que nous allons faire à présent, en voyant ce qu'il en est de la situation du marché du médicament dans les trois pays du Maghreb.

Depuis l'acquisition de leur indépendance, les trois pays du Maghreb se sont dotés d'une véritable industrie pharmaceutiques en vue de la fabrication de leurs propres médicaments ou dans le cadre de partenariats avec les grands groupes multinationaux. On compte ainsi une trentaine d'usines pharmaceutiques en Tunisie et au Maroc, et une douzaine en Algérie.

L'Algérie

Depuis son indépendance et jusqu'en 1997, l'Algérie s'est isolée vis-à-vis des grands groupes pharmaceutiques, ce qui a eu des conséquences néfastes sur son système de santé.

Ainsi, les seuls accords de fourniture de médicaments concernaient des pays comme la Jordanie, la Pologne ou la Bulgarie. Ces médicaments étaient des copies de médicaments occidentaux, moins chers mais aussi de mauvaise qualité. On a même déploré quelques cas de contrefaçons, avec les risques que l'on peut imaginer (pas de principe actif dans le médicament).

Tableau 4: Le secteur pharmaceutique au Maghreb (2003)

Pays	Chiffre d'affaires 2003 (progression)	Consommation de médicaments 1998	Pharmacies nombre	1 pharmacie pour x habitants	Nombre d'usines	Couverture des besoins nationaux
Algérie	590 M$ (+2%)	9,3 $/hab	1 752	17 800	12	20%
Maroc	570 M$ (+ 6%)	16,4 $/hab	1 351	22 000	28	80%
Tunisie	270 M$ (+ 8%)	20,3 $/hab	1 264	7 500	30	43%

Source: Ministères de la Santé publique.

Par ailleurs, les statistiques sur les maladies et la consommation de médicaments étaient pratiquement inexistantes, ce qui rendait impossible une gestion de stocks « *normale* ». Les ruptures de stocks étant fréquentes, il n'était pas rare de voir des Algériens dévaliser les pharmacies des aéroports de Tunis ou de Paris.

Enfin, les quelques usines pharmaceutiques du pays étaient mal encadrées et tournaient mal.

Depuis 1997, avec l'arrivée du nouveau gouvernement, la situation semble avoir changé, et les autorités ont donné 2 ans à tous les importateurs de médicaments du pays pour mettre en place des projets industriels en vue d'assurer une partie au moins de la consommation nationale de médicaments.

Aujourd'hui, 6 usines fabriquent des produits pharmaceutiques et 6 autres les conditionnent dans des conditions acceptables. Malgré ces efforts, 80% des besoins en médicaments sont toujours importés, et notamment de France (2/3 des importations).

L'Algérie dispose actuellement de l'industrie pharmaceutique la plus en retard, mais c'est également celle qui suscite le plus d'intérêt de la part des groupes multinationaux, étant donnée la taille du marché naissant.

Le Maroc

Au Maroc, 28 usines pharmaceutiques couvrent 80% des besoins de la population, le reste étant importé de France. Cependant, elles tournent à seulement 40% de leur capacité de production, et leur avenir reste incertain dans le contexte de mondialisation que l'on connaît.

La voie que tente de suivre le Maroc est celle de l'exportation d'une partie de la production, ce qui permettrait de relancer la production dans des conditions meilleures. Actuellement, le pays exporte 8% de sa production pharmaceutique vers l'Afrique subsaharienne, la Chine, la Russie, la Suisse, l'Allemagne et la Belgique.

La Tunisie

En Tunisie, une trentaine d'usines pharmaceutiques assurent 43% des besoins de la population, une partie de celle-ci étant exportée. De ce point de vue, c'est le pays qui semble détenir l'industrie pharmaceutique la plus performante.

L'approvisionnement en eau potable

Selon les normes retenues par l'OMS, l'accessibilité à l'eau potable en milieu urbain signifie que: « *de l'eau non contaminée est disponible à des fontaines publiques à moins de 200 mètres du foyer d'habitation* ».

En milieu rural « *un accès raisonnable implique que les membres de la famille ne passent pas un temps disproportionné de leur journée à se procurer de l'eau non contaminée à des sources ou des puits sanitaires protégés* ».

À partir de ces définitions, l'eau potable était en 1988 accessible à 85% de la population urbaine en Algérie, et à 100% de la population urbaine en Tunisie et au Maroc.

En milieu rural, il existe un contraste important entre les pays. Au Maroc, 18% de la population rurale seulement disposait d'eau potable entre 1988-1990, alors qu'en Tunisie cette proportion atteignit 99% dès 1990 et seulement 55% en Algérie.

L'apport Nutritionnel

En 1980, les trois pays avaient atteint un niveau d'apport calorique moyen supérieur au minimum requis selon les normes de l'OMS.

En 1965, pourtant, deux d'entre eux présentaient des insuffisances importantes: l'Algérie et la Tunisie. Depuis, les progrès tunisiens ont été particulièrement remarquables puisqu'en 1980, le minimum requis étant largement atteint. Mais en Algérie, il était tout juste atteint et restait inférieur au niveau moyen des pays à revenu intermédiaire.

Par ailleurs, la mesure de l'apport calorique moyen cache des différences sensibles entre différents groupes de populations, selon le milieu et le niveau de revenu. En Algérie, et surtout au Maroc où la moyenne reste relativement basse, il faut donc craindre qu'il existe encore des poches importantes de carence nutritionnelles avec des répercussions non négligeables sur l'état de santé.

L'amélioration de la consommation alimentaire a été dans tous ces pays l'objectif prioritaire des deux dernières décennies. Les politiques de subvention alimentaire ont été le principal levier pour atteindre cet objectif: elles ont consisté à distribuer à la population des produits alimentaires à des prix abordables, l'état prenant en charge la différence.

Aujourd'hui, et sous la pression des organismes financiers internationaux, ces politiques semblent remises en cause. Les critiques portent sur leur poids dans les déficits publics, sur le fait qu'elles n'ont pas ciblé avec précision les populations, réellement démunies, sur leurs effets pervers sur la production agricole et sur leur rôle dans l'aggravation de la dette.

Il reste à savoir à l'avenir si l'amélioration de l'état nutritionnel pourra être poursuivie, voire maintenue, en mettant en œuvre d'autres politiques moins coûteuses et plus axées sur l'offre.

L'éducation des filles

Les derniers travaux de la Banque mondiale renvoient à ce que H. Mosley a appelé le « *concept de synergie social* ». Il écrit à ce propos: « un seul déterminant social, tel que le niveau d'instruction des femmes, peut agir à travers plusieurs variables intermédiaires simultanément ».

Ceci permet du même coup de comprendre pourquoi de nombreuses techniques médicales modernes efficaces dans leur contexte d'origine le sont beaucoup moins dans le contexte de nombreux pays africains, si les femmes n'ont pas les capacités intellectuelles et matérielles d'y recourir.

Transposées à la région du Maghreb, ces conclusions donnent un nouvel éclairage et permettent de comprendre pourquoi la Tunisie, où les femmes bénéficient d'un statut relativement plus favorable que ses voisins, présente une meilleure et plus rapide évolution des principaux indicateurs sanitaires. Elles expliquent également en partie le décalage observé entre les ressources sanitaires importantes mises en place en Algérie et l'état de santé peu satisfaisant obtenu.

L'éducation des filles apparaît alors comme un facteur essentiel pour diffuser les gestes et comportements élémentaires permettant de prévenir les maladies, d'établir des diagnostics simples quand elles surviennent et de recourir à la médecine moderne.

Indépendamment de l'éducation, l'autonomie des femmes même non instruites est un élément capital dans le processus sanitaire et en particulier dans les sociétés où la charge des enfants est confiée exclusivement aux femmes.

La Réforme du système de santé en Tunisie

La révision du mode d'intervention de l'État d'une manière générale et la réforme du système sanitaire en particulier sont devenues l'un des thèmes centraux du débat politique en Tunisie.

La Nécessité d'une réforme

Le système de santé tunisien s'est trouvé confronté ces dernières années à de profondes mutations de la société, un boom technologique dans les sciences médicales, et une poussée inflationniste sans précédent, autant de défis qui ont rendu nécessaires certaines réformes en profondeur.

D'abord, sur le plan démographique, la population urbaine est sur le point d'achever sa transition démographique, ce qui se traduit par un début de vieillissement et donc une émergence des pathologies chroniques dégénératives telles que les maladies cardio-vasculaires ou certaines tumeurs.

Or, ce type d'affections nécessite des soins spécifiques où l'on n'a plus affaire à des omnipraticiens comme ce fut le cas jadis, mais à une multitude de spécialistes, chacun se devant d'être extrêmement pointu dans son domaine.

Cela rend nécessaire une vulgarisation des technologies médicales modernes et coûteuses, telles que l'hémodialyse ou la transplantation d'organes. Ces technologies de pointe posent à la fois le problème de la modernisation de l'infrastructure sanitaire urbaine, mais également celui du financement de l'acte sanitaire, qui devient dans certains cas prohibitif. L'écart grandissant entre les déboursements effectifs réalisés par les patients auprès des prestataires de services d'une part et les remboursements des frais de soins par les organismes d'assurance d'autre part montre d'ailleurs que le système d'assurance est aujourd'hui à bout de souffle.

Sur un autre plan, il semblerait que l'environnement socioculturel de la Tunisie soit favorable à toutes les formes de changement possibles, et notamment au niveau de l'éducation, de la santé et des loisirs. En effet, le profil du Tunisien moderne a radicalement changé: plus instruit, plus moderne, plus émancipé, il cohabite avec des sociétés, lointaines géographiquement, mais rapprochées par les nouveaux moyens de communication.

Le fatalisme qui caractérisait la population a été remplacé par une attente de résultats concrets, c'est-à-dire une guérison à plus ou moins longue échéance, et un rallongement de la vie. La relation patient/médecin a ainsi radicalement changé.

Toujours sur le même plan, il faut noter que le Tunisien adopte un comportement à risque, tant dans son alimentation que sa sexualité ou sa sédentarité et son manque d'exercice physique. Ce comportement à risque appelle également une adaptation du système de santé.

Sur le plan économique, les restrictions budgétaires et l'accroissement du coût des nouvelles technologies médicales ont entraîné une remise en cause de l'engagement de l'État dans le mode d'intervention et le financement systématique des soins. Ainsi, la part des dépenses publiques de santé sont passées de 6,6% du budget total de l'État en 1985 à 8,7% en 1999, soit un accroissement de seulement 2,1 points en près de 15 ans. La part des dépenses sanitaires publiques est passée, quant à elle, de 2,2% du PIB en 1990 à 2,1% en 1999.

D'un autre côté, l'éthique veut que la prise en charge des personnes sans ressources ou aux ressources limitées soit une forme indéniable de progrès social et un acquis à ne jamais remettre en cause.

Les réformes en cours du système de santé en Tunisie

Le gouvernement a pris conscience de l'ampleur des défaillances du système sanitaire et a engagé tout un train de mesures visant la réforme du système de santé:

- la modernisation des structures sanitaires publiques;
- la refonte du régime d'assurance-maladie;
- le rapprochement entre les différents régimes d'assurance actuels jusqu'à parvenir à un régime de base obligatoire et unifié;
- la compression des coûts des prestations médicales;

- l'utilisation des médicaments génériques (dont les brevets sont tombés dans le domaine public, environ 30% moins chers, et qui représentent actuellement 10% des médicaments consommés, contre 3% en Europe);
- la prise en charge par l'État des soins lourds, tels que la chirurgie cardio-vasculaire, la transplantation d'organes ou les hémodialyses.

Le financement des soins: le cas de la Tunisie

Abordons la question du financement des prestations médicales en Tunisie. À cet effet, nous commencerons par présenter les différents acteurs intervenant dans la prise en charge des soins, puis nous examinerons les défaillances du système d'assurance-maladie actuel, avant de voir ce qu'il en est de la réforme en cours.

Les intervenants du système de financement de soins en Tunisie

Le volume global des dépenses médicales des ménages en Tunisie s'élevait à environ 900 M$. Voyons comment se répartissent ces dépenses selon les différents acteurs économiques concernés par la santé.

En 1999, le financement des dépenses globales de santé se faisait de la manière suivante: en portant ces chiffres sur un graphique, nous pouvons mieux visualiser la répartition des dépenses en matière de soins.

Figure 2: Répartition des dépenses en soins en Tunisie en 1999 (%)

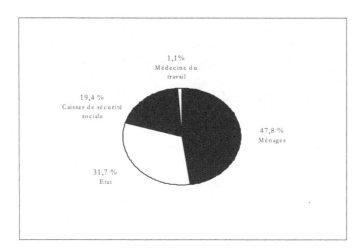

Source: Ministère de la Santé Publique.

On voit très nettement sur le graphique que près de la moitié des dépenses globales de santé est supportée par les ménages alors que l'État vient en second lieu, loin derrière. Les différents régimes de sécurité sociale représentent à peine le 1/5ᵉ du total.

Quant à la médecine du travail, elle est pratiquement inexistante dans le système de santé tunisien. Cela est regrettable, car les entreprises tunisiennes ont la capacité de participer davantage au financement des soins de la population active employée.

Les défaillances du système actuel d'assurance-maladie

La principale défaillance dans le financement du système de santé en Tunisie réside dans la multiplicité des régimes de remboursement des prestations médicales.

En effet, il existe actuellement de nombreux régimes assurant le remboursement des soins, chacun ayant son propre environnement juridique, et il est déplorable de constater la quasi-absence de coordination entre ces régimes.

Outre les régimes légaux qui couvrent 2.4 millions de travailleurs, il faut citer les assurances groupes complémentaires, qui couvrent environ 200 000 travailleurs, une cinquantaine de mutuelles (mutuelle des enseignants, mutuelle des magistrats,...) qui regroupe environ 130 000 personnes, et enfin les régimes spécifiques à certains corps de métiers, tels que le Ministère de la défense nationale, le Ministère de l'intérieur, la Société nationale de Transport (SNT), la Société tunisienne d'Electricité et de Gaz (STEG) ou la Société nationale du Chemin de Fer tunisien (SNCFT).

> À cela, il faut ajouter la médecine du travail, dont la législation prévoit l'existence d'une structure médicale interentreprises pour les entreprises employant entre 40 et 300 personnes, et une structure complètement autonome pour les entreprises employant plus de 300 salariés.[6] Cette structure particulière, encore peu présente comme on l'a vu supra, concerne surtout les actes médicaux courants ou préventifs.

Conclusion

Que conclure de tout cela, si ce n'est que nous avons sous les yeux trois systèmes de santé différents mais qui, à quelques nuances près, ont atteint des niveaux comparables.

Le défi qui se pose à présent dans la région est le suivant: après avoir réussi à contrôler sa natalité, le Maghreb se doit à présent d'achever définitivement sa transition démographique en parachevant l'œuvre engagée depuis les années 1960.

Pour cela, il faudrait tenir compte des changements observés dans la société maghrébine ces dernières années. Il faudra tenir compte, notamment du vieillissement en cours de la population, et de la transition épidémiologique dans lesquelles se sont engagées les populations. A titre d'exemple, le système sanitaire doit être prêt à offrir des services spécialisés aux seniors qui sont de plus en plus nombreux, en créant des services de gériatrie.

Notes

1. OMS.
2. Élisabeth Longuenesse, *Santé, médecine et société dans le monde arabe*, Paris, L'Harmattan, 1995, p. 42.

3. E. Bergsma, P. Jongejan, K. Schaapveled, *Sustainable development and health*, La Haye, 1992.

4. S. L. Cristopher Murray et Julio Frank, in *Bulletin de l'OMS*, 2000, Genève, p. 163.

5. Brunet-Jailly.

6. Code du travail.

9

La Lutte contre le Sida en Afrique du Nord

Sofiane Bouhdiba

Introduction

Le SIDA est-il, en Afrique du Nord, une épidémie ou au plus quelques cas isolés? Peut-on affirmer, que l'Islam, religion principale dans cette région du monde, a joué le rôle de frein dans la propagation du SIDA? Pourquoi cette nette dichotomie des deux côtés du Sahara, entre d'un côté une Afrique sub-saharienne minée par le mal, avec 2,3 millions de décès par SIDA en 2001,[1] et de l'autre une Afrique du Nord *apparemment* indemne, avec seulement quelques dizaines de milliers de décès[2] la même année?

Telles seront quelques-unes des questions auxquelles nous tenterons de trouver quelques éléments de réponse dans ce cours. Pour cela, notre réflexion s'articulera autour de trois grandes parties: nous ferons d'abord le point sur l'épidémie du SIDA en Afrique du Nord, en examinant quelques indicateurs-clés, nous verrons ensuite quels sont les grands axes du programme de lutte contre le SIDA en Afrique du Nord, et la dernière partie de ce cours se fera en termes de perspectives.

Le Sida en Afrique du Nord

En Afrique du Nord, on estime le nombre d'adultes (15-49 ans) vivant avec le virus du VIH/SIDA à 117 200 personnes en 1999, ce qui traduit un taux de prévalence du SIDA d'environ 0,05%.

Lorsqu'on sait que près de 24 millions d'adultes sont infectés par le virus, avec un taux de prévalence de 8,57%, et quand on sait que 2,2 millions de personnes en sont décédées en 1999, on se rend compte de la dichotomie existant entre les deux côtés du Sahara.

Voyons maintenant comment se présente la situation dans chacun des 3 pays d'Afrique du Nord.

État des lieux

L'Algérie

En Algérie, 110 000 adultes sont infectés par le virus du VIH/SIDA, ce qui indique un taux de prévalence de 0,07%.

On ne dispose pas d'informations concernant la séropositivité des femmes se présentant aux consultations prénatales, mais on sait que le taux de prévalence était de 1% en 1988 chez les professionnelles du sexe à Constantine et à Oran.

En Algérie, le Programme national de Lutte contre le Sida (PNLS) existe depuis 1988, mais n'a été officiellement coiffé par le gouvernement qu'en 1999. Les secteurs couverts par le PNLS sont les suivants: l'éducation, la santé, la police, l'armée, la fonction publique, le sport, le système pénitentiaire et l'immigration. Le monde rural reste donc livré à lui-même.

Il existe un comité interministériel national pour la lutte contre le SIDA, présidé par le Ministre de la Santé publique et de la Population.

Il n'existe pas de législation spécifique au VIH/SIDA, ce sont les dispositions légales générales sur la santé qui sont appliquées, en cas de discrimination pour cause de VIH par exemple.

On ne sait pas grand chose sur l'impact économique du VIH/SIDA en Algérie, mais on sait qu'au niveau des ménages et dans le secteur agricole, le virus est la cause d'une augmentation des dépenses de soins, et donc une diminution de l'épargne et un changement à terme des schémas de production.

Concernant l'éducation, le modèle mis au point par L'UNICEF et l'ONUSIDA montre qu'en Algérie, le décès ou l'élimination physique des enseignants infectés entraîne une grave perturbation dans le déroulement des cours.

Le Maroc

Au Maroc, 5 000 adultes sont infectés par le virus du VIH/SIDA, ce qui indique un taux de prévalence de 0,03%. Ce taux était de 0,02% en 1996 chez les femmes en consultation prénatales.

L'impact économique du VIH/SIDA au Maroc semble relativement faible, si ce n'est qu'au niveau des ménages il entraîne une diminution de l'épargne.

La Tunisie

Selon les services de la santé publique tunisienne, le premier cas de SIDA est apparu en Tunisie en 1985.[3] Entre cette date et 1990, 53 cas ont été recensés, dont 34 décès. Depuis, les cas recensés ont évolué de la manière suivante:

Il y aurait aujourd'hui 906 cas de personnes atteintes du SIDA en Tunisie: 635 hommes, 199 femmes et 72 enfants. Selon une autre source, 329 personnes atteintes de SIDA seraient décédées en Tunisie depuis l'apparition du virus.

Figure 3: Cas de SIDA chez les 15-49 ans en Tunisie

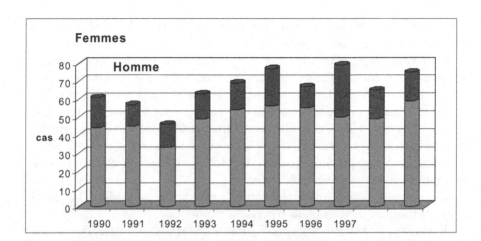

Selon l'ONUSIDA, la situation serait bien plus alarmante, puisqu'il y aurait 2200 adultes âgés de 15 à 49 ans infectés par le virus en 1999,[4] ce qui signifie un taux de prévalence du SIDA de 0,04%, et de 0,03% chez les consommateurs de drogue par injection.

Le SIDA touche davantage les hommes (80% des cas) que les femmes (20%), environ 25% des cas sont des jeunes de 15-29 ans, et 60% ont entre 20 et 40 ans.

Constatations

L'incertitude des chiffres

Le manque, pour ne pas dire l'absence d'informations locales, ainsi que l'incertitude des chiffres publiés par ONUSIDA, en disent long sur la difficulté de se rendre compte de la situation réelle du SIDA en Afrique du Nord.

La différence entre les deux sources officielles (les gouvernements respectifs et ONUSIDA) est également révélatrice quant aux difficultés à étudier une pathologie « *honteuse* » et passée sous silence dans un pays où les tabous restent malgré tout puissants.

La Localisation des cas

Quoiqu'il en soit, le SIDA semble être localisé exclusivement en milieu urbain (en Tunisie, tous les décès ont eu lieu en milieu urbain), dans les capitales et les grandes villes, et notamment le long de la bande littorale.

En Tunisie, par exemple, la moitié des cas sont concentrés autour de la capitale et ses banlieues, et 30% des cas concernent les villes du littoral Est.[5]

Figure 4: Mode de transmission du VIH/SIDA au Maghreb

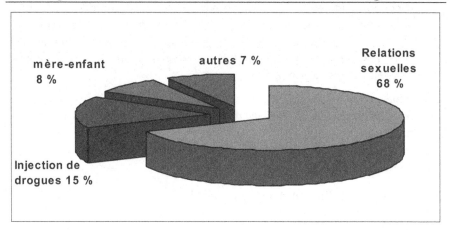

Le Mode de transmission du virus

Voyons sur le graphique suivant quels sont les principaux modes de transmission du VIH/SIDA au Maghreb: les facteurs exposant les individus au risque d'infection sont divers, les rapports sexuels représentant toutefois la principale voie de transmission.[6]

Concernant les vecteurs de la maladie, deux phénomènes majeurs sont en cause.

Il faut y voir d'abord les effets pervers de la mixité entre la population locale et les touristes. Cela expliquerait peut-être la concentration des cas de SIDA le long des zones balnéaires du Maghreb. En Tunisie, par exemple, les cas se concentrent dans une bande s'étendant du Nord-Est (régions de Tabarka et Bizerte) au Sud-Est du pays (région de Jerba).

Le retour des travailleurs émigrés à l'étranger constitue le deuxième vecteur de propagation du virus.

Dans les deux cas, l'infection peut être qualifiée d'exogène, puisqu'elle procède, non pas d'une pratique culturelle locale, mais bien d'un choc entre deux cultures.

Même si les statistiques publiées par le Ministère de la Santé ou l'ONUSIDA ne prennent pas en compte l'ensemble des décès par SIDA, il faut reconnaître que cette maladie est loin de représenter une cause majeure de décès urbains en Tunisie. Ainsi, selon l'ONUSIDA,

> Une étude réalisée en 1991 parmi des femmes en consultation prénatale à Tunis n'a trouvé aucun signe d'infection à VIH.

> Une étude effectuée en 1999 dans une région non précisée n'a relevé aucun signe d'infection parmi des femmes testées cn consultation prénatale.

Le dépistage du VIH parmi des professionnel(les) du sexe a relevé moins de 1% d'infections parmi les femmes testées pendant la plus grande partie des années 1990 et n'a trouvé aucun signe d'infection parmi les femmes testées entre 1998 et 1999.

Un pour cent des consommateurs de drogues injectables testés entre 1993 et 1996 étaient positifs pour le VIH. En 1997, 0,3% des consommateurs de drogues injectables testés étaient positifs pour le VIH.[7]

Cette faible prévalence du SIDA serait due en partie à la culture islamique qui condamne les rapports sexuels non légitimes, c'est-à-dire en dehors des liens sacrés du mariage.

La société tunisienne voit également d'un mauvais œil les changements trop fréquents de partenaires sexuels.

La Lutte contre le Sida en Afrique du nord

Les stratégies locales

La lutte contre le SIDA n'a pas encore réellement commencé à s'organiser au Maghreb, pour plusieurs raisons: d'abord, le gouvernement commence à peine à admettre l'idée que le virus du VIH/SIDA a pénétré les frontières physiques, d'une part, et la barrière érigée par l'islam, d'autre part.

Par ailleurs, les facteurs à l'origine de la transmission du virus sont encore mal connus, et le silence qui plane autour des personnes infectées ou décédées du SIDA n'est pas là pour arranger les choses.

La riposte au virus n'est donc que rarement fondée sur une compréhension claire des circuits de transmission et les stratégies des groupes à risque sont encore mal connues.

Toujours est-il qu'il se dégage progressivement une volonté politique d'élaborer et d'appliquer une stratégie de lutte contre le SIDA dans la région.

Parmi les points-clés des PNLS (Programmes nationaux de Lutte contre le SIDA), certains ont davantage retenu notre attention. D'abord, il s'agit de comprendre les différents modes de transmission de l'épidémie. À partir de là, les divers programmes peuvent mobiliser les forces en présence, de manière à faire intervenir les acteurs médicaux classiques, mais également la société civile, les ONG, le secteur éducatif, les scouts, etc.

Parmi les autres grands volets de ces programmes citons la vulgarisation, à travers un vaste programme de communication mettant l'accent sur les modes de transmission du virus et la nécessité de ne pas traiter les personnes infectées en *paria* de la société, ainsi que la détermination des groupes à risques, afin d'élaborer des stratégies spécifiques; les groupes à risque isolés pour l'instant sont les prostituées et, dans une moindre mesure, les consommateurs de drogue injectable.

Les PNLS intègrent également un vaste volet médical, qui comprend la mise en place d'une infrastructure médicale (locaux, médicaments, matériel), la surveillance épidémiologique, et notamment le contrôle systématique du sang et ses dérivés, la prise en charge médicale, sociale et psychologique par l'état des soins des personnes infectées, ainsi que la formation de médecins spécialistes du SIDA.

Les programmes ne négligent pas pour autant le volet social de la question, puisqu'ils s'intéressent aussi très largement à l'élaboration d'une stratégie en vue du changement des comportements sexuels des jeunes, l'intégration du volet SIDA dans les programmes de santé de la reproduction, en profitant du réseau de planification familiale (qui a déjà fait ses preuves du reste); ainsi que la promotion du préservatif masculin, dont le taux de prévalence n'est que de 9,4%.

Enfin, au niveau institutionnel, les pays du Maghreb ont procédé à l'ouverture de représentation nationales de l'ONUSIDA, à l'amendement de lois en vue de lutter contre les pratiques contribuant à la propagation du SIDA, et en particulier au niveau de la prostitution clandestine, ainsi qu'à la mise en place d'une cellule d'écoute pour les jeunes, c'est-à-dire un numéro de téléphone vert renseignant les jeunes sur les questions relatives au SIDA.

Les stratégies régionales

Au niveau régional, de nombreuses actions concertées ont été mise en place, comme par exemple la participation au HARPAS (HIV/AIDS Regional Program in the Arab States), créé en septembre 2002. Un premier atelier « *Leadership for an expanded response to HIV/AIDS in the arab region* » s'est tenu du 28 septembre au 1er octobre 2002. Cet atelier a abouti à la recommandation suivante: l'élaboration régulière de rapport-pays concernant l'épidémie de SIDA. Dans la pratique, il n'y a rien eu de concret, mais les travaux de cet atelier auront eu au moins comme résultat de rompre le silence qui régnait jusque-là autour de la question du SIDA dans les pays arabes et d'unifier les points de vue des décideurs.

Citons également la création du réseau RANAA (Regional Arab Network Against AIDS). Ce réseau a été créé par l'atelier « *Leadership, partnership and networking of civil society organisations on HIV/AIDS in the arab region* », qui s'est tenu du 9 au 13 décembre 2002 à Tunis et qui a réuni 14 États arabes.

Par ailleurs, les gouvernements essaient de se concerter autant que faire se peut, comme en témoignent la réunion des pays du Moyen-Orient et de l'Afrique du Nord (MENA) qui s'est tenue du 1er au 2 juin 2003 au Caire, avec pour objectif de clarifier les missions des ONG dans les pays respectifs, et en particulier dans la prise en charge des personnes vivant avec le virus. En témoigne aussi cette importante réunion qui s'est tenue le 5 mars 2003 au Caire afin de mettre sur pied une stratégie en vue de faire participer le monde des arts et du spectacle à la lutte contre le SIDA. Cette réunion a abouti à un atelier qui s'est tenu en juillet 2003 et qui a commencé à mettre en pratique les recommandations précédentes.

Enfin, citons pour clore ce chapitre le projet initié par le PNUD et l'UNESCO, qui a consisté en la traduction en arabe d'un kit publié il y a quelques années par ONUSIDA (HIV/AIDS, human rights and youth). Ce projet a été concrétisé par un atelier qui s'est tenu à Bhersaf (Liban) en juin 2003.

Les déterminants dans la lutte contre le Sida en Afrique du Nord

Nous allons examiner deux déterminants et essayer d'évaluer le rôle qu'ils ont joué dans la lutte conte le SIDA en Tunisie: le préservatif et la religion.

Le préservatif

La question que de nombreux experts ont posé a été la suivante: quel est le rôle joué par le préservatif dans la lutte contre le SIDA en Tunisie?

Voyons dans le tableau 5 dans quelle mesure sont utilisés les moyens de contraception en Tunisie:

Tableau 5: Prévalence des méthodes de contraception en Tunisie en 2002

Méthode contraceptive	Prévalence
Stérilets	57,6%
Pilule	42,2%
Calendrier	21,1%
Stérilisation féminine	10,4%
Coitus interruptus	9,5%
Condom	9,4%
Injections	8,4%
Crèmes	5,1%
Implants	1,3%
TOTAL	80,4%

Source: ONFP.

Figure 5: Méthodes contraceptives en Tunisie

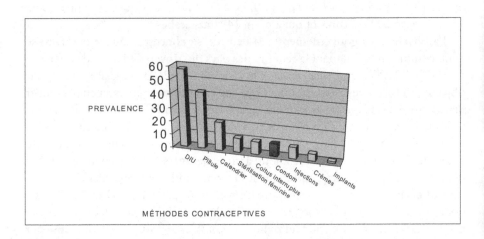

Comme on peut le voir, le préservatif masculin (condom) occupe le 6ᵉ rang. La vente des préservatifs a été autorisée par le gouvernement en 1961,[8] mais les premiers lots ont été utilisés en 1966, lorsque 5 000 condoms ont été distribués à la population. Le nombre de condoms utilisés a évolué de la manière suivante:

Tableau 6: Nombre de préservatifs utilisés

Année	Nombre de condoms utilisés	Nombre de condoms utilisés par homme âgé de 15–50 ans
1966	5 000	0,5
1978	1 800 000	1,3
1986	2 000 000	1,1
1992	3 450 000	1,6
1997	4 000 000	1,5

source: ONFP.

Figure 6: Nombre de condoms utilisés

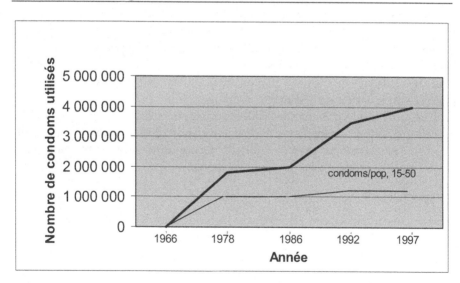

On voit que, malgré l'augmentation rapide du nombre de préservatifs utilisés, le nombre de préservatifs utilisés par homme âgé de 15 à 50 ans est resté relativement stable.

Le condom n'a pas joué un rôle important dans la stratégie de lutte contre le SIDA pour les raisons suivantes:

- dès le départ, le condom a été introduit dans une optique de planification familiale, son rôle de protecteur contre les MST n'est apparu que bien plus tard;
- la population ne lui fait pas confiance;
- les jeunes ne savent pas l'utiliser;
- il retarde l'érection et diminue le plaisir sexuel;
- les partenaires sexuels déclarent se connaître suffisamment pour ne pas avoir à l'utiliser dans un but de protection contre le SIDA;
- il est difficile pour un homme d'acheter un préservatif auprès d'une femme, et vice versa;
- les mères ne donnent pas de préservatifs à leurs filles, car ce serait encourager la perte de leur virginité.

La religion

La religion joue un rôle de protection contre le SIDA, de deux manières: le mariage et la circoncision. L'islam interdit les relations sexuelles hors du cadre du mariage, ce qui constitue une barrière contre les MST et le SIDA. En Tunisie, comme dans tout pays musulman, les jeunes garçons sont circoncis vers l'âge de 5 ans. Or, de nombreuses études ont démontré que les hommes circoncis avaient une probabilité moindre d'être infectés du virus du SIDA. Une récente comparaison entre 27 études portant sur le lien entre le risque de contracter le SIDA et la circoncision a démontré une probabilité diminuée de moitié.[9] La question que l'on pourrait poser ici est la suivante: y a-t-il effectivement un lien de cause à effet, ou faut-il plutôt y voir les effets de la sexualité islamique?

Une autre étude portant sur 6 800 hommes en milieu rural en Ouganda a montré que 16% des hommes non circoncis étaient séropositifs, contre seulement 7% chez ceux circoncis. Le seul risque d'infection réside dans l'utilisation d'un scalpel infecté entre deux circoncisions successives.

Perspectives

Il est vrai que le taux de prévalence du SIDA reste encore à un niveau relativement faible, autour de 0,03%. Cependant, on observe une augmentation du nombre de personnes infectées, ce qui signifie que la menace se précise dans la région.

L'observation nous montre une augmentation des taux de prévalence chez deux groupes à risque particulièrement vulnérables dans cette région du monde: les femmes et les enfants.

Par ailleurs, la médiocre qualité des informations cache en réalité une situation beaucoup plus alarmante que celle que nous livrent les statistiques publiées. Dans les pays du Maghreb, il s'agit davantage d'estimations que de données concrètes. De plus, les populations maghrébines sont aujourd'hui soumises à un tel bouleversement culturel qu'il faudra compter à l'avenir avec de nouveaux comportements, notamment en matière de sexualité.

Ainsi, l'âge aux premiers rapports sexuels est désormais de 17 ans en Tunisie. Comme, de plus l'âge au mariage a notablement reculé (30 ans), l'activité sexuelle hors mariage augmente, avec tous les risques qui lui sont attachés. Les jeunes constituent donc désormais un groupe à risque, et ce qui n'arrange rien, c'est qu'ils représentent une part importante de la population.

De même, la consommation de drogues injectables, phénomène de mode copié de l'occident, risque d'introduire une nouvelle classe à risque dans une société où les seules drogues consommées étaient le *takrouri* ou le *hachich*, qui, sur le plan épidémiologique du moins, ne jouent aucun rôle.

Enfin, si le virus du VIH/SIDA a pour la première fois touché les populations maghrébines par le Nord (Europe du Sud: Italie, France, Espagne), c'est au Sud que la menace gronde actuellement. En effet, l'ouverture du commerce aux pays d'Afrique subsaharienne (signature du protocole de Durban en juillet 2002) a accru les mouvements d'hommes d'affaires de part et d'autre du Sahara. Par ailleurs, l'installation de la BAD à Tunis a accru les déplacements des diplomates africains et leurs familles. Enfin, depuis quelques années, la Tunisie est devenue une véritable plate-forme migratoire, une sorte de relais, à travers lequel transitent des milliers de migrants clandestins, en vue d'atteindre dans une seconde étape l'Eldorado sud-européen. Il va sans dire que de tels flux d'individus provenant de zones à risque jouera certainement un rôle majeur dans la transmission du virus à l'intérieur des frontières du Maghreb.

Conclusion

On voit donc que l'Afrique du Nord se trouve actuellement dans une situation un peu particulière: d'une part, les indicateurs récents sont plutôt rassurants, et le SIDA ne semble pas constituer une menace de premier plan. D'autre part, tout porte à croire que la transition culturelle que connaissent les populations maghrébines va entraîner une flambée dans les 10 prochaines années.

Il s'agit donc à présent de rompre le silence, chose qui semble avoir déjà été faite, de comprendre les mécanismes de l'épidémie dans la région, puis de mettre en œuvre une stratégie réaliste qui se veut davantage préventive que curative.

En tout cas, le bouclier que constituait l'islam face à l'épidémie semble désormais relever davantage du mythe que du réel. Il faudrait donc se rendre compte que les pays d'Afrique du Nord doivent d'ores et déjà mettre en place des structures de prise en charge et passer d'une stratégie d'observation/prévention à une politique sanitaire curative.

Parmi les mesures à mettre en application en ce sens, citons la nécessité de créer des centres spécialisés dans le traitement des cas de SIDA, en les nommant ouvertement. En effet, jusqu'à ce jour, les cas de VIH sont traités plus ou moins confidentiellement dans les services infectieux des hôpitaux publics. C'est donc désormais ouvertement que les pays du Maghreb devront affronter l'épidémie du VIH dans les années à venir

Notes

1. ONUSIDA, *Le point sur l'épidémie de SIDA*, ONUSIDA/OMS, Genève, décembre 2001, p. 29.
2. 30 000 décès par SIDA en 2001 pour la région Afrique du Nord/Moyen-Orient, selon ONUSIDA, *Le point sur l'épidémie de SIDA*, ONUSIDA/OMS, Genève, décembre 2001, p. 29.
3. Le premier cas de SIDA dans le monde avait été observé en 1981 à Los Angeles, USA.
4. ONUSIDA, *Le SIDA en Afrique pays par pays*, ONUSIDA/CEA, Genève, décembre 2000, p. 229.
5. Ministère de la Santé publique.
6. ONUSIDA, *Le point sur l'épidémie de SIDA*, ONUSIDA/OMS, Genève, décembre 2001, p. 20.
7. ONUSIDA, *Le SIDA en Afrique pays par pays*, ONUSIDA/CEA, Genève, décembre 2000, p. 229.
8. Loi n° 61-7, 9 Janvier 1961, *JORT*, 3-6 Janvier 1961, autorisant la vente des produits contraceptifs.
9. ONUSIDA, AIDS epidemic report, June 2000, p.70.

Bibliographie

Livres

Association internationale des Démographes de Langue française (AIDELF), 1997, Actes du colloque *« Mortalité, morbidité: problèmes de mesure, facteurs d'évolution, essai de prospective »*, Paris, PUF.

Association internationale des Démographes de Langue française (AIDELF), 2002, Actes du colloque *« Vivre plus longtemps, avoir moins d'enfants: quelles implications? »*, Paris, PUF.

Benaicha, N., Gueddana, N., Jarraya, S., 1985, *Un enfant et deux Tunisies*, Tunis, ONFP.

Bergsma, E., Jongejan, P. and Schaapveled, K., 1992, *Sustainable Development and Health*, La Haye.

Camau, M., 1989, *État de santé*, Paris, CNRS.

Chevallier, L., 1947, *Le problème démographique Nord-africain*, éd. Presses universitaires de France, p. 194.

Commission scientifique de développement, 1995, *Population du sud et santé*, Paris, ORSTOM.

Dupaquier, J., 1997, *L'espérance de vie sans incapacité*, Paris, PUF.

Institut de Recherches et Études sur la Population (IREP), *Mortalité et santé de la population*, Tunis, IREP.

Longuenesse, E., 1995, *Santé, médecine et société dans le monde arabe*, Paris, L'Harmattan.

Salem, G., 1998, *La santé dans la ville*, Paris, Karthala-ORSTOM.

Seklani, M., 1966, *La mortalité et le coût de la santé publique en Tunisie* tomes 1 et 2, Université de Paris.

Vallin, J. et Locoh, T., 2002, *Population et développement en Tunisie: la métamorphose*, Tunis, CERES.

Articles

Ault, B and Olshansky, S. J., 1986, 'The fourth stage of the epidemiologic transition: the age of delayed degenerative diseases', *The Milbank Quarterly*, No. 64, 3.

Ben S., Olfa, C. et Nadia, 2001 « Réformes du système de santé tunisien et assurance maladie », *La Tunisie médicale*, vol. 79, n° 10, Tunis, octobre.

Ben Y. A., Phantan, T., Souissi, H. et Wessen, A. F., 1974, « Services de santé: couverture, facteurs et indices d'utilisation », *Bulletin de l'OMS*, n° 51.

Bouafif, N., Hajem, S., Ennigrou, S., Touati, M., Ben Hamida, A. et Zouari, Béchir, 2000, « Déclaration des causes de décès en Tunisie », *La Tunisie médicale*, vol.78, n° 12, Tunis, septembre.

Caselli, G., Mesle, F. et Vallin, J., 2001, « Les entorses au schéma de la transition épidémiologique », in *Actes de la XXXIVe conférence générale de la population*, IUESP, Salvador, Brésil, août.

Faculté des sciences humaines et sociales de Tunis, 1997, Actes du colloque *Développement et transition démographique en Afrique*, Tunis 26-28 avril 1995, Tunis.

Gaha, C., 1998, « Les déterminants de la santé selon les médecins tunisiens », *Correspondances*, n° 53 novembre, Institut de Recherches sur le Maghreb contemporain (IRMC), Tunisie, pp. 7 à 9.

Gonzalez-Quinones, F. and Reher, D., 2001, 'Mother's Death and Children's Death', in *Actes de la XXXIVe conférence générale de la population*, IUESP, Salvador, Brésil, août.

Jeannee, E. et Salem, G., 1988, « Urbanisation et santé dans le tiers monde », in « *Santé et médecine, l'état des connaissances et des recherches* », INSERM/ORSTOM.

IFORD, 1993, *Actes du colloque international sur la mortalité infantile et juvénile en Afrique: bilan des recherches et politiques de santé*, IFORD.

Kaddar, M., 1992, « Le financement de la santé au Maghreb: données et problèmes actuels. Communication », in *Actes du colloque Le financement des soins et la maîtrise des coûts*, Tunis, 27-30 juillet.

Legare, J., 1990, « Espérance de vie en bonne santé: construction et application », in *Population âgée et révolution grise*, Chaire Quetelet 1986, Université Catholique de Louvain, Belgique.

Mc Kee, M., 2001, 'Emerging Diseases: The Need for a New Research Framework', in *Actes de la XXXIVe conférence générale de la population*, IUESP, Salvador, Brésil, août.

Mc Nicoll G., 1990, 'Comments on Policy Aspects of Health-transition Researchs', in J. C., Caldwell, S., Findley, P., Caldwell, G., Santow, W., Cosford, J., Braid and D., Broers-Freeman eds., *What We Know About Health-transition: The Cultural, Social and Behavioural Determinants of Health*, Health Transition Series, Book Number 2, pp. 911–912.

Mosley W. H., Bobadilla J. L., Jamison D. T., 1993, *The Health Transition: Implications for Health Policy in Developing Countries*, Chapter 28 in D.T., Jamison, W.H., Mosley, A.R., Measham, and J-L., Bobadilla eds., *Disease Control Priorities in Developing Countries*, New York, Oxford University Press for the World Bank.

Newhouse J. and Phelps, C. C., 1976, *New Estimates of Price and Income Elasticities of Medical Care Services*, in *National Bureau Services*, No. 27, New York.

Njah, M., Mtir, N., Kacem, M., Ben Salem, K., Haj Frej, A. et Marzouki, M., 1993, « Pratiques de prévention et de promotion de la santé en médecine libérale », in *Tunisie médicale,* vol. n° 71, Tunis, janvier.

Omran, A., 1971, 'The Epidemiologic Transition: A Theory of the Epidemiology of Population Change', in *The Milbank Memorial Fund Quarterly,* No. 49, 4.

Picheral, H., 1989, « Géographie de la transition épidémiologique », in *Annales de géographie* n° 546, CNRS-Armand Colin, mars-avril.

Tabutin, D., *Avantages comparés des enquêtes à passages répétés et à passage unique pour la mesure de la mortalité dans les pays en développement,* Union Internationale des études en Sciences de la Population, Belgique.

Tabutin, D., 1991, « *La surmortalité féminine en Afrique du nord* », in Population n° 4, INED, France, août.

Tamouza, S., 1996, *Mortalité et systèmes de santé au Maghreb,* communication présentée au 2ᵉ *congrès régional arabe de population au Caire - 8 au 12 décembre,* Paris, CEPED, Paris, décembre.

Enquêtes

Institut national de la santé publique, 1996, *Enquête nationale médico-sociale sur l'état de santé et les conditions de vie des personnes âgées de 65 ans et plus vivant à domicile,* Tunis, décembre.

Ministère de la santé publique, 1999, *Enquête morbidité et mortalité hospitalière dans les hôpitaux régionaux,* Direction Etudes et Planification, Tunis, mars.

Ministère de la santé publique, 2000, *Enquête nationale sur la santé et le bien-être de la mère et de l'enfant,* Direction des Soins de Santé de Base, Tunis, décembre.

ONFP, 1985, *Enquête Mortalité et morbidité infantile,* Tunisie.

ONFP, 1988, *Enquête Démographie-santé,* Tunisie.

ONFP, 1996, *Enquête tunisienne sur la Santé de la mère et de l'enfant 1994-1995,* Tunisie.

ONFP, 2001, *Enquête tunisienne sur la Santé de la famille 2001,* Tunisie, octobre.

Publications Diverses

DHS, *DHS analytical reports* N° 4, 1997, DHS mortality indicators, USA.

DHS, *DHS comparative studies* N° 25, 1997, Maternal health care, USA.

FNUAP, 2003, *Rapport annuel Tunisie 2002,* Tunis.

League of Arab State, 1998, *PAPFAM Project document,* Le Caire.

Ministère de la santé publique, *Bulletin épidémiologique 2001,* Direction des Soins de Santé de Base, Tunis, septembre.

Ministère de la santé publique, 2002, *L'assurance de la qualité en première ligne: concepts, organisation et méthodes,* Direction des Soins de Santé de Base, Tunis.

OMS, 2000, *Rapport sur la santé dans le monde 1999,* OMS, Genève.

ONUSIDA, 2000, *Le SIDA en Afrique pays par pays,* Genève, décembre.

ONUSIDA, 2000, *Rapport sur l'épidémie mondiale de VIH/SIDA,* Genève, juin.

ONUSIDA, 2001, *Le point sur l'épidémie de SIDA,* Genève, décembre.

ONUSIDA, 2004, *Breaking the silence around HIV/AIDS in the Arab region*, Geneva.

PNUD, 2002, *Rapport sur le développement humain en Tunisie 2001*, PNUD, Tunisie.

USAID, 1995, Implementing reproductive health programs, New York.

IV

Les systèmes de santé et les maladies chroniques

10

Les maladies chroniques non transmissibles dans le système de santé au Sénégal: le cas du diabète dans la ville de Dakar[1]

Oupa Diossine Loppy

« On fait la Science avec les faits comme on fait une maison avec des pierres; mais une accumulation des faits n'est plus une Science qu'un tas de pierres n'est une maison » (Poincaré 1924).

Introduction

L'OMS[2] a défini la santé comme étant le bien-être physique, mental et social; ce n'est pas uniquement l'absence de la maladie. La santé n'est donc pas un luxe et c'est pourquoi elle fait partie des principes des droits humains. Tout être humain a droit à une santé saine.

Les Etats d'Afrique sont pauvres et c'est une lapalissade de le dire. Toutes les maladies ne sont donc pas prises en compte dans les priorités. C'est le cas du cancer, de l'hypertension artérielle et du diabète, au Sénégal. Alors que le cancer des enfants progresse très vite[3] et les autres maladies chroniques non transmissibles également.

Au Sénégal, le diabète, la drépanocytose, l'hypertension artérielle et le cancer prennent de plus en plus d'ampleur. Ce sont des maladies qui, très souvent, sont liées à l'hérédité et à une alimentation malsaine. Ces maladies chroniques non transmissibles sont devenues des maladies du siècle. Elles font des ravages et freinent le développement d'un pays. Ces maladies ne sont pas transmissibles c'est pourquoi elles ne sont pas prises en compte dans l'élaboration de la politique de santé publique alors que le paludisme (transmission indirecte) et le Sida (transmission directe) le sont. La politique de la santé des pays en développement vient d'ailleurs.

Le Sida comme le paludisme est une maladie très dangereuse et fatale. Toutes les deux font des ravages. Mais le Sida[4] au Sénégal, n'est pas la première cause de mortalité. Le nombre de personnes infectées par le VIH/SIDA est de 1,5% alors que les sujets atteints par le diabète sont de 2%.[5] Le Sida fait donc ombrage aux autres maladies surtout les maladies chroniques non transmissibles. Il y a un plan national de lutte contre le paludisme et un plan national de lutte contre le Sida mais il n'y a pas de plan national de lutte pour l'alimentation qui est la principale cause des maladies chroniques. Or, « sans une alimentation saine, on ne peut pas vivre en bonne santé ».

Malgré l'ampleur des maladies chroniques au Sénégal, surtout le diabète, elles sont négligées. Pourquoi ne font-elles pas partie des priorités de l'élaboration de la politique de la santé publique? Le choix vient-il de l'extérieur?

L'État est fournisseur du personnel et des moyens, régulateur et facilitateur du secteur de la santé; nous pouvons nous interroger s'il peut bien gérer le système sanitaire si sa politique est définie ailleurs. N'est-il pas pertinent de porter un regard critique aussi sur le budget du Ministère de la Santé comparé à celui de la Défense?

C'est l'État qui a la mission d'élaborer la politique de la santé publique et, de ce fait, il joue le rôle de régulateur en créant un cadre juridique et des agents pour appliquer des lois et règlements en vigueur.

La réforme hospitalière

La réforme intervenue en 1998 a pour but de revitaliser le service public hospitalier en améliorant la qualité et la sécurité des soins ainsi que le renforcement des capacités de gestion.[6] Ce n'est pas un désengagement de l'État car il va toujours apporter la subvention aux Établissements publics de santé (EPS). En juin 2001, déjà, dix hôpitaux nationaux se sont érigés en EPS.

L'hôpital principal de Dakar (HPD) a un statut particulier tandis que Abass N'dao est géré par la commune de Dakar. Même si l'hôpital principal reçoit une subvention de l'État, elle ne dépend pas du Ministère de tutelle mais de la Défense nationale.

Le système de santé au Sénégal a quatre niveaux: la région, le département, la communauté rurale et le village. Dakar compte sept hôpitaux et chacune des onze régions un hôpital régional; il y a quarante-sept centres de santé au niveau départemental (district), six cent cinquante-neuf postes de santé dans les communautés rurales et des cases de santé dans les villages.[7] Il y a un lit d'hôpital pour 1 298 habitants et un médecin pour 18 410 habitants.

« Le système de santé, et non le système de soins, sera défini par nous comme l'ensemble des pratiques sociales sur un espace donné qui expose de façon différentielle des espaces à un certain profil sanitaire ».[8]

Il y a, en 1998, quatre cent sept médecins, neuf cent trente-quatre infirmiers, quatre cent soixante quatorze sages-femmes, sept cent trente et un agents d'hygiène, deux mille cinq cents matrones et deux mille quatre cent vingt-quatre agents de santé.[9]

De manière générale, les infrastructures sont vétustes. Au CHU A. Le Dantec, tous les services sont asphyxiés: orthopédie, urologie, chirurgie générale, radiologie, biologie, biochimie et, seuls les cas d'urgence sont traités; la raréfaction des consommables et des médicaments est aussi des problèmes que rencontre, grosso modo, les infrastructures sénégalaises.[10]

Les déterminants d'un système de santé qui peut être efficace sont: la proximité de l'offre de santé, les prix des médicaments peu élevés, etc. Le taux de femmes adultes alphabétisées est de 25% et l'indice de fécondité est de 6,5 enfants. L'espérance de vie est de 47 ans.

Les recettes et les modiques subventions de l'État ne permettent pas de couvrir les dépenses. Les praticiens pensent d'ailleurs que le mode de gestion est inadapté. Pour sauver leur structure, les médecins ont diagnostiqué les maux et ont élaboré un document mais le ministère de tutelle reste encore indifférent à leur proposition.

Le manque du personnel qualifié est aussi l'une des difficultés que rencontre le système de santé au Sénégal. Selon un médecin, « sans formation continue et de pointe, on ne peut plus parler de CHU ».

À l'instar des autres pays en développement, le Sénégal connaît un déficit du personnel de santé. C'est ainsi qu'une politique de recrutement dans ce secteur a été initiée. Cinq mille agents ont été recrutés en 2003[11] et l'objectif est de recruter d'ici 2007 un total de quinze mille agents. Il y a un déficit de l'ordre de trois mille agents: médecins, infirmiers, sages-femmes, techniciens supérieurs de la santé et aides-infirmiers.

La région du Fleuve (Saint-Louis), Tambacounda, Ziguinchor et Kolda souffrent plus de cette situation. Par des raisons diverses, des postes de santé sont fermés à cause du manque de personnel (quand on veut punir un fonctionnaire on l'envoie à Tambacounda, Ziguinchor et Kolda ce qui est à cause du conflit casamançais mais pour Saint-Louis on ne dispose pas encore d'explication).

Les besoins sont très forts dans le domaine: il y a un manque de personnel qualifié. Selon un responsable du secteur, l'État ne totalise pas plus de six mille agents.[12] En 2003, l'État visait à recruter trois mille agents mais au bout du compte c'est seulement 672 qui ont été recrutés. Et la même poursuit en indiquant que le changement des ministres dans le secteur de la santé ne permet pas d'appliquer les conclusions issues de 2000 où les décideurs, les bailleurs de fonds, les collectivités locales, les syndicats se sont penchés sur la question (que disent les assises?).

Une source du SUTSAS[13] soutient que les problèmes du système de santé c'est « l'absence de transparence, d'équité et de démocratie ». Les agents, par la complicité de ceux qui gèrent le secteur, ne respectent pas les affectations car tout le monde veut travailler à Dakar.

Les questions politiques, culturelles et économiques sont des facteurs de réussite ou non d'un système de soins. L'étude de la santé est une perspective sociale et politique des problèmes de santé d'un État.[14]

La réforme hospitalière, même si elle est critiquée par certains, a pour objectif de donner plus d'efficacité aux systèmes de soins et de santé face à l'ampleur des problèmes de santé.

L'ampleur des maladies chroniques

Le cancer des enfants se développe très vite par rapport à celui des adultes mais les ¾ guérissent définitivement. Les plus fréquents: cancer du rein (facile à traiter selon les spécialistes), cancer des ganglions ou lymphome de Burkitt africain (plus répandu et plus difficile à traiter, toujours selon les spécialistes).

Face à cette situation, l'Association « Taxawu Sunnuy Doom »[15] a lancé l'opération « pièces jaunes », du 1er au 30 mars 2004, pour la campagne de lutte contre le cancer des enfants et pour l'assistance des enfants malades.

Cent onze millions d'enfants âgés de moins de quinze ans souffrent du cancer dans les pays francophones à travers le monde.

Le cancer fait des ravages au Sénégal, surtout celui des enfants. En effet, six cents en sont victimes par an. N'étant pas la priorité de la santé publique, le cancer a fait mobiliser des âmes charitables qui ont initié une chaîne de solidarité pour la prise en charge des patients à travers le parrainage. Madame Maïssa Diop et l'association Taxaw Sunnuy Doom ont créé la chaîne de solidarité grâce aux bonnes volontés dont le slogan est « N'oubliez pas que les enfants eux aussi … ont le cancer ».

L'objectif de cette chaîne de solidarité est « d'optimiser la prise en charge de ces petits patients afin d'obtenir des résultats analogues à ceux enregistrés dans les pays développés ».[16] En 1990, il y a un taux de guérison de 25% alors qu'il est de 9% en France. Le taux de rémission est de 66% sur trente quatre cas de prise en charge entre 2001 et 2003 grâce à l'appui du Groupe franco-africain d'oncologie pédiatrique.

La prise en charge complète d'un enfant atteint d'un cancer de rein gravite autour de 1 450 000 F CFA; pour le cancer des ganglions, le coût de la prise en charge tourne autour de 1 800 000 F CFA.[17]

S'il n'y a pas une politique de la santé qui englobe toutes les maladies dangereuses en matière curative et de prévention, les populations seront toujours exposées aux maladies comme le diabète.

Les facteurs de risque d'attraper le diabète

Une mauvaise alimentation et l'absence d'activité physique sont à l'origine de l'obésité et du surpoids. Une étude a montré que cette maladie pourrait être la première cause de décès aux États-Unis d'ici 2005.

En 2000, la mauvaise alimentation a fait quatre cent mille morts contre quatre cent trente-cinq mille décès liés au tabagisme, quatre vingt-cinq mille causés par l'alcool selon l'étude des Centres de contrôle et de prévention des maladies (CDC). Pendant que les décès causés par le tabagisme est en baisse, passant de 19% en

1990 à 18,1% en 2000, ceux liés à l'alcool sont passés de 5% à 3,5%.[18] Un changement de comportement peut largement diminuer le nombre de décès dus au diabète.

Entre 1990 et 2000, les décès dus à la mauvaise alimentation ont vu leur taux passer de 14% à 16,6% du total des décès soit la plus forte progression, note le rapport, parmi les causes de la mortalité aux États-Unis.

Le surpoids et l'obésité sont des facteurs de risque pour le diabète, la maladie cardiaque et certains cancers.

Les gens mangent mal. Ils ne savent pas manger car ils croient que bien manger c'est manger à sa faim. Ainsi, une bonne alimentation doit être un défi pour les pays en développement. Une certaine couche de la population n'a pas les moyens de varier son alimentation et n'a pas non plus l'éducation adéquate pour consommer plus ce dont le corps a plus besoin, donc même ceux qui ont des moyens ne savent pas équilibrer leur alimentation.

Au Sénégal, le cep bu djën[19] est le principal mets des Sénégalais. Le riz qui devrait accompagner le poisson et les légumes se trouve être la principale alimentation.

La mauvaise alimentation est donc liée aux facteurs économiques donc politiques et socioculturels. Si les gens n'ont pas les moyens d'appliquer une politique nutritionniste, la meilleure des politiques échouera nécessairement.

Le diabète est une maladie silencieuse qui ne fait pas beaucoup de bruit comme le paludisme ou le Sida mais il est massif car une importante partie de la population sénégalaise vit avec ce fléau.

L'ampleur du Diabète

Au Sénégal, on désigne le diabète par « la maladie du sucre ». En Ouganda, c'est « chu kali » qui signifie sucre et au Kenya « Suk Ari » en swahili veut dire également sucre.

Il y a plusieurs associations de diabétiques dans le monde. C'est le cas au Sénégal. Nous tenterons de voir si l'objectif de l'Association sénégalaise des diabétiques est de partager la douleur pour diminuer la souffrance ou c'est pour un apport en biens matériels, financiers, l'entraide ou encore s'unir pour avoir plus de force pour faire pression sur les autorités. Nous pouvons, d'emblée formuler l'hypothèse selon laquelle en écoutant les autres parler des mêmes maux, donc, tout un chacun peut se dire « je ne suis pas seul et il y a peut-être pire ailleurs ». Ce qui est une manière de se consoler un peu par la souffrance des autres.

Le seul centre spécialisé dans le traitement du diabète au Sénégal est le centre antidiabétique « Marc Sankalé » de l'hôpital Abass Ndao. Ce centre a accueilli à ses débuts deux cents patients[20] et le nombre de patients est passé à plus de vingt mille avec une progression de deux mille cas par an. Cette progression et les coûts de la prise en charge sont au centre des préoccupations de l'Association sénégalaise de soutien aux diabétiques (ASSAD) car il n'y a pas encore une politique de santé, au Sénégal, qui intègre les maladies chroniques comme faisant partie des priorités.

La progression de la maladie est inquiétante. Ce qui est plus inquiétant également c'est la non-prise en charge des malades, malgré la création d'une division des maladies chroniques non transmissibles au Ministère de tutelle. La progression vertigineuse du diabète peut s'expliquer par les mauvaise habitudes alimentaires, par la pauvreté, les tabous alimentaires et à l'analphabétisme.[21]

Le Centre est créé en 1965 par des médecins comme le Pr Marc Sankalé dont il porte le nom. Mais depuis 1975, le Centre n'a plus de budget de fonctionnement même si une partie des salaires du personnel est payée par le Ministère de tutelle et l'autre par l'ex-communauté urbaine de Dakar, aujourd'hui c'est la commune de Dakar qui gère et le Centre et l'hôpital Abass Ndao.

Le diabète est lié d'une part à la suralimentation et d'autre part à la malnutrition.

L'ASSAD est créée en 1982 et son but est « d'améliorer le sort des patients et d'en faire des personnes sans handicap ». Elle œuvre aussi pour avoir des pouvoirs publics de subvention des prix de l'insuline, la réalisation d'un centre qui répond à l'ampleur de la maladie au sein des populations car l'exiguïté et l'éloignement par rapport à certains patients est un handicap pour l'accès aux soins. L'ASSAD est une chaîne de solidarité assez large entre les diabétiques et aussi entre les personnes aisées et non nantis.

Elle apporte des moyens financiers grâce à ses adhérents pour le bon fonctionnement du Centre. Les membres de l'Association ont quelques privilèges par rapport aux diabétiques non adhérents: chacun va débourser quatre mille F CFA à raison de quatre visites annuelles; cette politique sociale est entretenue grâce à la coopération entre le Centre et l'ASSAD.[22] Le diabète est une « maladie nouvelle »;[23] elle fait partie des autres maladies émergentes.

L'augmentation du taux de sucre se fait de façon chronique. Ce qu'on appelle une hyperglycémie, c'est le diabète. Le diabétique est un sujet qui mange beaucoup sucré et gras, boit beaucoup, urine beaucoup et dans certains cas se met à maigrir.

Le diabète a des marqueurs génétiques, c'est une maladie familiale et à vie.[24] Il y a deux types de diabète: le diabète insulinodépendant ou de type 1 qui touche généralement les sujets jeunes et le diabète non insulinodépendant ou de type 2 qui touche le plus d'adultes.

Au Sénégal, 90% des diabétiques sont de type 2 et 10% seulement de type 1. Au Centre « Marc Sankalé », 70% des patients en traitements sont des indigents, 15% sont des malades nantis et 15% sont de la classe moyenne.

Comment prévenir le diabète?

Une cure d'amaigrissement pour des sujets obèses, avoir une alimentation équilibrée et moins sucrée et moins grasse, et avoir une activité physique. La campagne de sensibilisation n'est plus développée. Malgré l'organisation chaque année d'une semaine nationale du diabète, ce qui va en droite ligne de la journée mondiale du diabète, l'antenne à la télévision, un tranche hebdomadaire de vingt à trente minutes n'existe plus depuis 1985.

Pour faire face au mal, le Centre et l'ASSAD comptent sur l'éducation, la sensibilisation et la formation du personnel d'encadrement, l'information des populations et le dépistage.

Les diabétiques méritent, à l'instar des malades du Sida et du paludisme, que l'on leur accorde plus d'attention et de considération en allouant plus de moyens pour couvrir les frais de soins et la prise en charge psychosociale.

Compte tenu de la situation géographique et le manque de moyens chez certains patients, les malades éprouvent des difficultés pour se faire soigner.

Les difficultes d'accès aux soins

Dakar compte dix-neuf communes d'arrondissements (loi sur les collectivités locales de 1996) qui dépendent de la commune de Dakar. La région de Dakar est découpée en quatre villes: Dakar, Pikine, Rufisque et Guédiawaye. La ville de Dakar, malgré le nombre de ses habitants inférieur à celui de Pikine,[25] garde les prestiges, les fonctions et les privilèges de la première ville du Sénégal.[26]

Les accès aux soins et à une alimentation saine et équilibrée, à l'eau potable ne sont pas donnés à tout le monde dans les pays en développement. Les États ne satisfont pas la prise en charge médicale et psychologique et l'accès aux soins sur le plan financier et géographique.

L'accès équitable aux soins et l'accueil par un établissement hospitalier à tout malade est un droit garanti par la loi n°98-08 du 02 mars 1998 portant sur la réforme hospitalière au Sénégal. La discrimination est également interdite car refuser de soigner un malade quelle que soit la raison constitue le refus d'assistance à personne en danger; un délit prévu et puni par l'art. 49 al. 2 du Code pénal sénégalais.

Les malades du diabète ont des difficultés d'accès aux soins.[27] Compte tenu des coûts des soins et de l'intensité des traitements, la situation des diabétiques mérite une réflexion pour ne pas dire une attention particulière quand on sait qu'il y a parmi eux des sujets indigents. Les coûts, les conséquences dans la vie professionnelle et sociale sont des indicateurs qui doivent susciter une réflexion chez tout citoyen. Compte tenu du temps de l'institut, nous nous limiterons à la ville de Dakar. On pourrait schématiser les objectifs ainsi:

Une politique de la santé ne doit pas seulement se limiter à administrer des soins; elle doit aller au-delà car derrière la maladie il y a un malade, un individu qui tient à sa dignité.

La santé publique est un savoir et un savoir-faire; c'est une méthode et un état d'esprit. Elle renvoie à l'idée de l'hygiène publique.[28] La vente des médicaments en dehors des circuits normaux pose un problème de santé publique.

La violation des droits de la personne humaine est interdite par les normes internationales. En effet, la charte des Nations Unies oblige les Etats à respecter les droits des individus: « discrimination au regard du sexe, de la race, de la langue, de la religion, de l'opinion politique et autre statut ». Le concept de « santé pour tous » doit être traduit en actions concrètes.

Face à la dégradation du système sanitaire public, les populations nanties optent pour le service privé. Ce secteur offre-t-il les meilleurs services?

Certains se tournent vers la médecine traditionnelle même si elle n'est pas toujours la moins coûteuse.[29] D'autres préfèrent consulter un tradi-praticien.

La médecine moderne soigne les symptômes de la maladie et la médecine traditionnelle identifie les causes du mal et met les moyens nécessaires pour les combattre.[30]

Dans l'analyse du comportement des malades, il est important d'avoir à l'œil les enjeux sociaux de la maladie. Elle est vue en Afrique comme étant causée par un esprit maléfique et c'est la médecine traditionnelle (tradi-praticien, guérisseur ou sorcier) qui est sollicitée pour enrayer le mal ou le mauvais sort alors que la médecine moderne est convaincue qu'il faut chercher les causes naturelles de la maladie et d'agir sur elles. Ces deux conceptions sont contraires mais pas contradictoires et c'est pourquoi les deux médecines sont associées par les patients, la plupart du temps, dans les soins. De plus, dans les deux cas, les soins ne sont pas seulement physiques (le corps) mais la santé du corps est aussi importante que les soins mentaux (esprit). Le médecin comme le tradi-praticien soigne et le corps et l'esprit.

Quand la dimension humaine est oubliée, on n'est plus loin de la barbarie. C'est la rigueur scientifique dans toute sa dimension et le respect de l'autre qui sont des facteurs-clés dans ce processus. S'il n'y a pas ce respect, on assistera à la santé des riches contre la santé des pauvres. Laisser les diabétiques n'ayant pas les moyens de se faire soigner à eux-mêmes, c'est les conduire irréfutablement vers la mort.

Les enjeux sociaux de la maladie peuvent-ils bouleverser les stratégies de politique de santé ou obligent-ils une coopération entre la médecine moderne et la médecine traditionnelle? Si les patients se démarquent de plus en plus des structures étatiques, peut-être que cela aidera l'État à prendre plus de responsabilités en protégeant davantage le secteur de la santé.

L'État n'est pas le seul acteur dans la mise en place d'une politique de la santé. Le poids des bailleurs de fonds, le clientélisme de certains régimes politiques font que la gestion de la santé au niveau politique ne répond pas souvent aux attentes des populations.

La gestion politique de la santé

Lutter contre la pauvreté c'est améliorer l'équité, c'est redistribuer les richesses de manière rationnelle, c'est instaurer une politique d'allocation de chômage pour protéger les pauvres à ne pas devenir de plus en plus pauvres. En effet, l'état de pauvreté des Etats africains est un facteur aggravant du système sanitaire précaire et peu efficace. Les programmes de lutte contre la pauvreté doivent intégrer la dimension santé « Mens sana in corpore sano ».[31]

Le concept de bonne gouvernance invoque trois acteurs: l'État, le secteur privé et la société civile. La bonne gouvernance c'est « la manière dont est exercé le pouvoir pour gérer les ressources économiques d'un pays en vue du développement.[32] Pour le PNUD, « Elle [la bonne gouvernance] comprend les mécanismes, procédés et institutions par lesquels les citoyens et leurs groupes articulent leurs intérêts, exercent leurs droits légaux, remplissent leurs obligations et gèrent leurs différences ».

Nous considérons que la bonne gouvernance doit être vue comme la défense de la cause des pauvres et la bonne gestion des affaires publiques. Le Sénégal consacre 1,3% de son PNB à la santé contre 4,2% à l'éducation.

Les États sont « responsables en dernier ressort du bien-être de leurs citoyens dont ils doivent prendre le plus grand soin ».[33] La santé pour tous en l'an 2000, cet objectif de l'OMS, est de mener la planète à un niveau de santé socialement et économiquement productive; et il est clair que la santé est le moteur de tout développement.

L'efficacité d'un système de santé se mesure sur la qualité des soins et la satisfaction des malades, de la salle d'attente à l'hôpital à l'administration des soins.[34] Elle répond à plusieurs facteurs.

Quelle que soit la politique élaborée, si les praticiens ne sont pas bien formés les objectifs risquent de ne pas être atteints; la formation ne doit pas se limiter seulement à la biomédecine ou à la biochimie.

La formation du corps médical aux sciences sociales

Confrontés à la mort, c'est la peur, la colère et l'angoisse qui envahissent le malade et l'habitant. Il est donc nécessaire de lui donner la vie en lui apportant du réconfort, surtout des personnes qui souffrent de maladies chroniques.

La mission du corps médical et paramédical est de surveiller et de soigner, de prendre en charge. La confiance naîtra entre les patients et le personnel de la santé quand ceux-là se rendront compte que celui-ci a pour mission de résoudre ou d'atténuer leurs problèmes; et à défaut de bouter la maladie hors de leur cadre de vie, leur rapport atténuera alors la souffrance.

L'attitude à adopter varie d'un malade à l'autre: chacun vient avec ses maux et ses mots qui sont susceptibles d'être différents de ceux des autres; chacun vient avec ses sentiments. Il peut être angoissé ou replié sur lui-même ou être de mauvaise humeur et s'en prendre au corps médical et paramédical. Ce sont des réactions normales, elles sont normales parce que la personne est malade et qu'elle a besoin de l'aide du personnel de santé. C'est pourquoi les gestes simples, comme serrer la main, embrasser, sourire, incliner la tête en signe de salutation, sont très importants pour le patient.

Conclusion

La priorité est donnée à une maladie si elle présente un caractère commercial. Les maladies dont l'ennemi est clairement identifiable présentent plus d'intérêts que les autres. Pour le Sida c'est les rapports sexuels à risque qui sont pointés du doigt et pour ce qui est du paludisme c'est l'anophèle. Les donateurs, pour décaisser les fonds, posent des conditionnalités. C'est dire que ce sont eux qui élaborent et déterminent la politique de santé dans les pays qui n'ont pas les moyens de réaliser leurs objectifs en matière de santé publique. Les ministères de la santé ne font qu'exécuter une politique définie de l'extérieur. Alors, que faire?

Notes

1. Les diabétiques qui adhèrent à l'Association sénégalaise de soutien aux diabétiques (AS-SAD) ne sont pas tous de Dakar et tous les diabétiques de Dakar n'adhèrent pas à l'ASSAD.
2. Organisation Mondiale de la Santé.
3. On note 400 à 600 nouveaux cas de cancer chaque année et 10% seulement des enfants atteints du cancer sont traités.
4. Le premier cas de Sida est dépisté en janvier 1986 au Sénégal; à la fin de l'année il y a eu 15 nouveaux cas dépistés.
5. Les statistiques disponibles au Centre « Marc Sankalé » de l'hôpital Abass Ndao.
6. Le budget du Ministère de la Santé au Sénégal est de 8% en 1972-1973 et de 5,5% en 1981-1982.
7. Projet de prévention de la mortalité maternelle au Sénégal. Réf: Sen/86/007. Gouv. du Sénégal et le PNUD.
8. La santé dans la ville, p. 58.
9. Projet de prévention de la mortalité maternelle au Sénégal. Réf: Sen/86/007. Gouv. du Sénégal et le PNUD.
10. *Walfadjri*, 18/03/2004.
11. *Sud Quotidien*, 19/02/2004.
12. *op.cit.*
13. Syndicat unique des Travailleurs de la Santé au Sénégal.
14. La santé dans la ville, p. 302.
15. Au secours des enfants en wolof.
16. Pr Moreira.
17. 1 • = 655,7 F CFA.
18. *Walfadjri*, 11/03/2004.
19. *Journal of the American Medical Association* - JAMA -, 10/03/2004 cité par *Walfadjri* du 11/03/2004.
20. Le riz au poisson qui se trouve être le plat le plus prisé par les Sénégalais.
21. Certains documents mentionnent cent vingt-sept patients.
22. Pr Saïd N. Diop, *Le Soleil*, 15/11/2002.

23. Il est même prévu la création d'un coopérative qui aura pour objectifs de subventionner la vente de l'insuline: le coût à la pharmacie est de 1400 F CFA contre 1000 F CFA aux diabétiques qui adhèrent à l'ASSAD.
24. Pr Saïd Nourou Diop.
25. Les spécialistes ne préfèrent pas parler de maladie héréditaire.
26. 910.000 contre 800.000 habitants.
27. La santé dans la ville.
28. Les malades du sida sont traités gratuitement.
29. Critique de la santé publique, p. 8, Didier Fassin et Jean-Paul Dozon.
30. Une piste qui pourrait être explorée dans une autre étude.
31. La santé dans la ville, p. 76.
32. Un esprit sain dans un corps sain.
33. Banque mondiale.
34. OMS.
35. OMS.

Bibliographie sélective

Aguercif, M. et Aguercif-Meziane, F., 1993, « Le système de santé publique en Algérie: évaluation 1974-1989 et perspectives », *Les Cahiers du CREAD*, n° 35/36, pp. 97-102.

Antoine, P. et Bâ, A., 1993, « Mortalité et santé dans les villes africaines », *Afrique contemporaine*, n° 168, octobre-décembre, pp. 138-146.

Banque mondiale, 1994, *Sénégal: évaluation des conditions de vie*, Washington, Banque mondiale.

Brooks, D. D., 2002, *L'eau. Gérer localement*, CRDI.

Brownlee, A., 1993, *La recherche sur les systèmes de santé: un outil de gestion*, Ottawa, CRDI.

Centre international de l'enfance, 1976, *La santé de la famille et de la communauté*, Dakar, Saint-Paul.

Cichon, M. et Gillion, C., 1993, « Le financement des soins de santé dans les pays en développement », *Revue internationale du travail*, vol. 132, n° 2, pp. 193-208.

De La Moussaye, E. et Jacquemot, P., 1993, « Politique de santé: les trois options stratégiques », *Afrique contemporaine*, n° 166, avril-juin, pp. 15-26.

Dujardin, B., 2003, *Politiques de santé et attentes des patients: vers un dialogue constructif*, Paris, Karthala.

El Harti, A., 1988, « Le système de santé au Maroc entre les contraintes financières et les exigences sociales », *Afrique et Développement*, vol. XIII, n° 2, pp. 5-27.

Egrot, M. et Taverne, B., 1990, *Interventions sanitaires et contexte culturel: Actes de la deuxième journée d'anthropologie médicale de l'AMADES*, Marseille 28 avril, Toulouse.

Estrella, M. et al., 2003, *Apprendre du changement. Questions et expériences de suivi et évaluation participatifs*, Karthala, CRDI.

Fassin, D. et Defossez, A., 1992, « Une liaison dangereuse. Sciences Sociales et santé publique dans les programmes de réduction de la mortalité naturelle en Equateur », *Cahiers des Sciences humaines*, vol. 28, n° 1, pp. 23-36.

Fassin, D., 1996, *L'Espace politique de la santé*, Essai de généalogie, Paris, PUF.

Fassin, D., 2000, *Les enjeux politiques de la santé. Études sénégalaises, équatoriennes et françaises*, Paris, Karthala, 2000.

Fassin, D. (dir), 2001, *Critique de la santé publique*, Paris, Balland.

Fairhead, J. et Leach, M., 1994, « Représentations culturelles africaines et gestion de l'environnement », *Politique africaine*, n° 53 mars, pp. 11-24.

Grenier, L., 1998, *Connaissances indigènes et recherche. Un guide à l'intention des chercheurs*, CRDI.

Hours, B., 1992, « La santé publique entre soins de santé primaires et management », *Cahiers des Sciences humaines*, vol. 28, n° 1, pp. 123-140.

Hours, B., 2001, *Systèmes et politiques de santé: de la santé publique à l'anthropologie*, Paris, Karthala.

Jaffré, Y. et Olivier de Sardan, J. P., 2003, *Une médecine inhospitalière*, Paris, Karthala.

Klimek, C. Y. et Peters, G., 1995, *Une politique du médicament pour l'Afrique: contraintes et choix*, Paris, Karthala.

Michel, H., 1979, *Pour une éducation africaine de la santé*, Essai d'un manuel pédagogique adapté à l'Afrique [Thèse d'État], Université de Dakar.

Ndiaye, S., Diouf, P. D. et Ayad, M., *Santé familiale et population*. Région de Dakar: Résultats de l'Enquête.

Oufriha, F. Z., 1993, « Difficile structuration du système de santé en Afrique: Quels résultats? », *Les cahiers du CREAD*, n° 35/36, pp. 7-58.

Oufriha, F. Z., 1988, « Essai sur le système de soins en Algérie », *Économie appliquée et Développement*, n° 13, 1er trimestre, pp. 60-75.

OMS, 1975, *Comment répondre aux besoins sanitaires fondamentaux des populations dans les pays en voie de développement*, Genève.

OMS, 1981, *Élaboration d'indicateurs pour la surveillance continue des progrès réalisés dans la voie de la santé pour tous d'ici 2000*, Genève.

OMS, 1982, *Rôle des centres de santé dans le développement des systèmes de santé des villes*, Genève.

OMS, 1992, *Économie hospitalière et financement des hôpitaux dans les pays en développement*, Genève.

OMS, 1998, *Rapport sur la santé dans le monde*, Genève.

OMS, *Contrôle social des techniques hospitalières: une approche possible*, cahier SHS n° 10.

Pathmanathan, I., 1993, *Gestion de la recherche sur les systèmes de santé: un outil de gestion*, Ottawa, CRDI.

Plantes médicinales du Sahel, série Études et Recherches, n° 187-188-189.

Prescott-Allen, R., 2003, *Le bien-être des nations. Indice par pays de la qualité de vie et de l'environnement*, Eska/CRDI.

PNUD, 2001, *Rapport national sur le développement humain au Sénégal: gouvernance et développement humain*, New York.

Population et santé dans les pays en développement, vol.1: population, santé et survie dans les sites du réseau INDEPTH, Réseau INDEPTH, CRDI, 2003.

République du Sénégal, Ministère de la santé, 1989, *Programme de développement intégré du secteur de la santé*, avril.

Salem, G., 1998, *La santé dans la ville*, Karthala/Orstom.

Seck, M., 1991, « Une stratégie de promotion de la santé », Vie et Santé, n° 6, pp. 3-5.

Smith, G. et Naim, M., 2000, *Mondialisation, souveraineté et gouvernance*, CRDI.

Sy, A. B., 1991, « Quelle santé pour l'Afrique? », *Afrique-Espoir*, n° 2, pp. 2-7.

Wone, I., 1984, « Médecine et développement au Sahel, indicateurs de santé », *Cahier Medesahel*, n° 1, p. 298.

11

La gestion de maladies chroniques en Algérie: le cas du cancer

Farida Mecheri

Introduction

Selon les donnés récentes sur le profil de la morbidité dans le monde, publiés par l'Organisation mondiale de la santé (OMS 2003), les maladies chroniques connaissent une montée de plus en plus importante. Le rapport de l'OMS montre que la charge de morbidité due aux maladies non transmissibles est en augmentation et représente prés de la moitié de la charge mondiale de morbidité générale (tous âges confondus). Cela concerne aussi bien les pays développés que les pays en voix de développement. Selon le même rapport, alors que la proportion de la charge de morbidité imputable aux maladies non transmissibles se maintient à plus de 80% chez les adultes de 15 ans et plus dans les pays développés, elle dépasse déjà 70% dans les pays à revenus moyen.

Dans beaucoup de pays en développement, la progression de l'épidémie des maladies non transmissibles s'accélère sous l'effet du vieillissement de la population et des changements survenus dans la distribution des facteurs de risques.

L'une de ces maladies est le cancer qui a fait 7,1 millions de décès dans le monde en 2002, selon toujours le rapport OMS de 2003. 17% de ces décès sont liés au cancer du poumon en 2000. Cela coïncide avec l'apparition d'une épidémie de tabagisme dans les pays à revenu faible à moyen. Par contre, chez les femmes, c'est le cancer du sein qui entraîne le plus de décès dans les pays développés et dans les pays en développement. Mais selon le rapport de la santé (OMS 1998) dans les pays en développement le cancer du col de l'utérus est aussi répandu (les femmes interrogées dans mon travail sur la trajectoire des malades atteints d'un cancer avaient le cancer du sein ou le cancer du col de l'utérus et ces types de cancers ont une signification qui dépasse la logique médicale pour engendrer un explication socio-anthropologique).

Ces données recueillies sur la situation épidémiologique des maladies chroniques en général et du cancer en particulier dans le monde vont être revues avec quelques spécificités en Algérie. Ce pays connaît désormais une situation alarmante concernant la morbidité due aux maladies endémiques (non transmissibles). Le rapport récent de la ligue algérienne des droits de l'homme (Ladh 2003) a montré la résurgence de certaines de ces maladies liées à la pauvreté, au recul de l'hygiène et aux conditions d'existence dans les quartiers défavorisés. Grâce aux différents programmes nationaux instaurés lors des dernières décennies, on assiste à une véritable transition épidémiologique marquée par l'amorce de la transition démographique, l'augmentation de l'espérance de vie des personnes âgées, la transformation de l'environnement et les changements de mode de vie. Cette transition nous interpelle pour un déploiement vers de nouvelles pathologies. Les maladies chroniques commencent à poser de véritables problèmes de santé publique (Hamdi Cherif 2004), en l'absence d'une stratégie nationale de lutte contre ces maladies, que ce soit sur le plan préventif ou sur le plan curatif.

La prise en charge de ces maladies demeure encore très insuffisante en raison du manque d'infrastructures et de médicaments adéquats. Les établissements publics ne supportent pas les frais de traitement, la plupart des malades — surtout à faible revenu — finissent par l'abandon de traitement. Le non-remboursement et la suspension de l'importation de certains médicaments compliqueront davantage le problème des malades chroniques, toujours selon le rapport de la ligue algérienne des droits de l'homme.

Pour le cancer, les données des hospitalisations pour pathologie cancéreuse, ainsi que les résultats obtenus par les registres des cancers, mettent en évidence l'augmentation constante de l'incidence des cancers au cours de la dernière décennie. Les localisations pulmonaires et digestives chez l'homme et les localisations génitales chez la femme sont les plus fréquentes. Mais pour une maladie qui s'inscrit dans le rang des nouveaux besoins prioritaires en santé publique on trouve que la prévalence et l'incidence de la morbidité cancéreuse ont été toujours sous-estimées en Algérie, car peu d'études épidémiologiques ont été réalisées dans ce domaine. Actuellement, toutes les données d'incidence disponibles sont établies à partir des registres du cancer mis en place à l'ouest, à l'est et au centre du pays (ces points ont été relevés lors de la première journée d'étude qui réunissait les spécialistes en cancérologie pour donner un panorama sur l'épidémiologie des cancers solides en Algérie, 1999). Les résultats montrent que le cancer du sein est le premier cancer en Algérie; c'est le premier cancer féminin depuis 1990, avec une incidence régulièrement croissante, alors que l'incidence du cancer du col de l'utérus stagne avec une tendance à la diminution. Chez les hommes le cancer du poumon est le premier et il est en augmentation continue au fil des ans. Certaines localisations paraissent spécifiques à notre pays et parfois à certaines régions. Par exemple, le cancer des voies biliaires, qui est au 3e ou 4e rang des cancers féminins, le cancer du naso-pharynx qui paraît fréquent à l'est du pays, le cancer de l'estomac à l'ouest.

À titre indicatif, 2 270 nouveaux cas du cancer ont été enregistrés dans la wilaya d'Alger en 1999, ce qui donne une incidence moyenne de 100 cas pour 100 000 habitants. Rapporté à l'échelon national, cela représentait 30 000 nouveaux cas à prendre en charge annuellement. C'est dire l'importance des moyens humains et matériels à mettre en œuvre. Cette situation s'aggravera dans la prochaine décennie. Elle est liée au génie évolutif de certaines localisations mais aussi au retard apporté au diagnostic, aux difficultés de la prise en charge, au manque observé au niveau des centres anti-cancéreux, les plus anciens (Sétif, Oran, Alger étendu à Tizi-ouzou et Blida depuis 1997) aux plus récents (Tlemcen, Batna, Constantine) et la création de ceux de Sidi-bel-abbés et Annaba. Il n'existe pas suffisamment de couverture médicale en dehors de ces centres que ce soit dans le diagnostic ou le traitement avec l'impératif d'établir pour chaque région une carte des moyens humains et matériels de prise en charge. Cela confirme l'idée d'inadaptation des structures d'accueil et ajoutant à cela le nombre de malades en augmentation, l'insuffisance sinon l'absence de soins palliatifs, ces facteurs rendent encore plus pénible la détresse des malades et celle de leur entourage (ministère de la santé publique).

Ces données factuelles sur la prévalence des maladies chroniques en Algérie — surtout celles liées au cancer — et sur la prise en charge et la gestion montrent un grand déficit lié à la lourdeur de ces maladies. Selon M. Mebtoul (Directeur du groupe de recherche en Anthropologie de la santé), ce déficit est lié aussi au personnel de santé, aux usagers et gestionnaires, aux logiques de défiance dans les rapports noués entre les acteurs qui participent à l'activité de santé, illustrant ainsi leur profonde « insatisfaction » par rapport au mode de régulation actuel du système de santé. Ce mode de régulation (la façon dont l'État agence et organise les relations entre les agents de la santé) est fortement marqué par une dynamique verticale, uniforme et centralisée où prédomine une logique administrative opaque (Hours 2001).

Il y a en revanche un travail très approfondi dans les pays occidentaux afin de trouver de nouvelles mesures concernant la gestion des maladies chroniques dans ces pays. Avec l'hospitalisation à domicile ces pays parviennent à alléger les coûts de la santé. Ce projet prometteur est le résultat de constatations scientifiques très importantes et la valorisation du rôle de la famille par l'analyse des relations existantes entre les réseaux familiaux et la santé et aussi la spécificité des expériences des maladies chroniques qui s'étalent aux différentes sphères de la vie sociale. Pour ces chercheurs, l'influence de la famille sur la santé des individus prend des représentations différentes et le rapprochement entre la famille et la santé dépasse les situations limites comme le vécu d'une maladie chronique pour inclure aussi le travail domestique de la santé (Cresson 1991). Cette nouvelle perspective peut contribuer selon ses concepteurs à alléger le coût de la prise en charge dans les structures de soins. Elle aide à maintenir l'identité sociale du malade qui vit une maladie de longue durée ou chronique. Une pathologie transformée en un lent processus investit alors des espaces sociaux plus vastes (Menoret 1999) et là se pose une question très importante: est-ce possible l'application de cette politique qui est l'hospitalisation à domicile? On ne peux pas répondre dans l'immédiat car cela nécessite aussi des investigations qui prennent en compte les spécificités de notre société. Ces études doivent avoir un volet pluridisciplinaire, et c'est dans cette perspective que j'essaie d'inscrire ma réflexion. Bien sûr, je ne sais pas faire de la publicité pour appliquer l'hospitalisation à domicile, mais en fait prendre l'exemple d'une maladie chronique qu'est le cancer pour comprendre sa trajectoire en mettant bien l'accent sur les différents acteurs dans cette trajectoire, y compris la famille. Ici je m'inscris dans la logique de Mebtoul qui, en passant par les structures de santé, essaye de valoriser les autres acteurs surtout la famille considérée comme un groupe organisateur des soins. La famille joue un rôle actif dans le processus thérapeutique qui n'est pas seulement médical mais il prend aussi une dimension liée aux habitudes antérieures et à la capacité de pratiquer les activités quotidiennes (Mebtoul 1998).

C'est dans cette perspective que j'ai entrepris une étude exploratoire sur les trajectoires des malades atteints d'un cancer à Blida, l'une des régions où se trouve un centre anticancéreux. J'ai essayé dans mon travail de comprendre les bouleversements produits par l'avènement du cancer dans la vie des malades et de leur entourage. Le cancer est entouré d'images négatives liées à la mort et à la souffrance. J'ai voulu aussi ressortir le travail de gestion mené par les différents acteurs dans les différentes sphère de la vie sociale pour faire face à ces bouleversements en faisant un brassage de micro et de macro. Ces propositions sont encadrées par un ensemble de questions qui interpelle ma problématique et qui suscite une exploration théorique et empirique avancée en développant la réflexion sur d'autres maladies chroniques.

De là les questionnements principaux sont les suivants:

- Quels sont les changements produits par l'avènement du cancer dans la vie des personnes atteintes?

- La représentation sociale du cancer crée-t-elle une situation limite et quelles sont les images sociales liées au cancer qui influent le plus sur cette situation limite ou situation de crises?

- Les structures de soins constituent-elles seulement un champ thérapeutique pour traiter la maladie dans sa dimension biologique ou bien représentent-elles également un monde social spécifique – vu la spécificité de cette maladie chronique entourée d'incertitude et vu aussi la réalité sociologique de ces structures?

- Comment apparaît le travail de gestion des différents acteurs de la trajectoire (le malade, la famille, l'entourage, les professionnels de la santé…) et quelles sont les différentes négociations qui peuvent être entreprises pour faire face aux diverses situations rencontrées dans la trajectoire?

- Comment apparaît l'influence du type de cancer, de ces stades et des différents variables socio-anthropologiques (le sexe, l'age, le niveau d'instruction, le niveau économique, la culture sanitaire, le capital relationnel, la situation des structures de soins, les pratiques thérapeutiques parallèles et la conception profane de la santé et de la maladie…) dans les trajectoires des malades atteints d'un cancer?
- Comment peut-on évaluer le rôle de la famille dans la prise en charge du cancer?

À partir de ces questions, l'objectif principal de cette étude est d'essayer de comprendre, à travers une approche décentralisée, le rôle des différents acteurs dans la prise en charge du cancer en prenant en compte sa spécificité et en mettant l'accent sur le rôle de la famille. Cela ouvrira la voie sur d'autres atteintes chroniques pour améliorer, dans une perspective à long terme, la gestion des maladies chroniques dans le système sanitaire en Algérie.

Revue de la littérature

Dans la littérature récente sur la santé et la maladie, on constate un intérêt de plus en plus important pour l'étude des maladies chroniques et cela est lié, comme on l'a dit dans l'introduction, au profil de la morbidité dans le monde caractérisé par l'amorce des maladies endémiques, celles-ci créent selon Adam et Herzlich (1994) une transformation dans le statut des malades et dans les types de relations sociales tissées autour du malade. Cela montre les nouvelles tendances heuristiques pour encadrer les expériences des maladies chroniques qui dépassent le cadre classique de la maladie comme étant un comportement social déviant (Bourricaud 1995). Par contre, dans le cas des maladies chroniques liées à la durée, l'incertitude relève des perturbations répétées mais pas nécessairement homogènes. La construction de la maladie devient plus complexe car on gère la chronicité et non plus un traitement efficace (Cresson 1991); cette complexité est liée à des histoires personnelles, à un discours scientifique, au système de valeurs et à des structures de prise en charge des maladies (Aich 1998).

On comprend alors l'importance d'un cadre théorique adapté à la spécificité des maladies chroniques, ce cadre est celui du sociologue américain Ansalem Strauss. Comme interactionniste, Strauss s'est penché sur l'étude de l'action en essayant de joindre le niveau de l'acteur individuel à celui des microprocessus et finalement au niveau macrosocial et structural, en faisant ressortir les stratégies de l'interaction, à savoir le temps, l'espace, la culture et le statut économique et technologique. Ce cadre théorique appliqué aux maladies chroniques par Strauss permet de construire un modèle d'analyse qui dépasse le vécu de la maladie comme étant seulement une réalité biologique pour la découvrir aussi comme une réalité sociale, et il est difficile en fait de séparer ces deux aspects.

Le concept de trajectoire est un concept clé dans mon étude, car il permet d'introduire toutes situations créées par l'avènement de la maladie chronique, le cancer pris comme exemple. On a parlé dans l'introduction de la perception de la maladie ou, pour utiliser un concept sociologique, de la représentation sociale du cancer, qui véhicule la trajectoire de la maladie (Herzlich 1970). Elle est l'observation de la manière de penser, de vivre des gens dans la société à travers l'ensemble des valeurs, les normes sociales et les modèles culturels. Elle étudie la manière dont on construit ces objets sociaux qui sont la santé et la maladie.

La trajectoire se déroule dans des mondes sociaux définis comme des réseaux d'acteurs qui participent à faire certaines activités, et là on va répondre à un ensemble de questions: qui est l'acteur? avec qui il rentre en interaction? quel est l'objectif de l'action? comment est organisée l'action et selon quel compromis? Ces concepts appartiennent à un modèle d'analyse qui sert de fil conducteur dans l'étude des trajectoires des malades atteints d'un cancer. Les autres concepts comme la négociation, les processus de la normalisation, la famille et d'autres seront expliqués dans le rapport final.

Et pour mieux cerner mon terrain, j'ai essayé de consulter un ensemble de travaux faits sur le vécu des maladies chroniques (Kirchgasser et Edwards 1987, Hannes 1987, Kaufmann 1989, Gerard sd et Pedenelli 1988, Waissman 1995, Fassin 1996, Mebtoul 1998).

Ce qui caractérise ces études, c'est la reproduction des expériences des différentes maladies chroniques dans un cadre psychosocial et anthropologique en utilisant le cadre conceptuel cité auparavant mais retravaillé en profondeur selon le type de maladie et la spécificité de la société. Ce qui le rend plus opérationnel pour cadrer l'étude et pour expliquer ses résultats.

Pour cerner le niveau macrosocial et structurel, il est important de dresser un bref aperçu sur les résultats d'un ensemble d'études faites sur le système de santé en Algérie. Un tel aperçu montre pourquoi porter l'intérêt sur ce genre de questions. Il permet aussi de répondre à beaucoup de situations produites au courant de la trajectoire:

- la gratuité des soins n'a pas minimisé l'inégalité sociale face à la santé entre le rural et l'urbain, mais elle a accentué les différences sociales pour l'accès aux soins et la prévention;
- il y a un décalage entre les principes théoriques d'organisation du système sanitaire et sa mise en application. La société algérienne a développé un système sanitaire hétérogène qui s'éloigne d'un « système national de santé » (Azougli 1988);
- toutes les classes sociales refusent le système sanitaire, mais pour des raisons différentes qui sont l'image des divergences objectives et subjectives existant entre ces classes; les classes moyennes centralisent dans l'obtention des soins plus spécialisés « soins à l'étranger », d'un autre coté les usagers issus des catégories défavorisées vivent l'injustice de l'institution médicale à

travers la perception de leur difficultés d'accès au médecin, ne payant ainsi qu'à l'hôpital (Azougli 1988);

- malgré l'existence des structures de soins gratuits qui effectuent le rapport économique entre le médecin et le malade, on trouve une inégalité dans l'obtention des soins; des facilités d'accès aux soins pour les classes sociales dominantes, sans passer par le rouage de l'organisation sanitaire avec la possibilité d'accès à toutes les sphères de la couverture sanitaire, par contre les catégories défavorisées les plus touchées par la maladie trouvent des difficultés pour l'accès aux soins « gratuits » (Thebaud 1977);

- ne pas reconnaître l'importance du système explicatif produit dans la société (les jugements, les savoirs, les perceptions concernant les symptômes, les manières thérapeutiques et les institutions) explique les limites des programmes sanitaires effectués à partir seulement d'un savoir médical (Mebtoul 1998);

- la famille est considérée comme un groupe organisateur des soins et elle joue un rôle actif dans le processus thérapeutique qui n'est pas seulement biologique, mais il prend aussi une dimension liée aux habitudes antérieures et à la capacité de pratiquer les activités quotidiennes (Mebtoul 1998).

Discussions des résultats

La construction des trajectoires des malades atteints d'un cancer, l'exploration de leurs discours montrent la richesse sociologique de ce thème. Bien sûr je ne peux pas présenter tous les résultats de ma recherche mais seulement ouvrir l'appétit sur ce que peut donner l'écoute des acteurs dans les trajectoires des maladies chroniques. Perception et actions, effet et gestion sont des logiques qui apparaissent tout au long des discours. Le cancer va d'un état de bouleversement psychique chez le malade et son entourage à un indicateur sociologique qui reflète une fragilité de la logique institutionnelle; il peut apparaître aussi comme un mécanisme de contrôle social.

La représentation sociale du cancer dans les dits des usagers montre un brassage entre une image universelle du cancer liée à la mort, à la souffrance et au châtiment et une conception sociale et culturelle particulière (mort biologique et mort sociale, la référence religieuse comme une aide et un soutien pour accepter la maladie. Il a été démontré par des études antérieures sur les immigrants surtout (Dutour *et al.* 1989), que la cancérophobie (Kaufmann 1989) montre un va et vient entre la logique médicale et la logique sociale ou le type de cancer constitue un facteur très impressionnant, puisque j'ai travaillé avec des femmes atteintes du cancer du sein ou de celui de col de l'utérus. Cela montre la place du profane qui désigne la maladie (cancer du col) par sa liaison à la procréation. L'organe est appelé selon sa fonction sociale et non seulement comme organe biologique.

Venant aux stades de reconnaissance de la maladie (reconnaissance médicale et sociale) et là on trouve que la décision d'accès aux soins n'est plus une simple réponse à des symptômes biologiques, mais il s'agit d'une décision collective ou l'autrui joue un rôle prépondérant lié au degré d'implication sociale.

Bibliographie indicative

Adam, P. et Herzlich, C., 1994, *Sociologie de la maladie et de la médecine*, Paris: Nathan.

Azougli, I., 1988, « Système de santé en Algérie: perceptions de l'institution médicale dans deux quartiers d'Alger », thèse de doctorat en Sociologie, Paris: EHESS.

Baszanger, I., 1986, « Maladies chroniques et leur ordre négocié », *Revue française de Sociologie*, vol. XXVII, janvier-mars, pp. 3-27.

Benoist, J., 2002, *Petite bibliothèque d'anthropologie médicale*, Paris: AMADES.

Cresson, G., 1991, *Le travail sanitaire profane dans la famille: analyse sociologique*, Thèse de doctorat, Paris: EHESS.

Cresson, G., 1995, *Le travail domestique de la santé*, Paris: Harmattan, Coll. Logique sociale.

Dutour, O. *et al.*, 1989, « Aspects anthropologiques du diabète sucré », *ECOL* Hum. Paris, vol. II, n° 1.

Fassin, D., 1996, *Les effets sociaux des maladies graves*, Paris: Erasme, décembre.

Friedrich, H. *et al.*, 1987, « Faire face à une maladie chronique », *Sciences sociales et Santé*, vol. V, n° 2, juin, pp. 31-44.

Gerard, P., *Existe t-il une construction familiale sexuée de l'autonomie?*, Université de Nancy: LASTES.

Henrad, J. C., 1988, « Maladies chroniques invalidantes », *Sciences sociales et Santé*, vol VI, n° 2, juin, pp. 25-30.

Herzlich, C., 1970, *Santé et maladie (Analyse d'une représentation sociale)*, Layahe: Mouton, Coll. Les textes sociologiques.

Hours, B., 2001, *Systèmes et politiques de santé (de la santé publique à l'anthropologie)*, Paris: Karthala.

Kaufman, A., 1989, « Les malades face à leur cancer », in Aïch, P. *et al.*, *Vivre une maladie grave: analyse d'une situation de crise*, Paris: Éditions Méridiens Klincsieck, Coll, Réponses sociologiques.

Kirchgässler, K., Matt, E., 1987, « La fragilité du quotidien », *Sciences sociales et Santé*, vol. V, n° 1, février, pp. 93-113.

Mebtoul, M., 1998, *Les significations attribuées par les médecins et les malades à la prise en charge de deux maladies chroniques (diabète et hypertension) dans la ville de Tlemcen*, Université d'Oran, 43 p.

Ministère de la Santé et de la Population, 1998, Système national de santé: éléments de réflexion, Assises nationales de la santé, 27 et 28 mai.

OMS, 1998, *Rapport sur la santé dans le monde*.

OMS, 2003, *Rapport sur la santé dans le monde (façonner l'avenir)*.

Parsons, T., 1995, « Structures sociales et processus dynamique: le cas de la pratique médicale moderne », in: Bouricaud, F., *Eléments pour une sociologie de l'action*, Paris: Plon.

Pedinelli, J. L., 1988, *Conduite et représentation des familles et des patients atteints de maladies graves et soumis à des thérapeutiques de suppléance*, Paris: C.N.R.S.

Strauss, A., 1992, *La trame de la négociation (Sociologie qualitative et interactionnisme)*, Paris: Éditions l'Harmattan.

Thebeaud, A.,1977, « Besoins de santé et réponse de l'institution sanitaire en Algérie », *Cahiers de Sociologie et de Démographie médicale*, n° 4, octobre-décembre, pp. 170-183.

Waissmen, R., 1995, « Interactions familiales et impact de la technologie dans la gestion d'une maladie chronique », *Sciences sociales et Santé*, vol. XIII, n° 1, mars, pp. 81-100.

Journée d'étude, 1999, Épidémiologie des cancers solides en Algérie, juillet.

12

Situation des malades tuberculeux en cours de traitement perdus de vue au Centre antituberculeux de Brazaville (Congo): une revue

André Mbou

La lutte contre la tuberculose est l'un des objectifs du millénaire fixé par les Nations Unies. Au regard de la mise en œuvre du Programme national de Lutte contre la Tuberculose, on constate un certain nombre de faiblesses telles que, le non suivi des malades à domicile, la non-intégration à grande échelle de la stratégie du traitement direct par observation du personnel de santé (DOTS) qui se fait au niveau du Centre de Santé, la formation du personnel, la rupture des stocks des médicaments.

Cette résistance soulève d'autres facteurs dont:

- l'accessibilité aux services de santé,
- le faible niveau de revenu des familles,
- la durée du traitement qui varie entre 6 et 8 mois,
- la résistance de certaines souches à certains médicaments.

C'est ainsi que la prise en charge du malade tuberculeux reste une préoccupation pour le Programme national de Lutte contre la Tuberculose. Ce denier devrait se préoccuper de la mise en œuvre du DOTS et sa décentralisation au niveau périphérique.

Introduction

En République du Congo, le droit à la santé est garanti par la loi fondamentale à savoir: droit à la protection de la santé des individus, droit à l'accès aux soins de santé. Au Congo Brazzaville, le département de la Santé, par le biais de sa Direction de la lutte contre la maladie, a mis en place un Programme national de

Lutte contre la Tuberculose (PNLT). Le programme assure les soins au tuberculeux à travers le Centre antituberculeux à Brazzaville. Le CAT a pour tâches:

- le dépistage des cas,
- le traitement et le suivi des malades,
- la surveillance épidémiologique.

Le PNLT a pour mission la mise en œuvre du programme d'élaboration des stratégies, la formation du personnel et la supervision des activités au niveau des centres.

La tuberculose est un problème socio-économique ayant des implications médicales et sanitaires considérables. Les approches de lutte devraient être faites en fonction des tendances de développement socio-économique et ethniques. Il est important de regarder les problèmes de résistance des malades au traitement antituberculeux avec pertinence. La stratégie DOTS s'avère indispensable surtout de son efficacité.

Problématique

La recrudescence des maladies endémiques reste une préoccupation pour les services de santé. Il a été constaté que la morbidité est encore élevée dans l'ordre de 23%. Cette morbidité est due, en grande partie, aux maladies transmissibles dont la tuberculose et d'autres infections respiratoires.

Les tuberculeux à macroscopie positive ou TPM+ sont responsables de l'extension de la maladie dans la population. Lutter contre la tuberculose consiste en leur détection, leur traitement et leur guérison bactériologique. La guérison d'un tuberculeux dépend de sa responsabilité dans la prise de son traitement jusqu'à la fin et son arrêt dépend de l'avis du personnel de santé qui soigne.

La tuberculose connaît une recrudescence inquiétante associée à l'infection VIH/SIDA et aux perturbations qu'a connues le Programme national de Lutte contre la Tuberculose durant les conflits sociopolitiques qui ont secoué le Congo de 1997 à 2001.

En 2002, la tuberculose demeure la quatrième cause de morbidité au Congo, dont le taux de mortalité est de 11%.

Dans le cadre de nos activités de surveillance épidémiologique et de gestion de l'information des malades, nous avons constaté à partir des données statistiques les faits suivants:

- une augmentation des cas de tuberculose référés à l'hôpital dans l'ordre de 10%, surtout dans les périodes des troubles sociopolitiques;
- la stratégie DOTS n'est pas intégrée effectivement au Centre de Santé dans leur paquet minimum d'activités;
- cette situation de non intégration du DOTS explique des problèmes de mauvaise mise en œuvre du programme. Cela aussi pose des problèmes d'accessibilité des malades aux soins;

- la tuberculose est toujours reconnue comme une maladie de la pauvreté accentuée par le mauvais état de santé chronique et aggravée par la co-infection tuberculose et VIH/SIDA;
- de 1998 à 2001, 13 253 cas de tuberculose ont été enregistrés au Centre antituberculeux (CAT) avec un taux de létalité de 0,70%;
- le taux d'abandon dans l'ensemble est dans l'ordre de 19%. Par contre en 2001, il a été de 16,10% et le risque de contamination reste encore élevé.

Certains facteurs tels que: la force de travail, le faible niveau de revenu de familles, le comportement des parents et celui du personnel de santé, le coût des services affectent l'état de santé et le comportement des malades dans la prise du traitement.

Au regard de tous ces faits, je me suis posé les questions suivantes:

- Quels sont les déterminants économiques, sociaux, culturels et éthiques dans le traitement de la Tuberculose?
- Quels sont les facteurs qui favorisent cet abandon?
- Quelles sont les difficultés rencontrées par le programme dans la mise en oeuvre du DOTS?

De ces questions découlent des objectifs:

- Identifier les facteurs d'abandon,
- Déterminer les difficultés de mise en œuvre du PNLT.

Notre hypothèse de travail se traduit par la non-observation du traitement par les malades tuberculeux.

Revue de la littérature

Le problème de la prise en charge et le suivi des malades tuberculeux dans les centres de santé ont donné lieu à des travaux de recherche qui ont été effectués aussi bien au Congo qu'ailleurs en Afrique. La littérature consécutive à ces travaux est peu abondante et n'est souvent connue que des spécialistes. Pour ce travail, nous nous sommes penchés sur les travaux effectués par des universitaires ou des spécialistes des questions de santé publique.

Dr Ibrahim M. Samba, Directeur de l'AFRO, dans son message à l'occasion de la journée mondiale de la santé sur la Tuberculose, à déclaré que 35% des États sur 46, ont assuré la mise en œuvre de la stratégie DOTS avec une couverture thérapeutique suffisante. Par contre la capacité de notification des cas reste encore faible soit 44%.

Dr Eugène A. Nyarko, dans son étude sur l'aperçu de la situation de la Tuberculose dans la région africaine, rappelle que l'engagement des gouvernants demeure insuffisant dans l'allocation des ressources pour la lutte contre la tuberculose. La faiblesse des systèmes de santé explique la mauvaise couverture des services de santé.

Wilfred C. Nkhoma, dans ses écrits sur la maîtrise de la double épidémie Tuberculose et VIH/SIDA, relève l'insuffisance des infrastructures de santé destinées à appuyer la mise en œuvre des programmes de lutte et le manque de coordination des efforts de traitement des cas communs (malades de Tuberculose et VIH/ SIDA).

Dr E. N. L. Browne explique l'impact socioéconomique de la Tuberculose. Au premier plan, il démontre que le taux de notification de la Tuberculose qui est de l'ordre de 10 à 15% intéresse plus la tranche d'âge économiquement productive (15-54 ans). Certains facteurs qui contribuent à l'accroissement des cas de tuberculose et aux décès sont: la croissance démographique et l'inefficacité des programmes de lutte contre la Tuberculose.

Concernant la difficulté de retrouver les malades ayant abandonné leur traitement, nous avons trouvé une réponse dans l'étude sur la situation réelle des patients tuberculeux à frottis positifs, au Malawi, réalisée par M. L. Kruytet et son équipe de recherche. Dans cette étude, ils ont en effet démontré que les fausses adresses données par les patients constituent un réel problème dans le suivi. Il est souvent difficile de les retrouver après constat d'abandon (Kruyt 1999:6).

Fanjosoa Rakotomanana et L. P. Rabanijoana se sont penchés sur le rapport entre le genre et la lutte contre la tuberculose. En effet dans leur étude sur les perdus de vue en cours de traitement dans le Programme national de lutte contre la tuberculose à Madagascar, ils montrent que le sexe masculin reste prédominant sur l'ensemble des malades (21,9%). Ils pensent que les hommes fréquentent moins les centres de traitement après dépistage, ceci à cause de certaines occupations et aussi de l'ignorance (F. Rakotomanana et L. P. Rabarijoana 1999:225-229).

Dans son étude sur la prise en charge des tuberculeux, J. Ndi-Ndi constate que les activités d'information, d'éducation et de communication (IEC) sont peu performantes. Les malades n'ont pas des informations suffisantes sur la maladie. Le personnel n'insiste pas trop sur cette activité.(Ndi-Ndi 1998:6).

Pour N. Bidounga, le problème majeur est celui du manque de ressources financières et l'insuffisance du personnel évoluant dans le Programme. C'est ce qu'il décrit dans son étude *sur la prise en charge de la tuberculose et évaluation du programme.*

Sur cette même question de prise en charge, S. Thiam nous donne l'expérience du Sénégal, au niveau de la population infantile de Dakar (Thiam 1997:15). Il indique que les enfants restent une population très vulnérable à cette pathologie, dont près de 15%. Cela est redevable aux mauvaises conditions de vie et de proximité.

La question de la prévalence a été abordée par Mafouana-Nsala et Aboubacry Fall. Dans son étude intitulée *La prévalence de l'infection à VIH/SIDA chez les tuberculeux hospitalisés au service de pneumologie du CHU-B.*, M. P. Mafouana-Nsala démontre la corrélation entre l'infection à VIH et la tuberculose pulmonaire. Cette association pose un problème réel dans la prise en charge de ces malades (Mafouana-Nsala 1998:16). Aboubacry Fall, quant à lui, a étudié la question de la prévalence de la tuberculose au niveau du district de Mbacké au Sénégal (Fall 1996:2). En 1991, dans son mémoire de fin cycle à l'Institut national des sciences de la santé (INSSA), Cyr Tchicaya se penche lui aussi sur la question du dépistage et de la prise en charge de la tuberculose dans les services de soins de santé primaire (Tchicaya 1992:95). Dans leurs travaux, les deux auteurs démontrent l'inexistence de l'intégration du programme de lutte contre la tuberculose dans les centres de santé intégrés. La mise en place des postes sentinelles pour la surveillance épidémiologique devrait permettre un dépistage systématique et un suivi régulier de malades.

Conclusion

Il est clair que la capacité actuelle de lutte efficace contre la tuberculose et le VIH/ SIDA est infime. Le Programme national de Lutte contre la Tuberculose (PNLT) devrait améliorer les services dans les centres de santé intégrés en accélérant la stratégie DOTS en vue d'améliorer la prise en charge des malades, les attitudes, les connaissances et les pratiques du Personnel. Formuler des stratégies à base communautaire pour rendre les services plus accessibles aux malades, susciter la volonté des gouvernants dans l'allocation des ressources est une nécessité qui relève des pouvoirs publiques.

Références

Bidounga, N., 1990, *Prise en charge de la tuberculose et évaluation du programme à Brazzaville*, Mémoire de fin de cycle au Centre Inter-État de Santé publique d'Afrique centrale, Brazzaville.

Baniafouna, C., 2001, *Congo démocratie, vol. 4. Devoir de mémoire. Congo - Brazzaville (15 octobre 1997-31 décembre 1999)*, Paris: l'Harmattan.

Constitution de la République du Congo adoptée au référendum de janvier 2002.

Fall, A., 1996, *Prévalence élevée des cas de tuberculose dans le district sanitaire de Mbacke (Sénégal), Mémoire de fin de cycle*, Institut de santé et développement.

Kala, R., 1985, *Considération épidémiologique à propos de l'étude rétrospective des tuberculeux à l'Hôpital Général de Brazzaville*, Thèse de doctorat de médecine, INSSA, Brazzaville.

Kruyt, M. L. et al., 1999, « La situation des patients tuberculeux à frottis positifs K au Malawi dans les cas d'abandon du traitement », *Bulletin de l'OMS*, pp. 386-391.

Loi 121/92 portant mise en place du Plan national de Développement sanitaire (PNDS).

Mafouana Nsala, M. P., 1998, *La prévalence de l'infection à VIH chez les tuberculeux hospitalisés au service de pneumo-phtisiologie du CHU-B*, mémoire fin de cycle en Santé publique.

Ndi-Ndi, J., 1998, *Prise en charge des malades tuberculeux à l'hôpital Jamot de Yaoundé*, Mémoire fin de cycle de santé publique, Université de Yaoundé.

OMS, 1996, *Prendre en charge la tuberculose au niveau national*, Genève, pag. mult.

OMS, 1996, *La tuberculose en Afrique: un continent de 46 pays, un combat incertain couronné de succès*. AFRO: Brazzaville.

OMS, 1997, *Guide pour la surveillance de la résistance bactérienne aux médicaments antituberculeux*.

OMS, 1998, *TB at crossroads: Who report on the global tuberculosis epidemic*, Geneva.

OMS, 2001, *Observation de la santé en Afrique*, volume 2, n°1.

ONU-SIDA, 1997, *Tuberculose et SIDA. Point de vue.*

Programme national de lutte contre la tuberculose, 2000, *Analyse épidémiologique de 1992 à 1994*, Brazzaville, Congo.

PNUD, 2002, *Rapport national pour le développement humain*, Brazzaville.

Rakotomanana, F. et al., 1999, « Profil des malades perdus de vue en cours de traitement dans le programme national de lutte contre la tuberculose à Madagascar », *Cahier de la santé*, vol. 9, n°4, juil.- août, pp. 225-229.

Razakazo, 1999, *Situation épidémiologique de la tuberculose à Madagascar*, Mémoire de fin de cycle, Ecole de santé publique, Madagascar.

Rathonina, 1998, *Etude épidémiologique et la lutte contre la tuberculose de la circonscription, médicale de Vakinakotia à Madagascar*, mémoire de fin de cycle, École de santé publique, Madagascar.

Thiam, S., 1989, *Prise en charge des enfants tuberculeux à Dakar*, Mémoire de fin de cycle, Institut de Santé et développement, Dakar.

Rakotomizao, J. R. et al., 1998, « Facteurs d'abandon du traitement antituberculeux à Antananarivoville et Antsirabe », *Int J. Tuber Lung Dis 2*, pp. 891-892.

Société des Nations (SDN), 1923, *Rapport provisoire sur la tuberculose et la maladie du sommeil en Afrique équatoriale*, Genève.

Tchicaya, C., 1992, *Intégration du dépistage et de la prise en charge de la tuberculose: service de soins de santé primaires*, Mémoire, INSSA, Brazzaville (Congo).

V

Priority Setting and Policy Making

13

Retirement Stress in Nigeria: A Psycho-political Analysis

Jane-Frances Agbu

Introduction

Retirement means different things to different people. Typically and like most English words, the meaning it takes depends on the context in which it is used. The context in which retirement is described here concerns 'giving up a regular job or regular activity with consequent cessation of the enjoyment of fringe benefits or other benefits associated with it'. Retirement could also be viewed as being outside the workforce, receiving some income from a previous job and having time to do the things the individual desires. Technically, retirement can begin anytime an individual has amassed enough capital to provide a living without holding a job. Retirement is not necessarily a dichotomy: retired versus not retired. It is a process that begins when the individual realises that some day he or she will leave a job, and ends when the individual becomes so feeble and impoverished that they can no longer play the retirement role (Atchley 1976). This then indicates that retirement is a process through which the retirement role is approached, taken up, learned, mastered and relinquished. When retirement is viewed as a social role, it undergoes the following phases: pre-retirement phase, honeymoon phase, disenchantment phase, re-orientation phase, stability and termination phase. The pre-retirement phase is divided into the two phases of remote and near, with the remote phase beginning when the individual takes a job and finishing when the individual ends his career. The near phase begins when the individual becomes aware that he or she will take up the retirement role very soon, with the attitude towards retirement becoming negative, probably because the realities of retirement become clear. The honeymoon phase is rather a euphoric stage in which individuals wallow in their newly found freedom of time and space, with many trying their hand at things they never had time for before. After the honeymoon is over and life begins to slow down, some people experience a period of disenchantment.

This depends on a lot of factors: few alternatives, little money, poor health etc. The re-orientation phase is then necessary for those whose honeymoon either did not get off the ground or landed with a crash. Here, the retiree tends to explore new avenues for involvement and to develop more realistic views about alternatives. The stability phase ushers in a relatively well-developed set of criteria for making choices while in the termination phase, people tend to lose their retirement role through illness and disability, which sometimes accompany old age. At this point, the individual ceases to retire and becomes dependent.

Retirement, seen as one of the biggest changes in the life cycle, can be a stressful period; no matter how prepared you may think you are, as there can be something that has not been planned or foreseen to upset things. With increased rate of early retirement, the experience of retirement can be very difficult. It may be an opportunity for increased leisure time for those with adequate pensions, but for those retiring through ill health and with a low or no pension, retirement may bring despair and limited opportunities. Indeed, there is a sense in which psychology as a state of mind and political economy of care, as perceived and experienced by the retirees, underlie the whole process.

This paper intends to critically examine retirement stress from a multi-disciplinary perspective with the emphasis on the psychological and political contexts. It is clear today that no comprehensive study of social issues could be done without recourse to the interrelated factors causing or influencing events. In this case, the focus is in analysing the various dimensions of retirement stress in Nigeria as they relate to both the political and social dynamics.

However, this study is basically a review of the state of discourse of retirement stress and relevant literature in Nigeria. It does not lay claim to any systematic survey for information gathering. However, extensive person-to-person interviews and primary documents were used as reliable sources of first-hand information on the plight of retirees and the state of retirement policy in Nigeria.

For a better understanding of the discourse, the paper raises the following questions:

a) To what extent can retirement stress be said to be a problem in Nigeria?
b) What are the political structures for managing retirement in Nigeria?
c) Is the financial architecture for managing pensions in Nigeria adequate?
d) What are the possible psychological implications of unchecked retirement problems on the national psyche?

Theoretical Underpinnings

Two theories, which dominated social gerontology in the 1950s, were Disengagement and Activity theories. Both postulate not only behaviour changes with age and retirement but also imply how that behaviour would change (Powell 2001). Disengagement theory, associated with Cumming and Henry (1961), proposed that a gradual withdrawal of older people from work roles and social relationships is both an inevitable and rational process. For this variant of functionalism, this process benefits society, since it means that the death of an individual member of society does not prevent the ongoing functioning of the social system. This theory argues that it was beneficial for both the retired individual and society that such disengagement takes place in order to minimise the social disruption caused by an ageing person's eventual death (Neurgarten 1998). A number of critiques exist: first, this theory condones indifference towards retirement, old age and social problems. Secondly, it represents a threat to the promotion of a positive and involved lifestyle for ageing persons across the lifespan (Powell 1999).

Activity theory, a counterpoint of Disengagement theory, claims a successful retirement can be achieved by maintaining roles and relationships. Any loss of roles, activities or relationships within old age, should be replaced by new roles and activities to ensure happiness, value consensus and well being. Thus, 'activity' was seen as an ethical and academic response to the disengagement thesis which recast retirement as joyous and mobile (Powell 2001). Nevertheless, Activity theory tends to neglect issues of power plays, inequality and conflict between age groups. An actual 'value consensus' may reflect the interests of powerful and dominant groups within the society who find it advantageous to have age-power relations organised in such a way (Phillipson 1998).

As an intellectual background against such functionalist theoretical dominance, the political economy of old age emerged from Marxist insights in analysing the capitalist complexity of modern society and how old age and retirement were socially constructed to foster the needs of the economy. The political economy approach desired to understand the character and significance of variations in the treatment of the aged and to relate these to polity, economy and society. For Ester (1979), political economy challenges the ideology of older people as belonging to a homogeneous group unaffected by the dominant structures in society. Political economy therefore focuses upon an analysis of the state in contemporary societal formations. Here, we can see how Marxism is interconnected to this theory. Ester (1979) also looks at how the state decides and dictates who is allocated resources and who is not. This impinges upon retirement and subsequent pension schemes. As Phillipson (1982) pointed out, the retirement experience is linked to the timing of the reduction of wages and enforced withdrawal from work, and has made many older people financially insecure. Hence the state could make and break the fortunes of its populace.

From this perspective, the nature of the Nigerian state as presently constituted, the state of its democracy, and the character of the political class, all serve as important constituents in examining social security and retirement. The suspicion is that the not too efficient Nigerian state characterised by official corruption and poverty has been instrumental in generating retirement stress for a significant percentage of its citizenry.

Retirement as Stressors

The question that most people often ask the newly retired person is: 'What do you do now?' I have watched most retirees literally torn between eagerness and reluctance to answer when asked this familiar question, probably followed by another: 'How do you pass your time?' Surprisingly, many fumble for an answer, with their thoughts turning from family responsibilities to pensions and concern about how to make ends meet. Faced with their problems, accentuated by a nagging wife or uncaring children, they are unlikely to seek comfort in retirement.

Stress is as much part of retirement as of any other period in life, however the impact of some sources of stress seems to intensify during retirement. Retirement, whether voluntary or involuntary, is a transition that requires tremendous adjustment. Most people take it for granted that they will retire someday, while some express dread of retirement. Attitudes towards retirement could be seen as a function of health, ageing, income, roles and expectations, relocation, changes in identity, and position held at retirement. Others could include educational background, versatility of the retiree, government's economic and political policies on retirement, gender, death of spouse, attitude to life, and emotional predisposition.

The concept, stress, was originally used in physics, primarily to describe tension or force placed on an object to bend or break it. When applied to the human condition, it was described as the non-specific response of body to demands placed on it (Selye 1956). Stress can also be understood as a life event that causes physical and psychological reactions in the individual. Today, the word stress is frequently used to describe the level of tension people feel because of the demands of their jobs, relationships and responsibilities in their personal lives (Seaward 1994). In eastern philosophy, stress is considered to be an absence of inner peace. In western culture, stress is viewed as a loss of control, while psychologically speaking it is described as a state of anxiety produced when events and responsibilities exceed one's coping abilities. To the disbelief of some, not all stress is bad. In fact, there are many who believe that humans need some degree of stress to stay alert. When stress serves as a positive motivator, it is considered beneficial, but beyond this optimal point, stress does more harm than good. Notable side effects of stress include high blood pressure, heart attacks, irritable bowel movement, aches and pains, ulcer, dizziness, sleeping difficulty, poor vision, headache, tiredness and in the extreme, death. Psychological effects include depression, anxiety, lack of concentration, tiredness and misery, irritability, negative mood, restlessness and suspicion. Others could lead to reduction in coping capabilities, low self-esteem and self-image, absolutist and dichotomous thinking, fear, hopelessness and helplessness. Other negative impacts of stress could also present themselves in the form of family and marital difficulties, disruption in effective communication, interpersonal difficulties, child abuse, wife battering, political alienation, corruption and greed, etc.

The question that arises when these definitions and side effects are examined closely is: Is stress the event itself or must it be defined in terms of certain reactions to an event? It does seem that stress must be defined in terms of the individual's reaction to the event, which in this case is retirement. Thus, experiences of retirement could also aid in the disruption of the ego and a sense of self worth, when people who have been seeking you dwindle; subordinates, followers, admirers become conspicuous by their absence. It is difficult to accept the fact that you have to wait now instead of people waiting on you. (Dhar 2004). Dhar also reported the case of a retiree whose nagging wife was almost invariably found deriving some sort of vicarious pleasure, bordering on perversion, in shouting at and humiliating her husband, even in the public gaze. Following his retirement, the situation had gone from bad to worse, leaving him with a bout of self-doubt, and loss of confidence. He of course became worried and apprehensive of the uncertainties of the future and lost his sleep and his health. The big fear is usually, who will take care of him now? Will he be a burden to their children? Other difficulties could come in the form of a loss of control over key positions of responsibility with a resultant feeling of frustration and anxiety. A very serious problem is having too much time to spend. Suffice to note that a good number of retirees, immediately after retirement, usually wallow in their newfound freedom of time and space. Here, most try to do all the things they never had time for before. When the 'honeymoon' is over and life begins to slow down, most experience bouts of disenchantment and isolation. Disruption in the usual waking-up routine of the retiree is also a huge challenge, because when not adequately overcome, it could trigger boredom and isolation. Retirement can also trigger marital stress and adjustment in couples. Mein (1998) for example, in his study found that men felt adjusting to a new role and relationship with their wives was the most difficult and unexpected part of retirement. Although retirement might be a way to get rid of the stressors and strains of work, surprisingly, it seems that spending the golden years with a wife is not the recipe for joy either. In another report by Jungmeen et al. (1999), men sometimes complained that retirement tended to reduce their wives respect for them, especially when the wives were not retired. Jungmeen et al. in another study stated that men who retired while their wives were still working showed a higher level of marital stress and distrust. The happiest men were the ones who found another job and whose wives were not working, and they reported the highest morale and the lowest depression and suspiciousness.

This brings us to this important question, 'Why do people work?' Some work for the money and they are most likely to continue even when the income is no longer needed. Some for the social interaction it provides, while others work for the sense of accomplishment it gives. However, when work defines a person: what you are, what you do and where you work, the retiree is very likely to feel disenchanted and restless when this identity tied to his working life seems to have fallen apart.

Perhaps a peep into life events associated with old age could also explain some sources of retirement stress. Such old age events could come in the form of physiological (medical) complications like the loss of energy, vulnerability to diseases due to wear and tear of the body over the years, and the fact that most non-communicable diseases like cancer, diabetes, high-blood pressure etc., manifest themselves at this critical period. Of course, none of these changes begins suddenly at old age; gradual decline in some kind of functioning starts earlier. However, it is during old age that these changes become more apparent. Also, along with the multiplicity of health problems of old age, physiological disturbances are usually chronic and are more difficult to detect. This is due to the fact that symptoms may not have the same characteristics as that of the same disease in a younger person.

Politically and economically, in other words, in terms of its political economy, retirement stress could be caused by inability of workers to obtain their gratuity on time and the hiccups experienced in the payment of pension benefits, as complained by many retirees from both public and private sectors of the economy. The experience is almost universal, the only exemption being perhaps the oil industry and some major organisations in the manufacturing sector. Other sources of stress include waiting endlessly for hours or days to be paid, while in some cases most go home dejected without receiving their pension, others end up carving an almost permanent niche at the payment centres. Also the erroneous assumption that the traditional, extended family, informal welfare institution is a substitute for a well-articulated social security for the aged and retired needs to be re-thought.

Prolonged stress is believed to weaken the immune system, leading to susceptibility to diseases. Inadequate social support and retirement policies could hasten the triggering of stress reactions in the elderly and retired, and invariably complicate most of their physiological changes. It is therefore obvious that the aged and retired would experience much more difficulty in coping with stress and diseases, coming from a more disadvantaged position.

Problems of Retirees in Nigeria

It suffices to note again that retirement in Nigeria is no longer a stage to which people look forward. Gone are the days when retirees, especially those from the public services were assured of regular pensions. Today, they live from hand to mouth and more especially, their days on earth appear numbered. Pension scheme meant to provide succour to retirees do not seem to be working, and retirees from the public sector know better the negative effect of labouring for the fatherland. From different sectors, they have gory tales to tell. A case in point is the tragic state of retirees of the Nigerian Railway Cooperation who were owed their pensions for twenty-four months (*The Guardian* Nigeria, 2004). Several of the military retirees were reported to have turned the streets of Abuja and Lagos into homes begging for survival following the failure of relevant authorities to pay their pensions. The worst scenario is that of the retired primary school teachers.

This class of pensioners according to reports have not been paid for decades and their case is worsened by the fact that they do not know which tier of government to turn to for their stipends. The literature is rife with the woes that retirees go through in Nigeria, both in the public and private sectors (*The Guardian* Nigeria, 2000, 2003, 2004). For most civil servants and top directors, retirement may mean relocating from government quarters to a private residence, which is usually made worse if the retiree is unable to afford an alternative residence or to access funds from financial institutions. Coupled with the poor financial status of the retiree and the fact that there is no organised package on health care, retirement is far from satisfying for many. Retirement is satisfying for most people if they have a decent income, enjoy good health and were not forced to retire (Foner and Schward 1981). Mein (1998) also observed that health and income were frequently mentioned as sources of stress and depression among retirees, especially among those from lower civil service grades, while Benjamin, Idler, Leventhal & Leventhal (2000) in another study assert that health and income put together lead to a more successful retirement. The following lamentation of Godson, a retired captain would probably speak the mind of millions of retirees:

> Not many people know what retirees go through in this country. On a personal experience, I retired as a Captain due to ill health. For my poor condition, I had hoped to collect my benefit soonest so that I can give myself a good treatment. At the pension directorate in Lagos, I met a brick wall, no one was ready to assist. Besides being tossed about for days and weeks, my file was declared missing. I was told to start afresh.

In an attempt at interrogating the architecture for the management of retirement factors and pensions in Nigeria, perhaps another example could drive this point home more strongly:

'50 Retired Teachers die while waiting for pension':

> They are honourable senior citizens, notwithstanding how badly emaciated some of them appeared, who had put in their entire productive years in the service of their fatherland. But what a price to pay, now at the twilight of their own lives, when they need all the help they can get, the country which they had served so conscientiously had turned its back on them. They are subjected to deprivation, hardship and death. The chairman of Retired Teachers' Association for example, claimed that in the last 6 months, 50 of their members had died, due to inability to get their entitlement. He also reported that one of them, a treasurer of the association, died recently, because he could not get 50,000 Naira, needed for medical treatment whereas the government owed him over 150,000 Naira unpaid pension arrears. They therefore demanded, among other things, for upward review and prompt payment of their pension arrears and most importantly, for a welfare package like free medical care in government hospitals.

They also claimed that a governor in one of the Eastern states in Nigeria was unfair in a statement credited to him that 'our children should take care of us'.

They went further to state that while it is the duty of their children to take care of them, the government should not claim ignorance of the fact that most of their children cannot find jobs and are still liabilities for parents (*The Guardian* Nigeria, 2004).

Many African governments, including Nigeria's, certainly find it convenient to assume that the extended family in Africa continues to adequately meet all the needs of its members even in retirement. This assumption may be convenient for government to make since it appears to provide a basis for a minimal role for the state in ensuring old age and retirement care. The extended family that is presumed to be taking adequate care of the elderly is not living up to its expectations. The contributory factors include: the serious problem of economic survival faced by the young, the presumed caregivers in the context of prolonged economic crisis and depression; the span and speed of social change associated mainly with urbanisation, industrialisation and exposure to foreign ideas, and the value crisis now prevalent in most African countries (Akeredolu-Ale 2001).

This then paints a clear picture of what retirees in most of the developing world go through every day due to inadequate or poorly managed retirement benefits and policies. When compared with their counterparts in the developed world, they are certainly having a rough deal. This is a bad signal for the retirees as well as millions of younger Nigerians who see in what is happening a frightening reflection of their own future.

Retirement Policy and Retirement Management

Until the mid 1980s, there were no widespread instances of retirement of old people from work in Nigeria; rather, they continued to work until they were compelled to leave due to ill health. However, it was during the Buhari regime of the mid 1980s that the retirement rule became very effective in the Nigerian public and private sectors. During this period, many workers who were above the official retirement age of sixty were compelled to retire and since then, retirement has become a planned phase and programmed aspect of employment in Nigeria. Today, the retirement age in Nigeria is sixty years or thirty-five years in service, while for university lecturers and judges it is sixty-five years and fifty-five to sixty years for the private sector. A person is qualified for a gratuity when he or she has put in five years of service while eligibility for a pension is ten years of service. The public sector, prior to the recent pension reform in 2004 in Nigeria, operated a non-contributory pension scheme, (pay-as-you-go scheme), while that of the private sector is contributory. Pension benefits in Nigeria are reviewed from time to time in order to meet with the social and economic changes in the country.

On the situation in the Africa region, the ILO assessed as 'weak' the coverage and effectiveness of existing social protection schemes relating to the contingencies of retirement, invalidity and death. It concluded that 'many African schemes have failed to provide effective social protection, even for the small minority of the population that they cover' (ILO 2000). North Africa has the oldest and most comprehensive schemes, with pension schemes based on social insurance principles operating in Algeria, Egypt, Libya, Morocco and Tunisia since the 1950s. In Francophone sub-Saharan African countries, priority has been given to employment injury schemes while many of the countries have similar schemes with pension provisions based on social insurance principles which guarantee a defined benefit determined by reference to length of service and average earnings. In Anglophone Africa, the emphasis has been placed on employment injury schemes, while the development of social insurance schemes has been much slower than in Francophone countries. Pension schemes have been restricted in most cases to permanent public servants, though national provident funds have been provided in some cases to cover non-pensionable public servants and employees of big firms in the organised private sector (ILO 2000).

The fact that the Nigerian government is not living up to expectations as regards pension and retirement is very obvious. Nothing could be more horrifying for the retired than to be owed money when other sources of income are closed. Solanke (2004) observed that government has a problem of funds. They do not fund as and when due, and when it is time to pay, they find it difficult to pay. For some, very few parastatals are trying to put money aside for pensions, it is either the trustee who does not manage the funds properly or the funds are lost in the process of management, or worst still, such funds are stolen out-right. And when this happens, the pensioners are subjected to untold hardship. Solanke concluded that the major problem bedevilling pension funds in Nigeria is outright corruption. Other problems associated with government pensions include arbitrary and sporadic retirement and retrenchment of 'under-aged' officers, thus expanding the population of young pensioners, the over-centralization of pension administration, inefficient record keeping, and the lethargic attitude of government employees which causes delays in effecting payments. Most importantly, there is the dishonesty and the phenomenon of ghost pensioners. Pension problems in Nigeria are also bedevilled by the lack of seriousness in addressing the problem by successive governments, money trapped in distressed banks and bureaucratic bottlenecks experienced by pensioners in a bid to access their pension. *The Guardian*, Nigeria (2004) observed that the pension crisis arose largely because the public service ballooned without control, under the belief that government money was inexhaustible. The situation of unpaid and irregular pensions clearly encouraged indolence, corruption, divided loyalty and inefficiency in the system. Such irregularities and deformities also have a tendency to discourage originality, creative hard work and patriotism. All these necessitated the cry for pension reform in Nigeria.

In the past, Nigeria initiated reforms with the setting up of committees. First was the Ajibola-led committee in 2002 which was mandated to harmonise the public-private sectors' pensions, while the privatisation agency in the country also set up a steering committee on the pension reforms with certain objectives. There was also an insurance industry committee on pensions set up to provide technical advice to the government on pension reform. The other was the Fola Adeola-led committee charged with the responsibility of pension reform in the country. The common denominator in all the committees' recommendations and resolutions was a call for reform based on the unanimous conclusion that the public sector, unfounded, pay-as-you-go defined benefit pension system has failed woefully. This led to President Obasanjo's call in his May Day speech for a contributory public sector pension scheme. The latest effort by the Federal government to address the issue is now generating a lot of controversy. The controversial pension reform bill sought to merge the separate private and public sector pension schemes into one, scrapping every other system in the country including the Nigerian Social Insurance Trust Fund (NSITF), among other things. One criticism is that the bill will not solve the existing problem in the public sector, but will rather infect the private sector with the same virus that rendered the public sector scheme unmanageable. However, the report of the Senate ad-hoc committee, after several deliberations, suggested the separation of the public sector contributory pension scheme from the private sector. In addition, the Nigerian Social Insurance Trust Fund (NSITF) was also retained despite the government's proposal that it should be scrapped. To ensure that operators and administrators do not abuse the scheme, the committee endorsed the idea of a regulatory body to be called the National Pension Commission (*The Guardian*, 16 February 2004).

The Pension Reform Bill was finally passed on the first of July 2004, two hundred and seventy- four days after it was sent to the National Assembly. President Obasanjo reiterated the fact that the bill was set to eliminate the embarrassing situation where workers give their best in productivity, and receive no pension. The Act, which harmonises public and private sector pensions, has the following as its highpoints:

- Any organisation that has more than five staff is duty bound to run a pension scheme;

- The Act preserves the existing private sector scheme, but lays down a framework within which they must operate to protect the welfare and rights of the beneficiaries;

- Although the bill repealed the Nigerian Social Insurance Trust Fund (NSITF) Act, the committee, after considering stakeholders' views, came to the conclusion that the NSITF be retained as a platform for delivering social security services to Nigerians. This is in consonance with the ILO convention.

- That the concept of Pension Fund Administrator (PFA) and Pension Fund Custodian (PFC), as introduced by the bill, was found desirable since it contains the most refined techniques for effective checks and balances. The qualifications of custodians were modified to ensure that only the most credible finance institutions could provide the services;

- The Act makes it mandatory for pension fund administrators to open savings accounts for pension beneficiaries;

- Pension fund administrators may also invest in real estate to protect funds against inflation and other economic hazards;
- The Act provides opportunities for Nigerians covered to make additional contributions and receive additional benefits, and for those not covered to willingly join the scheme.

On the speculation of what will become of the viable contributory pension scheme on the ground, the Senate stated that government parastatals like the Nigerian National Petroleum Corporation (NNPC), the Central Bank of Nigeria (CBN), and the Bureau of Public enterprises (BPE), which had pension funds of one billion and above will be allowed to set up their own funds management system. Other government organisations with pension schemes not as successful as CBN, NNPC, and BPE, will not be allowed (*The Guardian,* 30 June 2004). Some amendments made by the Senate include: the adoption of the House of Representative version to replace section 9 (1) (a) (i) & (ii), which provided for a minimum of 7.5 percent employee contribution and 7.5 percent employer contributions. Another amendment was in section 4(2) where the withdrawal of a lump sum by the retirees was reduced from 50 percent to 25 percent.

With the signing of the Bill into law, the Pension Act of 1990 expired.

After the review of the nation's new pension law, the Nigerian Labour Union observed that the new Act excluded certain pensioners like the Nigerian Railway Cooperation, Primary Schools and the Military. An enraged labour leader, Adams Oshiomhole, remarked that there was nothing to celebrate about the Act, as far as those pensioners who die daily in the queues waiting to collect pensions are not provided for. He lamented the fact that it was in response to their plight that the pension reform came up, and pitiably, there was no mention of their plight. Labour also lamented that the new Act put the pensioners at a disadvantage and many of them at risk of losing their savings to failed fund administrators. It also queried the measures put in place to guarantee savings of the pensioners in case of default by the pension administrator (*The Guardian,* 16 July 2004).

Organised labour also disagreed with the provision regarding the contribution ratio between the employer and employee in both the private and public sectors, observing that the harmonised position of labour submitted to the National Assembly was for 12.5 percent contribution for the employer and 5.5 percent for the workers. Similarly, the Senior Staff Association of Nigerian Universities (SSANU) also frowned at the contributory ratio of 1:1 saying that it negates the 3:1 internationally accepted norms of contributory pension schemes. (*The Guardian,* 3 February 2005). However, the Senate, in a bid to amend the new Pension Bill, is currently asking that government contribute an extra 2 percent of the monthly wage bill to its workers to the Redemption Fund. This is to ensure that the 'living standards of the employee are reasonably brought in conformity with that of their counterparts who occupy the same position in future and also by harmonizing the earnings of a previously retired person to rank pari-passu with that of his counterparts who have just retired and is payable under the law' (*The Guardian*, 30 January 2005).

On the lingering issue of pension arrears, President Obasanjo noted that the issue will require the government to come up with viable strategy and policy that will assure those who are owed arrears of pension that they will be paid. He therefore apologised for the pain and deprivations caused because of irregular and unpaid payments.

Conclusion

In concluding this article, one thing is obvious – that we all must retire one day and that each of us will react differently to our retirement situation. Some will find it easy to accept, while others will find it really traumatic. Though our ability to choose a rosy retirement may be a mirage, it is still very important to plan for retirement to avoid the pain and depression that normally accompany unplanned retirement. In the face of rapidly disintegrating joint family structure and inefficient government policies, people walking into retirement are likely to turn greyer and lonelier by the day, the more so if they do not have financial security. Perhaps this paper may sound stern if it suggests that individuals should try to take personal responsibility for the retirement problem that afflicts them, and perceive pensions and gratuities as an additional resource. If the government is finding it difficult to pay the working employees, it is certain that they may find it almost impossible to make the case of the pensioners a priority, unless there is sincerity and empathy. Even the corporate giants may not be prepared to discuss the need of retired persons due to dwindling income and profit coupled with suffocating demands for higher pay as a result of crippling inflation. Of course, the plight of retired teachers, railway workers, military personnel and a host of other pathetic stories about pensioners should serve as red signals for the working class and a constant reminder that 'the only person who should be concerned about your retirement is you'.

On the new pension contribution scheme in Nigeria, I feel that there is a point to be made for the Nigerian Government to have a more human face by lightening the burden on the various institutions, both public and private, in terms of the percentage contribution to the scheme. The war against corruption by President Obasanjo's administration and the effort at sanitising the public service are a welcome development which hopefully will impact positively on the management of pensions, and hence the plight of retirees in Nigeria. Also for a happier retirement and old age status, government should think of providing free medical services for its retired citizens, as a thank you gift for serving the state diligently. This is also necessary because of the health complications of old age and thus, coming from a more disadvantaged position, retirees may experience more difficulty in coping with stress and disease.

On a lighter note, after retirement, since one is no more a slave to a fixed schedule, one can devote some time to introspection, to try and rediscover one's self and acquire new ideas or pursue unconventional hobbies and interests. Think of retirement as a new lifestyle not as the end of the road. Develop your sense of humour and laugh at difficult situations. Take your health as an item of the highest priority, take pride in who and what you are now, be enthusiastic about the present and optimistic about the future and take personal responsibility for your financial future. Since enthusiasm is caught and not taught, the secret of growing old gracefully is never to lose your enthusiasm in remaining active in life.

References

Akeredolu-Ale, E. O. and Aribiah, O., 2001, *Social Policy in Nigeria*, Monograph Series No. 2, Ibadan, Josywale Press.

Atchley, R. C., 1976, *The Sociology of Retirement*, New York, Wiley & Sons.

Benjamin, Y., Idler, E., Levental, H., and Levental, E., 2000, 'Positive Effect and Function as Influence on Self-Assessment of Health: Expanding Our View Beyond Illness and Disability', *Journal of Gerontology*, 55B (2), 107-116.

Dhar, J. L., 2004, *An Iinterview with Self: Simple Ways to Unravelling the Power Within*, New Delhi, Wisdom Tree.

Ester, C., 1979, *The Ageing Enterprise*, San Francisco, Jossey Press.

Foner, A. and Schwak, K., 1981, *Aging and Retirement*, Monterey, Brookes/Cole.

International Labour Organisation, (ILO), 2000, *Social Security, Pension*, Geneva, ILO.

Jungmenn, O., and Philimeon, 1999, 'Retirement Can Spark Depression', BBC Online.

Mein, G., Higgs, P., Ferre, J. and Standford, S. A., 1998, 'Paradigms of Retirement: the Importance of Aging in Whitehall Study', *Social Science Medicine*, 47 (4), 535-545.

Newgate, D., ed., 1996, *The Meaning of Age*, Chicago, University of Chicago Press.

Phillipson, C., 1982, *Capitalism and the Construction of Old Age*, London, SAGE.

Phillipson, C., 1998, *Reconstructing Old Age*, London, SAGE.

Powell, J. L., 1999, 'The Importance of a "Critical" Sociology of Old Age', Social Science Paper Pub. 3,1.

Powell, J. L., 2001, *Theories of Social Gerontology: The Case of Social Philosophies of Age*, Liverpool, Centre for Social Science, John Moore University.

Seaward, B. L., 1994, *Managing Stress: Principles & Strategies for Health and Well-Being*, London, Jones & Bartlett.

Selye, H., 1956, *The Stress of Life*, New York, McGraw Hill.

Solanke, D., 2004, 'Why You Must Start Planning for Retirement', *The Guardian*, Lagos, 27 March.

The Guardian, 2000, 'Lamentations of Pensioners Amid Government Palliative', 22 June.

The Guardian, 2003, 'The Pension Crisis', 2 October.

The Guardian, 2004, 'WHO's Ranking of Nigeria's Health System', 7 January.

The Guardian, 2004, '50 Retired Teachers Die Waiting for Pension', 29 January.

The Guardian, 2004, 'New Pension Law, A Boost to Economic Reform', 30 June.

The Guardian, 2004, 'Gray Areas of the Pension Act by Labour', 20 July.

The Guardian, 2005, 'Senate May Amend New Pension Bill', 30 January.

The Guardian, 2005, 'Our Plight by Lagos Pensioners - as University Senior Workers Fault New Pension Scheme', 3 February.

14

Prefinancement communautaire des soins de santé pour un meilleur accès des populations rurales aux services de santé de base:
une estimation du consentement à pré-payer des ménages au centre du Cameroun

Joachim Nyemeck Binam et Valère Nkelzok

Dans une procédure d'analyse à deux étapes, les tests statistiques nous permettront d'apprécier le degré de corrélation entre les différentes valeurs du CAP et certaines variables socioéconomiques et culturelles prises individuellement.

Les résultats de cette étude enfin nous donneront des indications sur le taux de cotisation individuelle des membres dans une perspective de la mise sur pied d'un système de préfinancement des soins de santé de type mutualiste en milieu rural. Par ailleurs, l'identification des facteurs affectant la valeur du CAP les soins permettra de définir le profil des futurs mutualistes en vue d'aider les acteurs du développement local à mieux asseoir leurs stratégies de mise sur pied du système de préfinancement des soins de santé de base dans la localité d'étude. En estimant les capacités réelles des ménages ruraux au financement des soins, cette étude nous situera enfin sur les objectifs d'équité de la politique de contribution des ménages au financement des soins de santé.

Introduction

Le Cameroun a enregistré d'excellentes performances économiques qui se sont traduites par un taux de croissance annuel moyen de 7% au cours des deux premières décennies qui ont suivi son indépendance politique. Ces performances lui ont permis de se doter d'infrastructures sanitaires appréciables. A titre d'illustration, le Cameroun disposait de 1 031 établissements sanitaires dont 1 Centre hospitalier universitaire (CHU), 2 hôpitaux généraux de référence (Hôpital général), 3 hôpitaux centraux, 8 hôpitaux provinciaux, 38 hôpitaux départementaux, 132 hôpitaux de district et 842 centres de santé (Republic of Cameroon 2000), avec un personnel médical d'environ 14 292 employés (Ministry of Health 1997). Toutefois, les difficultés économiques devenues insoutenables depuis le début des années 80, ont nécessité des réformes de politiques sous l'impulsion de la Banque mondiale et du Fonds monétaire international. Ces mesures ont imposé, entre autres, le désengagement de l'État et la réduction des dépenses publiques, notamment dans le secteur sanitaire, faisant passer les dépenses du secteur sanitaire de 35 817 millions F CFA en 1986/87 à 18 167 millions F CFA en 1995/96, soit une baisse globale de 49% en huit ans.

Contrairement aux prédictions théoriques, la dévaluation du Franc CFA intervenue en 1994 n'a pas provoqué un recul de la pauvreté au Cameroun en général et dans les zones rurales en particulier (Republic of Cameroon 2000). On estime que l'incidence, l'intensité et la gravité de la pauvreté ont augmenté au Cameroun au cours de la dernière décennie; ce qui signifie que non seulement la pauvreté s'est généralisée, mais elle est également plus profonde et plus grave. La pauvreté est considérable dans toutes les régions rurales. En 2001, 50,5% des Camerounais sont affectés par la pauvreté, soit environ 6 217 058 millions d'individus.

En milieu rural, la pauvreté est devenue plus intense avec un taux de paupérisation de 56,7% en 2001. Les nombreuses mesures d'ajustement entreprises par le gouvernement, même-si elles n'étaient toujours pas directement ciblées sur les populations rurales, ont toutefois eu des effets délétères sur leur bien-être. À titre d'exemple, la diminution du niveau de rémunération des employés du secteur public et privé formel a eu pour conséquence la baisse du niveau de demande des produits alimentaires offerts par les populations rurales d'une part, et, d'autre part, la baisse du niveau de transferts familiaux vers les populations rurales.

L'état de santé occupe une place de choix parmi les indicateurs de bien-être, dans le processus de développement économique de tout pays. La santé peut être appréciée non seulement en tant qu'indicateur de développement économique mais aussi comme forme de capital humain. Comme indicateur de développement économique, la santé permet d'apprécier le succès ou l'échec d'un pays dans sa tentative de procurer à sa population des moyens vitaux. En tant que forme de capital humain, c'est un élément important du développement futur d'un pays. La santé est aussi un indicateur de pauvreté humaine.

Au Cameroun le bien être des ménages pauvres et vulnérables repose essentiellement sur un bon état de santé. La faible capacité des ménages à payer les soins de santé les amène à recourir à des solutions diverses. Il est courant de s'abstenir de tout traitement ou de pratiquer l'automédication avec des remèdes traditionnels ou de recourir aux guérisseurs traditionnels.

Suite à l'initiative de Bamako en 1987 et devant les difficultés budgétaires, l'État a mis en place un nouveau système de santé basé sur le cofinancement et la cogestion des services de santé par les bénéficiaires de la communauté. En principe, cette politique dite de recouvrement des coûts ne pose pas de problème si elle est accompagnée d'une amélioration de la qualité de ces services (Shepard 1992, Diop 1994, Schneider *et al.*, 2000, Griffin 1998). Toutefois, cette politique de recouvrement de coût n'est pas toujours de nature à faciliter l'accessibilité aux services de santé de base des populations rurales généralement vulnérables au Cameroun.

D'après le rapport 2002 sur les conditions de vie et profil de pauvreté au Cameroun, le nombre de visites dans les centres de santé a considérablement diminué. Dans l'ensemble, parmi le nombre de personnes ayant déclaré avoir été malades en 2001, moins de 48,7% ont été capables de s'offrir des soins médicaux dans un centre de santé, pendant que parmi les populations les plus vulnérables, seules 36,1% ont pu se rendre à un centre moderne de santé. En ce qui concerne les dépenses en soins de santé proprement dits, la somme dépensée par an par personne s'élève à 13 000 F CFA, soit 5 600 F CFA par personne chez les ménages pauvres contre 37 000 F CFA chez les autres (DSCN 2002).

Il apparaît dès lors clair que le paiement individuel direct, comme forme d'expression de « recouvrement des coûts », présente plusieurs inconvénients:

- il ne permet pas le partage des risques entre malades et bien-portants;
- il bute très rapidement sur la capacité des individus à payer et, face à des événements de santé très coûteux, ne permet de récupérer qu'une partie des coûts;
- il maintient souvent des individus dans une gestion au coup par coup des événements de santé et n'incite pas à l'anticipation des dépenses;
- les différentes solidarités, horizontales entre malades et bien-portants et verticales entre groupes sociaux, sont difficiles à prendre en compte.

Le caractère aléatoire de la maladie, la lourde charge que représentent pour les individus les frais inhérents à une hospitalisation ou à une maladie grave et, plus largement, l'origine sociale et économique des grands problèmes de santé militent en faveur d'une couverture collective des principales dépenses de santé surtout dans nos sociétés traditionnelles.

Il est grandement reconnu que les systèmes communautaires de partage de risque tel que le pré-financement pour utilisation future des services de santé sont en mesure non seulement, d'améliorer l'équité dans l'accès des populations rurales aux soins de santé de qualité, mais, en mesure également d'inciter les pourvoyeurs de ces soins, d'améliorer la qualité et l'efficacité des services offerts ainsi que l'implication des populations locales dans leur mise en œuvre et leur gestion (Atim 1999, Schneider *et al.* 2000). À cet effet, les systèmes de préfinancement de type mutualistes, avec une gestion décentralisée, peuvent constituer une voie originale, alternative et à la portée de nos communautés rurales.

En théorie lorsque l'on est en face de plusieurs catégories de demandeurs d'un bien ou service, la question d'équité nécessite de procéder à une segmentation du marché; de sorte que ceux qui ne sont pas capables de payer puissent payer le montant maximum qu'ils consentent payer. Il est donc important de connaître les montants que les populations rurales, généralement moins nanties, sont capables de payer et de comprendre les facteurs qui expliquent ces velléités à payer.

Comment peut-on résoudre le sempiternelle problème de disparité dans l'accessibilité aux soins de santé de base des populations rurales au Cameroun ? Quelle stratégie mettre sur pied afin de leur permettre de recourir facilement aux services de santé modernes en cas de maladie ? Quelles peuvent être leurs contributions pour la réussite d'une telle stratégie ? C'est à ces différentes préoccupations que ce projet de recherche tente à apporter quelques éléments de réponses.

Cette étude a donc pour objectif d'apprécier les possibilités réelles de participation des ménages ruraux au préfinancement collectif des soins de santé. De façon spécifique, il s'agit d'estimer, d'une part, la disposition à pré-payer des ménages et, d'autre part, à identifier les facteurs qui l'influencent.

Revue de la littérature

Elle porte essentiellement sur les systèmes de préfinancement de santé volontaires, les typologies généralement rencontrées en Afrique, le consentement à payer et les déterminants du consentement à payer.

Les systèmes de préfinancement de santé volontaires et à but non lucratifs

La dernière décennie a fait l'objet d'un intérêt croissant dans l'introduction et l'expansion des systèmes de solidarité basés sur le financement des soins de santé en Afrique (Abel-Smith 1986, World Bank 1987, 1993, Vogel 1990a, b, Shepard *et al.* 1992, WHO 1993, Ahrin 1995, Schneider *et al.* 2000). Les raisons souvent invoquées dans la promotion de ces systèmes est leur potentiel comme source de revenus stables et additionnels au financement des structures de santé, leur capacité à réduire les barrières financières à l'utilisation des services de santé ainsi que leur effet redistributif (Schneider *et al.* 2000).

Il est apparu évident que l'engouement d'un regain d'intérêt national dans la promotion des systèmes traditionnels de financement des soins de santé en Afrique au sud du Sahara n'est ni une forme équitable, ni efficace comme option de politique de financement en ce sens que dans la majorité des cas, seuls les employés du secteur formel sont pris en compte dans ce genre de système. Vogel (1990b) a parcouru les systèmes de financement des soins de santé dans 23 pays en Afrique au sud du Sahara et a abouti à la conclusion que ces systèmes ne promouvaient pas une grande équité dans l'accès aux soins de santé par les pauvres. Gruat a confirmé ce résultat en analysant l'allure et les problèmes de système de sécurité sociale en Afrique (Gruat 1990).

Il existe une littérature abondante sur les systèmes volontaires et à but non lucratifs de financement des soins de santé ces dernières années, attestant par là même, l'intérêt des chercheurs et du politique dans ce domaine. Cet intérêt a été conforté en reconnaissant en partie que les frais de santé affectent négativement le but important de la politique de santé d'équité et de plus grande accessibilité des pauvres aux services de santé (Gilson 1988, De Bethume *et al.*1989; Waddington and Enyimayew 1989, Abel-Smith 1993, Shaw and Griffin1995, Criel 1998, Schneider *et al.* 2000).

De Ferranti (1985) a examiné la faisabilité du recouvrement des coûts des soins de services de santé par les usagers en Afrique. Son étude a fait ressortir de nouvelles possibilités de politiques de financement des soins de santé qui sont devenues assez courantes aujourd'hui dans l'environnement sanitaire africain, spécialement, en ce qui concerne les frais de santé. De Ferranti (1985) a réalisé que la contribution des usagers aux coûts de santé pourrait prendre non seulement la forme de recouvrement direct au point de la réception des soins amis, également, la forme d'un préfinancement pour une utilisation future des services de santé. La dernière option selon lui a un potentiel assez élevé de recouvrement en ce sens que les charges de couvertures sont relativement moindres. Une croissance rapide et une participation entière de la communauté pourraient donc être source de revenus substantiels.

Dans ce même ordre d'idée, Carrin (1987) a examiné l'opportunité de préfinancement des systèmes communautaires de financement des soins de santé pour l'Afrique subsaharienne, au travers desquels les communautés en milieu rural et urbain contribuent au financement de leurs soins de santé soit directement dans les centres de santé, soit indirectement. Néanmoins, il insiste sur le fait que le financement communautaire entraîne une certaine implication de la population dans l'organisation du système. Il a mis en exergue deux avantages tant pour les systèmes de financement décentralisés que communautaires dans ce sens que le contrôle local des revenus aurait un impact positif sur l'incitation du personnel de santé dans la collecte des revenus tandis que, la conservation interne de ces revenus aurait pour conséquence de stimuler le personnel de santé à l'implication dans le système de financement. Le second avantage était que le système répondrait bien aux préférences et demandes des populations locales de sorte qu'ils acceptent en retour les mesures de recouvrement de coûts.

Kutzin et Barnum quant à eux, ont examiné les effets des programmes de financement des soins de santé sur les services de santé des pays en développement à travers une revue des principales caractéristiques institutionnelles de quatre systèmes y compris le système de financement des services de santé communautaire de l'Hôpital de Bwamanda en RDC (ex-Zaïre) et l'évaluation de leur impact tant sur l'équité que sur l'efficacité du secteur de santé (Kutzin and Barnum 1992). Les résultats de cette analyse ont montré que le système de financement de Bwamanda a atteint ses objectifs dans l'augmentation de la mobilisation des ressources des services de santé dans cette région mais, par contre, la principale faiblesse de cette approche était qu'elle a entraîné un accès inéquitable aux soins de santé entre les membres et les non-membres du système. Bien plus, il est apparu des possibilités de hasard moral en ce sens que les membres du système avaient tendance à une surconsommation des services offerts dans la mesure où le coût inhérent à un tel comportement était assez moindre pour eux comparativement à celui que pourrait supporter les non-membres. Il est également apparu la possibilité que le risque de sélection adverse existe: c'est à dire, la tendance pour les personnes malades de s'intéresser beaucoup plus au système comparativement aux personnes bien portantes.

Une étude récente de Creese et Bennett va plus loin sur la question de savoir dans quelles mesures les systèmes de préfinancement en milieu rural tels que discuté par Atim (1999) sont réellement en mesure de contribuer à l'accroissement des revenus des structures de santé ou à l'augmentation de l'équité dans l'accessibilité aux soins de santé; deux des principales raisons qui militent en faveur de la promotion des systèmes de pré financement des soins de santé (Creese and Bennett 1997). Sur la base d'une enquête mondiale sur les systèmes de pré financement, ces auteurs aboutissent à la conclusion que les systèmes mis en place dans les pays à faible revenu ont généralement une couverture très limitée, un taux de recouvrement des coûts très faible et une assez faible habilité à protéger les pauvres. Cependant, les auteurs ont atténué ce pessimisme en mentionnant que plusieurs des systèmes étudiés ont été très mal conçus. Par conséquent, il était possible qu'avec une bonne organisation et une bonne prise en compte des expériences d'ailleurs, la plupart des problèmes identifiés pourraient être résolus.

Par ailleurs, des études menées par Shepard *et al.* (1992) puis, Shneider *et al.* (2000) sur le développement et l'implantation des systèmes de pré financement au Rwanda ont montré que les systèmes de pré financement des soins de santé apparaissent comme des outils viables dans l'augmentation de l'autonomie financière des structures de santé et dans l'amélioration de l'accessibilité aux services de santé de ces communautés.

Par contre les réseaux de solidarité traditionnels tel que celui étudié au Cameroun par Atim (1999) n'a pas eu un intérêt similaire dans le contexte du débat sur le financement des soins de santé.

Typologies de systèmes de financement de santé volontaires et à but non lucratif

Il existe en Afrique, au moins cinq types de systèmes de financement des services de santé volontaires à but non lucratif tels qu'ils apparaissent dans la littérature et les observations. Le premier groupe est constitué des réseaux traditionnels sociaux de solidarité basés sur les liens tribaux (clan ou ethnie) du groupe cible, mais ces réseaux sont généralement basés en milieu urbain. Tel est le cas au Cameroun comme le mentionne Atim (1999). Le deuxième groupe se compose de mouvements ou association mutualistes de santé très inclusifs qui sont basés dans les communautés rurales ou urbaines, les entreprises, les syndicats, les associations professionnelles, etc., et qui ne sont pas restreintes aux critères ethniques ou autres facteurs similaires. Le troisième groupe forme un modèle de financement communautaire simplifié ou à faible participation, généralement organisé par les pourvoyeurs de soins de santé eux-mêmes dans un contexte de recouvrement de coûts et dans lequel, l'implication des membres dans la gestion du système est faible voire inexistante. Le quatrième groupe est un modèle de financement communautaire complexe ou à grande participation dans lequel la communauté participe à la gestion, tout au moins, au premier niveau des soins (centre de santé), habituellement, en partenariat avec le pourvoyeur des soins de santé. Le cinquième groupe est constitué de « sociétés d'aide médicale ». Ce sont en pratique les formes les plus avancées et développées des mouvements mutualistes, organisés à grande échelle en terme de membres et qui nécessitent un staff professionnel et certaines techniques de gestion empruntées aux compagnies commerciales d'assurance. Ces systèmes sont généralement rencontrés au Zimbabwe et en Afrique du Sud (Atim 1998).

Consentement à payer (CAP)

Il s'agit ici des montants que les personnes interrogées consentiraient à pré-payer dans le cas de la création probable d'une mutuelle de santé.

Dans la littérature, cette technique d'évaluation du consentement à payer tire son fondement dans la méthode d'évaluation contingente (CVM). Le principe fondamental de cette méthode est que les préférences des individus doivent servir de base à l'évaluation des gains et des pertes des biens et services qui n'ont pas de marché. Il revient alors aux individus d'exprimer leurs préférences à travers le concept de consentement à payer. Du fait qu'elle repose sur l'auto rapport, les économistes en particulier restent sceptiques à propos de la valeur de cette méthode, dans la mesure où les intentions déclarées ne correspondent pas souvent au comportement des individus. De plus, du fait de sa nature hypothétique, plusieurs biais peuvent survenir au cours de l'enquête (Mitchell and Carson 1989, Neill *et al.* 1994, Whittington 1998, Frykblom 1998, Bateman and Willis 1999, Smith 2001) entre autre:

> le biais stratégique qui survient lorsque le répondant pense aux conséquences ultérieures de l'enquête. Alors, il adopte un comportement stratégique et ne révèle pas sa vraie préférence: on dit qu'il joue au « passager clandestin ». Certains biais sont liés au manque d'information au niveau du répondant, ces biais potentiels sont appelés biais de l'information, dans cette catégorie on distingue en général, le biais du point de départ, la valeur proposée par l'enquêteur peut servir de point de repère au répondant.

Dans la littérature, l'on a assisté à un foisonnement de la recherche sur la méthode d'analyse contingente, et notamment plusieurs de ces études ont été faites dans le secteur de l'environnement. Les études dans le domaine de la santé sont à notre connaissance, très rares. Munasinghe (1996) et Smith (2001) fournissent plusieurs exemples de la méthode d'évaluation contingente pour évaluer la qualité des ressources environnementales dans les pays en voie de développement. Whittington *et al.* (1990) ont utilisé cette méthode pour évaluer la contribution financière des populations dans la fourniture de l'eau potable dans les pays en voie de développement et plus spécifiquement au Sud de Haïti.

En Afrique subsaharienne, Wasikama (1998) a utilisé cette méthode pour évaluer la contribution financière de la communauté internationale pour la préservation de la forêt de Taï en Côte d'Ivoire. Houdégbé (1999) a utilisé cette méthode pour évaluer le coût économique de la dégradation des ressources naturelles au Bénin et la valeur monétaire des aires protégées dans la zone cynégétique de la Djona au Bénin respectivement. De plus, Treiman (1993) cité par Pokou (1998) a utilisé cette méthode pour estimer également les aires protégées de la Pendjari. Par ailleurs, cet instrument a également été utilisé dans divers domaines socio-économiques outre qu'environnementaux: c'est le cas des travaux de N'guessan (1997) et Pokou (1998) où il a servi à estimer respectivement la valeur du moustiquaire imprégné dans les régions de Memni et Montézo en Côte d'Ivoire; et la contribution financière des populations pastorales dans la lutte contre la trypanosomiase animale dans le Nord de la Côte d'Ivoire.

Les déterminants du consentement à payer

Dans cette littérature, certains auteurs ont conclu que le consentement à payer était influencé par des caractéristiques économiques, socio-démographiques et les caractéristiques du bien en question (Whittington *et al.* 1990, Coffie 1997, Flores and Richard 1997, Pokou 1998, Houdégbé 1998, Bloom and Shenglan 1999, Atim 1999, Criel *et al.* 1999).

Tshinko *et al.* (1995) dans une évaluation ex-post, regroupent ces facteurs en trois catégories distinctes à savoir: les facteurs de prédisposition, les facteurs facilitateurs et les facteurs de renforcement.

Outre les variables socio-démographiques telles que l'âge, le niveau d'éducation, le genre, la religion, la taille du ménage, les facteurs de prédisposition découlent généralement de l'environnement socioculturel des répondants. Il s'agit généralement de la tradition d'utilisation des services de santé par les répondants, de la tradition locale d'entraide (expérience associative) et l'ouverture d'esprit des répondants.

Les facteurs facilitateurs sont essentiellement issus des conditions économiques des répondants: dans ce cas, le niveau de revenu des ménages est souvent considéré comme un indicateur pertinent de ce facteur. Et, enfin, les facteurs de renforcement synthétisent les caractéristiques propres au bien proposé: il s'agit souvent dans ce cas de l'expérience sanitaire vécu par le répondant (accueil, disponibilité des médicaments, qualité du praticien, etc.).

De cette revue de littérature, il apparaît que non seulement très peu d'études sur l'analyse du Consentement à Payer ont été entreprises dans le secteur de la santé en général et au Cameroun en particulier, la plupart d'entre elles entreprises dans le domaine du pré financement des soins de santé sont des études ex-post. Aucune étude à notre connaissance n'a abordé le problème dans le sens de la disposition des ménages à payer pour participer à un système de préfinancement des soins de santé et les facteurs qui la détermine. Une étude de cette nature, qui vise à évaluer le consentement à payer des populations surtout pauvres, en vue de favoriser l'émergence des systèmes de préfinancement communautaires des soins de santé est donc justifiée tant sur le plan scientifique que social.

Méthode d'analyse

Échantillonnage et données de l'étude

Les données relatives à cette étude proviendront principalement de l'enquête de base effectuée par le Mouvement d'Action d'Aide aux Initiatives locales de Développement (MAILD) dans le cadre du projet: « *Accessibilité des populations vulnérables aux soins de santé de qualité: quelles opportunités pour la création des systèmes de préfinancement des soins de santé de type mutualiste au centre Cameroun ?* »

Cette enquête a été conduite sur la base d'un échantillon aléatoire de 1500 ménages ruraux. La procédure d'échantillonnage suivante a été utilisée: il a été procédé dans un premier temps à l'identification des services de santé dans différentes localité rurales de la Province du Centre, après quoi, différents villages ont été choisi de façon raisonnée. À l'intérieur de chaque village, il a été procédé une identification des principaux groupements ruraux d'action communautaire ainsi que la liste des membres adhérents. Un tirage aléatoire a donc été opéré en vue de constituer un échantillon de 1500 ménages.

Le questionnaire et le guide d'entretien ont constitué les principaux outils de collecte des données sur:

- les caractéristiques socio-démographiques et culturelles telles que l'âge, le genre, le statut matrimonial, le niveau d'éducation, la taille du ménage, le nombre d'individus actifs dans le ménage, le nombre d'enfants de moins de 15 ans dans le ménage, la tradition d'utilisation des services de santé modernes;
- les caractéristiques socio-économiques telles que l'appartenance à un groupement d'intérêt économique comme proxy du capital social, le niveau de revenu des ménages;
- la valeur du consentement à payer, c'est-à-dire, les montants que les individus consentiraient à pré-payer en vue d'être membre d'un système de préfinancement pour une consommation future d'une certaine catégorie de soins de santé.

L'évaluation de la disposition à payer

La contribution des ménages au financement des soins de santé soulève le problème de la fourniture et de la tarification des biens et services publics tel que discuté par Kahneman and Knetsch (1992), Diamond (1994), Whittington (1998), Kriström (1993), Li and Fredman (1994), Jordan (1994), Li and Fredman (1994), Frykblom (1997), Brox *et al.* (2003).

Deux approches théoriques principales sont disponibles pour l'estimation fiable des velléités à payer des ménages. La première, l'approche indirecte, se sert des informations sur l'utilisation des biens ou services pour évaluer les réponses des consommateurs. Parmi ces méthodes, on note les modèles de coût de transport (travel cost), la méthode du prix hédonique (hedonic property value). La seconde, l'approche directe, consiste simplement à demander aux individus combien ils sont prêts à payer pour l'utilisation d'un bien ou l'amélioration d'un service. Cette méthode est appelée la méthode de l'analyse contingente. L'analyse contingente cherche à construire des marchés hypothétiques pour les biens publics. C'est une méthode d'enquête originairement utilisée pour attribuer des valeurs monétaires aux biens et services pour lesquels les prix de marché n'existent pas ou ne reflètent pas leur valeur sociale réelle.

Cette approche cherche donc à construire des marchés hypothétiques pour les biens en vue de permettre l'estimation de la demande de ces biens. Cette méthode qui a été appliquée à divers domaines s'est révélée appropriée pour évaluer les ressources non marchandes et les biens publics. Elle sera utilisée pour élucider la velléité à payer pour l'accès aux soins de santé.

L'un des problèmes majeurs liés à la technique de l'évaluation contingente est que pour certaines raisons, les personnes enquêtées ne répondent pas correctement aux questions et donc ne fournissent pas leurs vraies velléités à payer. Les deux variantes les plus utilisées dans l'analyse contingente sont la méthode de questionnaire ouvert et la méthode de questionnaire fermé ou la technique à choix dichotomique (bidding-game). Dans le questionnaire ouvert, il est demandé au répondant d'exprimer sa volonté maximale à payer. Par exemple, « quel est le montant maximum que vous serez prêts à payer pour participer à un système de préfinancement des soins de santé ? ». Le deuxième type de questions consiste à partir d'un montant de départ et de demander au répondant s'il est prêt à payer ce montant ou non (« bidding game »). Par exemple, « seriez-vous disposé à payer x Franc CFA pour participer à un système de préfinancement des soins de santé? ».

Pour les besoins de notre étude, nous nous servirons de la technique à choix dichotomique dans la mesure où elle répond mieux aux stratégie de marchandage pratiquées dans nos marchés locaux.

Les déterminants de la disposition à payer

Plusieurs techniques peuvent être utilisées pour identifier les déterminants du consentement à préfinancer les soins des ménages à savoir:

- les techniques économétriques où la valeur du CAP à payer est exprimée comme fonction d'un certain nombre de variables socioéconomiques et culturelles;
- les techniques statistiques où l'on procède à des mesures de corrélation entre la valeur du CAP et un certain nombre de variables socioéconomiques et culturelles.

L'utilisation des techniques économétriques certes plus complexes, nous permet d'apprécier l'effet de ces différentes variables sur le CAP prises globalement alors que les techniques statistiques permettent d'apprécier cet effet des variables prises individuellement.

Pour des raisons de simplicité nous nous servirons uniquement des techniques statistiques où il sera procédé à l'aide des tableaux de contingence à des tests statistiques des différents effets des variables socioéconomiques et culturelles sur la valeur du CAP.

Résultats attendus

Cette étude qui a pour objectif d'évaluer et d'analyser le consentement à préfinancer les soins de santé par les populations rurales vise une triple ambition: d'abord, l'estimation des différentes valeurs du consentement à préfinancer les soins de santé servira comme base de cotisation individuelle dans une perspective de la mise sur pied d'un système de préfinancement des soins de santé de type mutualiste en milieu rural. Ensuite, les résultats de cette étude permettront aux décideurs d'apprécier le niveau de disparité dans l'accès aux soins de santé de base des populations rurales en mesurant l'écart entre les coûts pratiqués dans les services de santé et les aptitudes réelles des ménages à payer. Enfin, l'identification des facteurs affectant la valeur du consentement à préfinancer les soins permettra de définir le profil des futurs mutualistes en vue de permettre aux acteurs du développement local de mieux asseoir leurs stratégies de mise sur pied du système de préfinancement des soins de santé de base dans la localité d'étude.

Références

Abel-Smith, B., 1986, 'Health Insurance in Developing Countries: Lessons from Experience', *Health Policy and Planning* 7(3), pp. 215-226.

Abel-Smith, B., 1993, 'Financing Health Services in Developing Countries: The Options', *NU Nytt om U-landshälsard* 2, 93, vol. 7.

Ahrin, D.C., 1995, 'Health Insurance in Rural Africa', *The Lancet* 345, pp. 44-45.

Atim, C., 1998, *The Contribution of Mutual Health Organisations to Financing, Delivery and Access to Health Care: Synthesis of Research in Nine West and Central African Countries.* Abt Assocs/PHR, Bethesda, MD.

Atim, C., 1999, 'Social Movements and Health Insurance: A Critical Evaluation of Voluntary, Non-Profit Insurance Schemes with Case Studies from Ghana and Cameroon', *Social Science and Medicine* 48, pp. 881-896.

Bloom, G., Shenglan, T., 1999, 'Rural Health Prepayment Schemes in China: Towards a More Active Role for Government', *Social Science and Medicine* 48, pp. 951-960.

Brox, J. A., Kumar, R. C. and Stollery, K. R., 2003, 'Estimating Willingness to Pay for Improved Water Quality in the Presence of Item Nonresponse Bias', *American Journal of Agricultural Economics* 85 (2), pp. 414-428.

Carrin, G., 1987, 'Community Financing of Drugs in Sub Saharan Africa', *International Journal of Health Planning and Management* 2, pp. 125-145.

Chabot, J., Boal, M. and Da Silva, A., 1991, 'National Community Health Insurance at Village Level: The Case of Guinea Bissau', *Health Policy and Planning* 6 (1), pp. 46-54.

Creese, A., Bennett, S., 1997, 'Rural Risk-Sharing Strategies in Health', Paper presented to an International Conference sponsored by the World Bank, *Innovations in Health Care Financing*, March 10-11, Washington D.C.

Criel, B., 1998, *District-based Health Insurance in sub-Saharan Africa*, Parts I and II: *Studies in Health Services Organization and Policy*, Antwerpen.

Criel, B., Van der Stuyft, P., Van Lerberghe, W., 1999, 'The Bwamanda Hospital Insurance Scheme: Effective for Whom? A Study of its Impact on Hospital Utilization Patterns', *Social Science and Medicine* 48, pp. 897-911.

De Bethume, X., Alfani, S. and Lahaye, J. P., 1989, 'The Influence of an Abrupt Price Increase on Health Service Utilization: evidence from Zaire' *Health Policy and Planning* 4 (1), pp. 76-81.

De Ferranti, D., 1985, 'Paying for Health Services in Developing Countries, An Overview' *World Bank Staff Working Paper*, No. 721.

Diamond, P. A. and Jerry, A. H., 1994, 'Contingent Valuation: Is Some Number Better than No Number?', *Journal of Economic Perspectives* 8(4), pp. 45-64.

Diop, F. P., 1994, 'Evaluation of the Impact of Pilot Tests for Cost Recovery on Primary Health Care in Niger, Technical Report No. 16', Bethesda, MD: Health Financing and Sustainability (HFS) Project.

DSCN, 2002, *Conditions de vie des populations et profil de pauvreté au Cameroun en 2001: premiers résultats. Direction de la statistique et de la comptabilité nationale*, mai, Yaoundé-R.C.

Flores, N. E. and Richard, T. C., 1997, 'The Relationship Between the Income Elasticities of Demand and Willingness to Pay', *Journal of Environment Economics and Management* 33(3), pp. 287-95.

Frykblom, P., 1998, 'Questions in the Contigent Valuation Method – Five Essays', PhD. Thesis, Acta Universitatis Agriculturae Sueciae Agraria 100, Swedish University of Agricultural Sciences, Uppsala.

Gilson, L., 1988, *Government Health Care Charges: Is Equity Being Abandoned?*, EPC Publication No. 15, London.

Gruat, J. V., 1990, 'Social Security Systems in Africa: Current Trends and Problems' *International Labour Review*, 129 (NE4), pp. 405-421.

Houdégbé, J., 1998, « Rentabilité économique des politiques de conservation des aires protégées au Bénin: cas de la Zone cynégétique de la Djona ». Thèse de Doctorat en Économie rurale, Cires-Université d'Abidjan.

Jordan, E., 1994, 'Differences in Contingent Valuation Estimates from Referendum and Checklist Questions', *Journal of Agricultural and Resource Economics*, 19 (1), pp. 115-128.

Kahneman, D. and Knetsch, J. L., 1992, 'Valuing Public Good: The Purchase of Moral Satisfaction', *Journal of Environmental Economics and Management* 30, pp. 57-70.

Kanbur, R., 1990, *La pauvreté et les dimensions sociales de l'ajustement structurel en Côte d'Ivoire. Les dimensions sociales de l'ajustement structurel en Afrique subsaharienne*. Document de travail No. 2. Banque Mondiale, Washington D.C.

Kriström, B. 1993, 'Comparing Continuous and Discrete Contingent Valuation Questions', *Environmental and Resource Economics* 3, pp. 63-71.

Kutzin, J., Barnum, H., 1992, 'Institutional Features of Health Insurance Programs and their Effects on Developing Country Health Systems', *International Journal of health Planning and Management* 7, pp. 51-72.

Li, C.-Z. and Fredman, P., 1994, 'On Reconciliation of the Discrete Choice and Open-Ended Responses in Contingent Valuation Experiments', in Li, C.-Z., *Welfare Evaluations in Contingent Valuation – An Econometric Analysis.* PhD Thesis, Umea Economic Studies No. 341, Department of Economics, Umea University.

Mills, A., 1983, 'Economics Aspects of Health Insurance', in: K., Lee, A., Mills Eds., *Health Economics in Developing Countries*, Oxford University Press.

Ministry of Public Health, 1997, National Health Management Information System: Annual Activity Report, Yaoundé. R.C.

Mitchell, R. C. and Carson, R. T., 1986, *Using Surveys to Value Public Goods: Contingent Valuation Method,* Washington D.C.

Mitchell, R. C. and Carson, R. T. 1989, *Using Surveys to Value Public Goods: The Contingent Valuation Method. Resources for the Future,* Washington D.C.

Munasinghe, M., 1996, *Environmental Economics and Sustainable Development.* World Bank Environmental Paper No. 3, Washington D. C.

N'guessan Coffie, F. J., 1997, 'Estimation de la demande des soins de santé antipaludéens et des Méthodes Préventives en Milieu Rural Ivoirien: le cas des villages de Memni et Montezo'. Thèse de Doctorat en Economie rurale. Cires-Université d'Abidjan.

Neill, H. R., Cummings, R. G., Ganderton, P. T., Harrison, G. W. and MacGuckin, T., 1994, 'Hypothetical Surveys and Real Economic Commitments', *Land Economics* 70, pp. 145-154.

Noterman, J. P., Criel, B., Kegels, G. and Isu, K., 1995, 'A Prepayment Scheme for Hospital Care in the Masisi District in Zaire: A Critical Evaluation', *Social Science and Medicine* 40 (NE7), pp. 919-930.

Qaim, M. and De Janvry, A., 2003, 'Genetically Modified Crops, Corporate Pricing Strategies, and farmers' adoption: the case of BT cotton in Argentina', *American Journal of Agricultural Economics* 85 (4), pp. 814-828.

Randall, A., Hoehn, J. P. and Tolley, G. S., 1981, 'The Structure of Contingent Markets: Some Results of a Recent Experiment', Paper presented at the American Economic Association annual meeting, Washington D. C.

Republic of Cameroon, 2000, *Interim Poverty Reduction Strategy Paper,* Cameroon, August 23.

Schneider, P., Diop, F. P. and Bucyana, S., 2000, *Development and Implementation of Prepayment Schemes in Rwanda.* Technical Report No. 45, Bethesda, MD: Partnerships for Health Reform (PHR) Project.

Shepard, D., Vian, T., Kleinau, E. F., 1990, *Health Insurance in Zaire. Policy, Research and External Affairs Working Papers,* WPS 489, Africa Technical Department, The World Bank. Washington.

Shepard, D. S. et al., 1998, 'Household Participation in Financing of Health Care at Government Health Centers in Rwanda', in A., Mills and L., Gilson, 1998, *Health Economics for Developing Countries,* London School of Hygiene and Tropical Medecine.

Tshinko, B. L., Constandriopoulos, A. P. et Fournier, P., 1995, « Plan de paiement anticipé des soins de santé de Bwamanda (Zaïre). Comment a-t-il été mis en place », *Social Science and Medicine* 40 (8), 1041-1052.

Vogel, R. J., 1990a, 'An Analysis of Three National Health Insurance Proposals in Sub-Saharan Africa', *International Journal of Health Planning and Management* 5, pp. 271-285.

Vogel, R. J., 1990b, *Health Insurance in Sub-Saharan Africa: A Survey and Analysis.* Policy, Research and External Affairs Working Papers, WPS 476, Africa Technical Department, The World Bank, Washington.

Waddington, C. J., Enyimayew, K. A., 1989, 'A Price to Pay. Part 1: the Impact of User Charges in Ashanti-Akim District, Ghana', *International Journal of Health Planning and Management* 5, pp. 287-312.

Wasikama, T. M. C., 1998, « Utilisation alternative des terres: une analyse économique de la préservation des forêts tropicales primaires (cas du Parc national de Taï, sud-ouest de la Côte d'Ivoire) ». Thèse de Doctorat en Economie Rurale, Cires-Université d'Abidjan.

Whittington, D., Briscoe, J., Mu, X., Barron, W., 1990, 'Estimating the Willingness to Pay for Water Services in Developing Countries: A Case Study of Contingent Valuation Surveys in Southern Haiti', Economic Development and Cultural Change.

Whittington, D. 1998, 'Administering Contingent Valuation Surveys in Developing Countries', *World Development* 26, pp. 21-30.

World Bank, 1993, *Report of the World Bank Africa Technical Department: Better Health in Africa, Human Resources and Poverty Division*, The World Bank, Washington.

World Bank, 1987, *Financing the Health Sector: An Agenda for Reform.* The World Bank, Washington.

World Health Organization, 1993, *Planning and Implementing Health Insurance in Developing Countries: Guiding Principles*, Macroeconomics, Health and Development Series.

15

The Impact of Structural Adjustment Programmes (SAPs) on Women's Health in Kenya

Damaris S. Parsitau

Introduction

The late 1970s and early 1980s were a difficult period for many developing countries because of high inflation, slow rates of economic growth, and declining earnings from exports. These factors affected national incomes and resulted in large government deficits, which in turn caused deterioration in the standard of living of families in the developing world.

During the 1980s, stabilisation and adjustment packages were introduced in many developing countries in an attempt to stop further deterioration in standards of living (Dixon et al. 1995, Barhin 1998). The term 'adjustment' refers to a range of macro-economic and structural measures that were promoted in the first instance by the Bretton Woods institutions - the World Bank and the International Monetary Fund (IMF) - to restore internal balances and increase the role of market force in the economy. Adjustment policies therefore denote the various mechanisms designed to reduce imbalances in Third World economies, both on external accounts and in domestic resource use. Adjustment frequently involved cutbacks in government expenditure. Consequently, real government expenditure per capita fell in over half the countries of the developing world in the period 1980-1984 (Cornia et al. 1987).

The impact of adjustment measures on local economic conditions varied widely as did the degree and consistency of their implementation. In sub-Saharan Africa, SAPs were implemented in only a handful of countries during the late 1970s, but by the end of the 1980s, most countries were formally involved (Streefland et al. 1998). In Africa, economic restructuring was a major component of the process of globalisation. Globalisation is a post-Second World War phenomenon that has become manifest in the last three decades. This is a process involving the construction of a world system (Aina 1996). Globalisation entails the restructuring of the global, national, local and household economies, as well as social structures and livelihood strategies. It has transformed the international and local division of labour, changed relations of production, employment, the provision of social services, cultures and so on. These processes have affected communities in rural and urban Africa (Aina 1996). SAPs were an important aspect of globalisation.

In Africa, the restructuring process, coupled with the implementation of SAPs, has had a devastating effect on the provision of social services such as healthcare and education. Cutbacks in government expenditure have created constraints in the provision of these services, leading to a decline in social welfare. Since SAPs touched on every facet of life in the relevant countries, it affected governance in a way no other policy package had done before.

This paper examines the impact of SAPs on women's health in Kenya. It argues that the reforms brought upon by SAPs led to a decline in the health of most women in Kenya. It further argues that SAPs, an imposition on developing countries by the Bretton Woods institutions, violated the rights of Third World societies through the denial of access to healthcare, which is a basic human right. Since women were the most affected group in Kenya, the paper calls for the engendering of health services in the country in order to meet the health needs of women.

Health Services in Post-independence Kenya

From the 1950s through to the 1970s, Kenya, and indeed most African countries, made substantial progress in healthcare delivery. In the 1970s, relatively high prices for Kenya's exports, which are mainly agricultural produce like coffee and tea, coupled with low interest rates, made increased spending in healthcare provision possible. Healthcare related projects, as well as the number of state medical personnel, also increased during this period. Consequently, there was a dramatic decline in infant and maternal mortality rates as well as a rise in life expectancy. In Kenya, the overall mortality rate dropped from 20 per 1000 persons in 1963 to 13 in 1987. Similarly, life expectancy increased from 49 years in 1960 to 58 in 1987. Immunisation also rose to 70 percent by the 1980s and early 1990s (Republic of Kenya Development Plan 1997-2001).

From the 1980s, however, the situation began to deteriorate. The early 1980s saw large drops in national income as the prices of coffee and tea in the world market fell to record low levels. This situation was compounded by increased interest rates on government borrowing, making debt servicing a problem for many African countries. This was largely responsible for the introduction of SAPs, which exacerbated the situation.

The economic crisis in many African countries, coupled with SAPs, undermined the health of many people in a number of ways. First, the removal of farming subsidies and the resultant rise in food prices threatened the ability of families to feed themselves and thus remain healthy. The increasingly harsh socio-economic conditions also affected many people's access to health services outside the public sector. Secondly, the reduction in government expenditure in the public health sector reduced both the quantity and quality of healthcare available to the general populace. Thirdly, SAPs brought about the introduction of user fees or cost-sharing in Kenya's social services sector in order to relieve the government of the financial burden of providing healthcare and education. The Bamako Initiative, which introduced user fees in the public health sector, meant that the beneficiaries of public health services, who hitherto received free medical care, would henceforth contribute to the financing of healthcare delivery. This meant transferring the cost of healthcare services to people who were already too poor to afford it.

At independence in 1963, the government of Kenya took the responsibility for financing public health services, thus relieving beneficiaries of the financial burden. But the cutbacks in government expenditure through SAPs hurt the poor and the vulnerable groups most because they were dependent on the previously subsidised social services. The negative effects of the SAPs were borne by the low-income population, the majority of who are women (Nzomo 1995). A World Bank study has shown that the poor suffered disproportionately from the effects of the economic decline of the 1980s and structural adjustment measures (World Bank 1991). Specific vulnerable groups, such as female-headed households, can be identified in both rural and urban environments.

Living conditions for urban and rural populations have clearly deteriorated since 1975. Public expenditure on health services has been low amidst increasing demand for these services. For instance, annual spending on health services per capita in Kenya declined from US $982 in 1980/81 to about US $6.2 in 1996 (Owino and Munga 1997). Today, the state can only cater for 50 percent of the total recurrent health expenditure. Meanwhile the majority of Kenyans are located more than eight kilometres from any form of health facility, and 40 percent of the rural population has no access to health services. There is also a general lack of quality healthcare due to under-staffing, under-stocking of medical supplies, corruption, and poor public health infrastructure.

Women and Health

The World Health Organisation (WHO) defines good health as a state of complete physical, mental and social well being of the whole person and not merely an absence of disease and infirmity. Good health is a human right that should be enjoyed by all. Moreover, a society's investment in the health of its citizens is essential for economic, social and political development.

Women play a crucial role in society. Besides their economic importance, they are educators as well as healthcare givers. It is therefore imperative that their health be taken seriously if the health of the rest of society is to be enhanced. It is the mother who first notices a cold, cough, a rise in temperature, or a gastro-intestinal condition that may arise in any member of the family (Wallace 1990). Besides, women have multiple roles as wives, bearers and minders of children, food producers, fetchers of water and fuel, nursing the sick and elderly, part of the paid labour force, etc. This visibility of women in every facet of life makes it imperative to focus on their health (Kamara 2000).

Yet, available information indicates that women as a group are the least healthy population in Kenya. Compared to men, women in Kenya have less access to medical care, are more likely to be malnourished, poor, and illiterate, and even work longer and harder. The situation exacerbates women's reproductive role, which increases their vulnerability to morbidity and mortality. Furthermore, women's roles as mothers and wives make them the primary health seekers and caregivers, which exposes them to infections. Women's economic dependence, exposure to violence, limited power over their sexuality, poor nutrition, inadequate access to safe water, sanitation facilities and fuel supplies, particularly in rural areas, all have negative effects on their health (UN 1996). As a group, women therefore need healthcare more than men do.

Discrimination against girls, often resulting from favouritism to sons in access to nutrition and health services, endangers their health and well being. Girls need but often do not have access to necessary health and nutrition services as they mature (UN 1996). There are also conditions that force girls into harmful practices such as female genital mutation, early marriage and childbearing. This is perhaps what forced Kenyan female members of parliament to call for the distribution of free sanitary pads to all adolescent girls in Kenya's rural areas in 2004.

Furthermore, women are subjected to peculiar health risks through childbirth. The lack of services to meet health needs related to sexuality and reproduction during pregnancy and childbirth is among the leading causes of mortality and morbidity of women of reproductive age in Kenya and the developing world. Maternal problems are preventable through access to healthcare, including safe and effective family planning methods. In many countries, Kenya included, the neglect of women's reproductive rights severely limits their opportunities in public and private life, including opportunities for education (UN 1996).

It is clear that provision of adequate healthcare, particularly to women, is critical to a nation's development. But how is the provision of healthcare services in Kenya? What has been the impact of SAPs on women's health in Kenya? What effect has the introduction of user fees in Kenya had on women's health?

SAPs and Women's Health in Kenya

A 1992 World Bank Report shows that the implementation of SAPs had a negative impact on a variety of groups. These groups include women who form the majority of the poor in society, but who are paradoxically the critical providers of health at home. This is particularly the case among female-headed households in both rural and urban areas. It is evident that the poor have suffered disproportionately from the effects of economic decline and the structural adjustment measures (Wallace 1991).

Economic decline and SAPs hit women harder than men. Being responsible for the well being of their families, women found it difficult to cope with increased burdens of disease and hunger. The retrenchment policies resulting from implementation of the SAPs also affected women more than men as women dominate the less skilled work force. As a group, women are less educated and their participation in formal employment is low. With SAPs came the rationalisation of formal sector employment, leading to the retrenchment of the less skilled cadres, mainly women. Cost-sharing policies in education and the healthcare sectors also affected women adversely. The removal of subsidies in the agricultural sector, and the resultant high cost of inputs as well as low returns on farm products, also adversely affected the living standards of women and children (Aina 1995).

A 1992 situational analysis by UNICEF shows that for every maternal death, about a hundred women suffer serious physical and mental complications (UNICEF 1989). Indeed, cases of such complications go unreported. During pregnancy, many women not only suffer infections, injuries and disabilities, but also receive no medical care, no special diet, no lighter workload or other considerations. SAPs worsened this situation.

Kenya has high rates of maternal and infant mortality. Reliable data are lacking but estimates based on the 1989 national census are at 74 per 1000 persons. Indications are that maternal and infant mortality increased with the economic recessions of the 1980s and the introduction of SAPs. A report by UNICEF points to a clear relationship between poor health among women and the introduction of SAPs (UNICEF 1990).

Family planning services help in reducing the rate of infant and maternal mortality. One of the immediate causes of major complications in pregnancy and childbirth is many or frequent births. Before the introduction of SAPs, family planning services were free of charge but that is now history. There is also the poor accessibility to medical facilities and essential services. The majority of rural women trek long distances to and from health facilities. Before the introduction of SAPs, health facilities were on average 6-7 kilometres away from most households, but many of them closed down while those that remained open lack basic amenities. At Nakuru District Hospital in Kenya, for example, expectant mothers are required to buy gloves, surgical blades, disinfectants and syringes in preparation for childbirth. In addition, they have to bribe hospital personnel in order to be attended to. This is usually too expensive for many women and they opt for traditional birth attendants.

Maternal mortality poses a major threat to women of reproductive age in Kenya. Data on maternal mortality are scanty, but in 1992 it was estimated to range between 150 and 300 per 100,000 births. The positive achievements in reducing mortality rates between 1960 and 1980s appear to have been reversed. Breman and Shelton (2001) have demonstrated the relationship between SAPs and the deterioration in healthcare services. There is a direct relationship between reduced government spending on healthcare because of structural adjustment policies and increased rates of child and maternal mortality as well as malnutrition.

One of the major causes of maternal and infant mortality in Kenya is lack of prenatal care. Statistics indicate that the majority of the women who die in childbirth, or whose children die before, during, or shortly after birth, had not been visiting prenatal clinics. For example, a study of maternal deaths at Pumwani Maternity Hospital in Nairobi shows that 66 percent of these deaths occurred in women who received no prenatal care or received it late. One of the major reasons why women do not visit prenatal and postnatal clinics is lack of resources. As already noted, while there was a steady improvement in reproductive health in the 1970s, the introduction of user charges in government hospitals in the 1980s has led to a decline in reproductive health (Kamara 2000).

Besides, many government hospitals lack essential amenities. Once machines and equipment such as incubators break down, they are rarely repaired. A fee is required from patients who are already too sick or poor to afford it. As a result, many turn to traditional birth attendants (TBAs) who are cheaper. Moreover, drugs are either unavailable or corruption makes them difficult to get as corrupt medical personnel sell public hospital drugs to private clinics. Cases of drugs in government hospitals expiring before use are also common. All these problems have led to the search for alternative therapies as people lose faith in public health facilities.

Family planning services also help in reducing infant and maternal mortality. One of the major causes of complications in pregnancy and childbirth is many or frequent births. Closely related to this issue is abortion, which causes a significant number of deaths in Kenya. Suffice to say that abortion is a thorny issue in Kenya today. Induced abortion, for example, accounts for 50 percent of all maternal deaths recorded at Kenyatta National Hospital in Nairobi. Illicit abortions in Kenya are carried out by quacks in backstreet clinics because of the lack of reproductive health facilities and the fact that abortion is illegal in Kenya.

Besides problems related to reproductive health, there are other health problems among women in Kenya. Women, like other social groups, require healthcare if they are to remain healthy. But a Kenya Demographic Health Survey (1998) shows that a significant portion of the gains made during the first 25 years of independence rapidly eroded in a short period due to the introduction of SAPs. The factors undermining women's health included deterioration in the quality and quantity of health services, decline in nutritional status, increased poverty, and impact of the HIV/AIDS pandemic.

Other factors include inadequate facilities and poor service. The physical set up of any health facility determines patient flow. Most of the facilities in public hospitals are rundown and the privacy of patients, especially in maternity wards, is lacking. Overcrowding and congestion increases the risk of infections. Health establishments also lack basic equipment. Where equipment is available, it is non-functional. Supplies such as protective clothing, cotton wool, and surgical gloves are inadequate.

Recent studies have shown that women are the major users of health services. They are also the main providers and promoters of preventive and curative healthcare. However, they do not make optimal use of the existing health services. The factors contributing to this include the inadequate quality and quantity of services, increasing cost, long distance to the medical facilities, negative attitude of medical personnel and lack of time and heavy workload. Furthermore, women bear the social and health burdens of their family. They cope with the increased burden of disease and hunger. SAPs resulted in increased burdens on women.

The Impact of Cost-sharing on the Health of Women

The Bamako Initiative introduced user fees or cost-sharing in many developing countries. This aimed at relieving governments of the financial burden of providing public services. This resulted in cutbacks in budgets for social services, including healthcare. Given the centrality of healthcare to a nation's well being, the introduction of cost-sharing would definitely hurt the poor and other vulnerable groups such as women and children. This would be the case in Kenya where women form the majority of the unemployed and are thus outside the scope of insurance schemes. How were women in Kenya expected to cater for their health needs?

Decline in government spending on healthcare means a decline in well being, especially for the poor who cannot afford the services offered by private healthcare providers. Studies have shown that the introduction of cost-sharing in the public health sector led to a decline in the utilisation of formal health services. In a situation of deteriorating service delivery and worsening household budgets, the question of introducing user fees is difficult. There is a need to ask consumers to supplement government expenditure on health services. But in a situation of low household incomes, user fees for health services can bar many people from such services. In the rural health centres studied, the utilisation of services remained substantially low. When discussing the utilisation of government clinics, the cost of the services is cited as an important determinant for the quality, accessibility and acceptability of the services available. Similarly, availability of drugs and outreach services are important considerations. Low morale among health personnel due to poor motivation is also an important factor in the quality of services provided in public heath facilities.

This situation makes the introduction of user fees a double-edged sword, potentially affecting service delivery as well as utilisation of the services. In January 2004, Kenyatta National Hospital, the largest public health facility in Kenya, introduced user fees for children under five years of age. This has had serious consequences. It has been reported that after the introduction of user fees at Kenyatta National Hospital, utilisation of services has gone down (*Daily Nation*, January 2004).

It is clear that the introduction of user charges in the public health sector has had negative effects on the poor, the majority of who are women. The partial privatisation of public healthcare, through the introduction of user fees, constitutes an assault on both the physical well being and dignity of poor women. Kamara (2000) reports that since the introduction of user fees in Kenya, there has been a dramatic drop in the number of hospital visits, while the infant mortality rate has risen and life expectancy has dropped. The introduction of user charges in the public health sector is in many ways a retrogressive measure. It makes healthcare cease to be a basic human right. Since these measures came with SAPs, the programmes may be considered to have been unjust and unethical.

Engendering Women's Health

In view of the impact of recent changes on the health of women, there is a need to integrate gender into health research, both conceptually and methodologically. Research that analyses the health problems of communities anywhere in Africa can no longer afford to neglect gender issues. Since women play important roles as informal healthcare providers and educators, as they seek to meet the health needs of their families, their significance for social well being can never be underestimated. For women to be able to fully perform their social roles, it is necessary to focus on issues that affect their health (Kamara 2000).

The production and reproductive activities of women makes their role as providers and consumers of healthcare the most critical aspect in a debate regarding gender in health research. However, the prevailing concept of health is not gender-sensitive. Women's health is directly or indirectly related to their reproductive health status. McFadden (1992) argues that women are often assumed to have no specific health needs outside of their mothering roles, an assumption borne out by most of the existing health programmes that target women only during their reproductive years. The safe motherhood initiative (SMI), mother and child health (MCH), primary healthcare (PHC), all include the mother because of her productive function vis-à-vis the survival and development of the child. When a woman is not expectant or lactating, she is essentially marginal to the health system.

Thus, women's reproductive roles largely serve as the basis for the definition of what health means for women at the personal, household, community and national levels. Consequently, the idea of health as a basic human right is rarely extended to women. Nor do women themselves perceive it in this holistic sense. Yet, African women as a group are the least healthy people in our communities. They are stressed, overworked, depressed, and generally unhealthy. As this paper has shown, the effects of SAPs on women's health went beyond reproductive health. There is therefore a need for a broad-based concept of health that goes beyond the narrow focus on women's reproductive health.

Women's health needs should be redefined to mean the totality of well being: reproductive health as well as other health needs. Health as defined by the WHO is a concept implying the totality of physical, emotional and psychological well being. For women, this concept means the right to a healthy existence as a human being whether one is lactating or not. The concept also empowers women as human beings. Health after all is a human rights issue and women everywhere are entitled to healthcare like everybody else.

Conclusion

This paper has tried to show the impact of SAPs on women's health in Kenya. It has argued that there was a direct link between the introduction of SAPs and deterioration in women's health as the SAPs led to a decline in public expenditure on healthcare.

The paper recommends that the following issues be urgently addressed in the quest for health for all, including women. First, there is a need for the evaluation of the existing medical facilities currently available in Kenya, and challenges to the government as a steward of the people to provide affordable healthcare for all. Secondly, medical services should be made both accessible and affordable to all, especially to poor rural women. Lastly, women's health needs, special or otherwise, should be given prominence.

Bibliography

Adebayo, A., 1990, *Structural Adjustment for Socio-Economic Recovery and Transformation: The African Alternative*, UNECA.

Aina, T., 1996, *Globalization and Social Policy in Africa: Issues and Research Directions*, Dakar, CODESRIA.

Antrobus, P., 1989, 'Women and Development: An Alternative Analysis', *Journal for International Development*, 1.

Baile, S., 1990, 'Women and Health in Developing Countries', *The OECD Observer*, December 1989/January 1990, pp. 18-20.

Bijlmakers, L., 2003, *Structural Adjustment: Source of Structural Adversity*, Leiden, African Studies Centre.

Cornia, G., et al., eds., 1987, *Adjustment with a Human Face*, Vol. 1: *Protecting the Vulnerable and Promoting Growth*, New York, Oxford University Press.

Denmark, 1995, 'Structural Adjustment in Africa: A Survey of the Experiences', Report prepared by the Centre for Development Research, Copenhagen, for the Danish Ministry of Foreign Affairs.

Giorgis, B. W., 1991, 'The Integration of Gender Analysis in Health Research', CODESRIA Workshop on Gender Analysis and African Social Science, Dakar.

Kamara, E., 2000, *The Effects of Structural Adjustment Programmes on Women's Health in Kenya*, ed., *Africa in Transformation*.

Kenya, Republic of, 1986, *The Seventh National Development Plan 1994-1996*, Nairobi, Government Printer.

Kenya, Republic of, 1992, *Women and Children in Kenya: A situational Analysis*, Nairobi, Mangra Phics.

Kenya, Republic of, 1994, *Kenya's Health Policy Framework*, Nairobi, Government Printer.

Kenya, Republic of, 1996, *Economic Reforms for 1996-1998: The Policy Framework Paper*, Nairobi, Government Printer.

Kimathi, W. and Omiya, P. J., 1994, 'The Growing Burden of Poverty on Women and Its Effects on their Reproductive Health Rights: An Analysis of the Kenyan Case', An IPPF Discussion Paper.

Macgregor, J., 1991, 'Towards Human-Centered Development: Primary Health Care in Africa', *African Insight*, Vol. 21, No. 3.

McFadden, P., 1992, *Health as a Gender Issue*, Centre for African Family Studies, (CAFS).

Nasirumbi, H., 1995, *Health Policies as They Affect Gender and Development in Kenya: A Case Study of HIV/AIDS Policies*, Mimeo, July.

Ngugi, R., 1999, *Health-seeking Behaviour in the Reform Process for Rural Households: The Case of Mwea Division, Kirinyaga District, Kenya*, Nairobi, African Economic Research Consortium.

Nzomo, M., 1995, 'Summary of Research Findings on the Impact of SAPs on Females and Gender in Kenya', in Kivutha, K., ed., *Women and Autonomy in Kenya: Policy and Legal Framework*, Nairobi, Claripress.

Olenja, J. M., 1991, 'Women and Health Care in Siaya', in S. Gideon, ed., *Development in Kenya: Siaya District*, Nairobi, Institute of African Studies.

Owino, W., 1998, *Public Healthcare Pricing Practices: The Question of Fee Adjustment*, Nairobi, IPAR.

Owino, W. and Munga, S., 1997, *Decentralisation of Financial Management Systems: Its Implications and Impact on Kenya's Healthcare Delivery*, Nairobi, IPAR.

Smyke, P., 1980, *Women and Health*, London, Zed Books.

Streefland, P., et al., 1998, *Implications of Economic Crisis and Structural Adjustment Policies for PHC in the Periphery*.

UNICEF, 1990, *The State of the World's Children*, Oxford University Press.

Wallace, H. and Kanti, G., 1990, *Healthcare of Women and Children in Developing Countries*, Oakland.

Werner, D., 1994, 'The Economic Crisis: Structural Adjustment and Healthcare in Africa', *Third World Resurgence*, No. 42/43, pp. 10-17.

World Bank, 1994a, *Adjustment in Africa: Reforms, Results and the Road Ahead*, Washington DC, World Bank.

World Bank, 1994b, *World Development Indicators*, Washington DC, World Bank.

16

Should We 'Modernise' Traditional Medicine?

Mugisha M. Mutabazi

Introduction

Traditional medicine plays a big role in the Ugandan health system, and the fact that government is committed to working with this sub sector to ensure good health for the population is a clear reflection of the good leadership the country has had for the last nineteen years. Efforts to bring the 'modern'[1] sector closer to the 'traditional'[2] health sub-sector began as far back as 1993, when reforms in the health sector were introduced. Available evidence suggests that important milestones in the search for a partnership between these two sectors have been reached (Birungi et al. 2001, Ministry of Health 2003, National Health Policy 1999, GoU 1995). Thus, the platform for partnership has been set. However, the form the partnership should take remains a bone of contention. While the government is of the view that this partnership should culminate in the integration of traditional medicine into the overall national health services, a close look at the dynamics in this sub-sector suggest otherwise. Moreover, there is clear evidence that unlike other actors in the private sector whose integration does not present immense bottlenecks, the traditional medicine sub-sector has unique circumstances and qualities that do not easily render it amenable to integration with modern health services, especially in the case of Uganda (Mugisha et al. 2004).

Nationally, the regime's aim at integrating these two sectors has for long been involved in a war of semantics as to what form this partnership should take. While some would prefer 'formalisation', others, want 'collaboration'. In fact, some have even talked of 'co-habitation' and 'co-existence' as if the two sectors have not always co-habited and/or co-existed. Hand in hand with other problems that afflict the country's health sector, the war of semantics on the form of partnership to be pursued has continued and the implications this issue may have on the entire health system are very obvious. In view of the above, this paper presents an alternative approach, which posits granting traditional medicine practitioners autonomous status, so as to drive the sub-sector towards 'modernisation'. The paper is divided into seven major sections: the introduction and background; the problem; the context of the public-private mix reform process, a critique of the existing model of integration; a review of empirical literature on challenges of integration; the model for the 'modernisation' of traditional medicine and practice, and lastly, conclusions and recommendations for the way forward are suggested. Where possible, the author has tried to capture local political issues pertaining to the sub-sector and how they fit in with the current debate on integration.

Background to the Problem

One third of the world's population still lacks regular access to affordable, modern, essential drugs. Traditional medicine is often the widely available and used alternative (Amai 2002). According to the World Health Organisation (WHO), 'traditional medicine' generally refers to ways of protecting and restoring health that existed before the arrival of modern medicine. 'African traditional medicine' has been conceptualised by the WHO Centre for Health Development as:

> The sum total of all knowledge and practices, whether explicable or not, used in diagnosis, prevention and elimination of physical, mental, or social imbalance, and relying exclusively on practical experience and observation handed down from generation to generation, whether verbally or in writing.[3]

Traditional medicine and traditional healers form part of a broader field of study classified by medical anthropologists as ethno-medicine. Ethno-medicine entails a study of the full range and distribution of health-related experience, discourse, knowledge and practice among different strata of the population; the situated meaning the aforementioned have for people at a given historical juncture; transformations in popular health culture and medical systems concordant with social change; and the social relations of health related ideas, behaviours and practices (Nichter 1992).

Traditional medicine therapy includes medication therapies, which involve the use of herbal medicines, animal fats and/or minerals, while non-medication therapies include acupuncture, manual therapy and spiritual therapy (Amai 2002). The Ministry of Health of the Uganda government has categorised traditional medicine practitioners into herbalists, spiritual healers, bone-setters, traditional birth attendants, hydro-therapists, traditional dentists and others. Of late, a number of non-Ugandan traditional medicine systems have been introduced such as Ayurvedic, Reiki, Chiropractic, Homeopathy and Reflexology and those who are involved in these practices are also recognised. However, traditional medicine practitioners do not include people who engage in harmful practices, such as casting of spells and child sacrifice (MoH 2004).

In Africa, up to eighty percent of the population use traditional medicine to meet their health care needs. In sub-Saharan Africa, the ratio of traditional healers to the population is approximately 1:500, while it is 1:40,000 for medical doctors (Abdol, K. et al. 1994). On the other hand, the ratio of traditional medicine practitioners to the population in Uganda is between 1:200 and 1:400, which significantly contrasts with available trained medical personnel for whom the ratio is 1:20,000 or slightly less (WHO 2001). These ratios underscore the importance of traditional medicine in the overall health care delivery system. However, compared to other parts of the world such as China where up to forty percent of both modern and traditional health care has been integrated, (Hesketh and Zhu 1997), traditional medicine in Uganda is still largely operating independently of the modern health services.

The government of Uganda formally recognised the importance of traditional medicine way back in 1997 when it initiated a project to integrate[4] it in national health services as part of the public-private partnership in health approach (PPPH)[5] (MoH 2004, MoH 1999, HSSP 2000). Through the public-private partnership, government aims at providing an enabling environment that allows for effective coordination of efforts among all partners, increase efficiency in resource allocation, achieve equity in the distribution of available resources for health, improve quality, ensure sustainability of health services and increases effective access by all Ugandans to essential health care. For this, a sector-wide approach (SWAP) has been adopted in which a common framework for health sector planning, budgeting, disbursement, programme management, support supervision, accounting, reporting, monitoring and evaluation is used according to agreed national development objectives and the main strategies for attaining them (MoH 2004). Strengthening the collaboration and partnership between the public and private sector in health is an important guiding principle of the National Health Policy of 1999.

Traditional medicine is gaining popularity in the country because it is easily accessible, affordable, sometimes free and there is a strong belief in its curative effect (Amai 2002).[6] Elsewhere, efforts to enhance collaboration between modern health services and traditional medicine are based on the fact that traditional medicine provides client-centred, personalised health care that is culturally appropriate, holistic and tailored to meet the needs and expectations of the patient. Traditional healers are culturally close to clients, which facilitates communication about disease and related social issues (UNAIDS 2000).

Despite all these efforts and recognition of its importance, traditional medicine has not fully been integrated into national health services and for some, it is even doubtful that the model of integration being pursued will yield the anticipated results.

The Context of the Public–Private Reform Process in Uganda

Before tackling the challenges of integrating traditional medicine into modern health services, it is warranted to comment on the context of the public-private partnership. Several factors have interacted in Uganda to present a complex context for a public-private partnership policy to evolve in. These factors include the dynamic changes that are ongoing in the health care system such as decentralisation, the weak revenue generating capacity of the public sector, and the breakdown of public health services. These factors were in turn a result of the following landmarks in the history of the country in general and the sector in particular: (i) political upheavals the country experienced in the years after independence up to the 1980s, which had profound implications for the health sector such as declining government expenditure on health care delivery, poor management, planning, control and massive brain drain from the health sector. These effects ultimately led to the proliferation of private profit-oriented health care providers who lacked regulation. Lack of proper management in the sector also culminated in the informalisation of public health care services and loss of public confidence in the system (Obbo 1991, Munene 1992, Birungi 1994, as reported in Birungi 2001), (ii) the establishment of a referral health institutional framework predominantly based on provision of curative health care, without corresponding capacity building measures for its management and staffing, also after independence; and (iii) the debilitating effects of the structural adjustment programmes of the international finance institutions, which further reduced government spending on health.

These problems led to the decline in public health care delivery in the country and encouraged the emergence of a weak but increasingly important private sector. The private sector that emerged was weak because it lacked any standards, had no policy to regulate its practice and was poorly funded. On the other hand, the sector was becoming increasingly important because it was providing a large percentage of curative health services compared to the public sector (Hutchison 1998). The private sector is composed, as already seen, by many actors, some of who were licensed and recognised by the government, while others were not licensed, but appreciated and legitimised by the communities. Despite the significant role played by the private sector, it remained isolated from district/national planning and information until recently - there were no programmes, official subsidies or incentives to influence the direction of private practice, and the relationship between government and the private sector was one of isolation interspersed with attempts at regulation and control (Birungi et al. 2001).

The Problem

Although the policy on public-private partnership is still in draft form, the public-private partnership approach to governance of the health sector in Uganda has been ongoing for some years. A partnership between the public and private sectors, which is deeply entrenched in the National Health Policy and the Health Sector Strategic Plan, is manifested in financial assistance, technical support, supervision and regulatory mechanisms, among others. While some actors in the private sector, notably the Private Not For Profit and Private Health Providers, have to a large extent been integrated (the above mentioned areas of collaboration affect these actors); traditional health practitioners are largely operating independently of the other actors in health delivery. Efforts to bring them on board have at best been implemented half-heartedly; they are still ridiculed, despised and treated with much cynicism.[7] Coupled with political interference and lack of support from outside the sub-sector, infighting, and the absence of meaningful involvement of traditional medicine practitioners in policy formulation has taken place, nursing some doubt as to how integration will be possible (Birungi et al. 2001).

The existing policy framework does not adequately acknowledge the diversity of traditional medicine, which, in fact is both heterogeneous and monolithic, that is, while there are different cultural groups and different cultural notions of healing, traditional medicine is a unique system of health care.[8] Traditional medicine has, as a result, remained fragmented, polarized and 'under developed', with serious negative implications for its future. This situation raises a number of fundamental questions, which this paper endeavours to address: (i) Is the existing model of integration relevant and applicable to traditional medicine and practice in Uganda? (ii) What are the challenges of trying to bring together modern and traditional medicine systems using the existing model of integration? (iii) Should we 'modernise' traditional medicine so as to make it more acceptable and competitive vis-à-vis modern medicine? (iv) What model of 'modernisation' is relevant in the prevailing context? Based on this analysis, solutions, which explore how traditional medicine and practice can be 'modernised' so as to make them acceptable to those who ridicule and undermine them on the one hand, and those who wrest life and a living from them on the other, are considered.

A Critique of the Existing Model of Integration

The current model of integration purportedly aims at bringing all stakeholders into national health services by providing an enabling environment that allows for effective coordination of efforts among all partners, increases efficiency in resource allocation, achieves equity in the distribution of available resources for health, improves quality, ensures sustainability of health services and increases effective access by all Ugandans to essential health care. However for this to succeed, an effective regulatory and institutional framework through which the various actors can collaborate is necessary.

Over the years, such a regulatory and institutional framework has evolved, although its content does not favour participation by all stakeholders in health and goes against the grain of some, particularly those in the traditional medicine sub-sector. The current regulatory framework does not consider the unique nature and diversity of traditional medicine. For instance almost every ethnic group in Uganda practices a particular form of traditional medicine, deeply entrenched in its cultural past and indigenous knowledge systems, but the current model of integration ignores this fact. Therefore the issue of standardisation becomes a daunting task, if not impossible, within the framework of integration and partnership being pursued in the country.

The question of who controls or regulates whom remains a big challenge to integration, given the fact that the values, philosophies and practices of modern and traditional medicine are in direct contrast with each other. Trying to regulate traditional medicine using the standards and principles of western medicine is a fundamental flaw in the existing framework and will not achieve its intended goals. According to the Secretary General of the National Council of Traditional Healers and Herbalists Associations (NACOTHA), in a workshop held in Kampala, the issue at hand is that those that are pursuing the current model of integration have:

> ... mixed cultural issues with religion. Cultural issues should not be mixed with religion or modern science. People should leave traditional medicine practitioners to explain these issues. For example, not everyone can explain things like 'ejjembe'[9] or 'emizimu'.[10] While these things are considered horrible, they are not necessarily bad as they are portrayed.

It seems from the above that efforts to incorporate traditional medicine into the cultural hegemony of western medicine will not be the best way forward for developing the sub-sector. Already, there is vehement opposition from practitioners to any attempts to streamline their practices into the fold of western medicine. Practitioners who attended a workshop held in Masindi town highlighted the extent of disagreement thus:

> This belief has taken long. It stems from colonialism. It was brought by the whites. They are the ones who branded everything African satanic. That is why our medicine is not developed, that is why we do not cooperate with modern practitioners. They emphasise tablets, but we insist on herbs and spiritual healing.

Although still in the doldrums, the public-private partnership has evolved in a reformed regulatory environment, which began in 1993, with the updating of the Uganda Pharmacy and Drug Act of 1970. These regulations have been reviewed relative to the private sector, and in a bid to increase its participation in health care delivery. In 1993, the National Drug Policy and Statute was passed, followed by the adoption of three professional bills in 1996 (now acts): the Uganda Dental Practitioners Bill, the Uganda Nurses and Midwives Bill, and the Allied Health Workers Professional Bill. The bills established for each category of health workers, a council - a public body to regulate and exercise general supervision and control over professionals and other provisions (Birungi, et al. 2001). However, this regulatory framework affects only health professionals in the public and 'formal' private sectors, but not traditional medicine practitioners. Failure to have an institutional and legal framework for traditional medicine means that it is difficult to regulate traditional medicine from the point of view of modern medicine, since the actors in this sector do not appreciate the dynamics of traditional medicine.

Other weaknesses in this regulatory framework have been raised by Birungi et al. (2001) and seem to emphasise the fact that the laws relating to traditional medicine and practice are old, archaic and have been overtaken by "events on the ground". Existing regulations treat traditional medicine practitioners as actors who are supposedly involved in wrong practices and must be controlled in the public interest. In an earlier study conducted in Kasese and Masindi districts (Mugisha et al. 2004), the views of the District Community Development Officer revealed the stark reality and extent to which traditional medicine practice is held in contempt. He noted thus:

> They have an association, which is not run well because these are illiterates. They are also recognised nationally. Given the support they have nationally, they would be strong, but sometimes, their activities undermine their strength, because some mix traditional healing with witchcraft. They would influence events because people believe in them, but poor management undermines them.

Thus, traditional medicine practitioners are very suspicious and sceptical of the intentions of public officials who have often victimised them. With this scenario, it is difficult to see how the much hyped partnership can work.

While collaboration between the public and private sectors has been ongoing, there is a lack of a comprehensive institutional framework enshrining this partnership in all matters of health service delivery such as planning, decision-making and resource mobilisation. In the present situation, the Ministry of Health is responsible for formulation, coordination and implementation of the national health policy, while districts, through the district health teams, implement policy and plan district health services. There is only a limited role played by 'formal' private sector actors through the expanded district health management teams, but not traditional practitioners.

Failure to not only consult but also provide for traditional medicine practitioners in these institutions at the district level means that big gaps exist, which could have strategic implications for the implementation of the partnership. Traditional medicine practitioners may oppose such structures, not because they do not want them but simply because they were not privy to their establishment and the fact that they do not cater for their interests. No wonder during workshops in Kampala and Masindi, practitioners expressed total disagreement with the proposed structures in the envisaged dispensation that will govern the sector. For example, members and the leadership of NACOTHA were of the view that instead of establishing a new council to oversee progress towards integration, their council should be formally empowered to take leadership through an act of parliament or be institutionalised in the policy being formulated.

Although traditional medicine practitioners have been encouraged to form associations and institutions through which they can articulate their interests, it appears these associations were not organised with regard to their terms and conditions. As has been the case in the past, government in collaboration with key individuals in this sector set the agenda on which these associations and institutions were hastily organised, 'supposedly to start benefiting from the new partnership that was going to evolve'. The associations did not evolve as indigenous people's organisations/associations with a local agenda aimed at improving the lives of members. There is no doubt that the majority of the traditional practitioners have shunned them, and those who operate within their framework do so out of necessity but not choice. Commenting on the need for locally initiated people's organisations, one of the participants in the workshop held in Masindi had this to say:

> When I was a teacher, we had a teachers' association. We would ask for salary increment and get it, but if we are not united as traditional medicine practitioners through an association, be it Kamengo, Uganda herbalists association or... we need to make an association whether we like it or not. We must unite and have objectives. How can we be assisted unless we are one?

Despite calls for unity made by some practitioners, it seemed as though others were sceptical about the intentions of the leaders of local associations. Local associations were said to have evolved into money-making ventures and extortion machines and their original aim of forging unity seemed to have been eroded. According to practitioners who took part in the workshop that was held in Masindi, 'There is a power struggle in the association (Uganda n'edagala lyayo). So this results in exploitation, whereby leaders connive with local defence force personnel to extort money from practitioners. A person may be asked to pay license fees for all the years he has operated as a TM practitioner at once'.

An important challenge posed by all these developments is the question of intellectual property rights that has taken centre-stage in the new development paradigm of promoting indigenous people's knowledge. In its document on the 'Protection of the Heritage of Indigenous Peoples', the United Nations Commission for Human Rights notes that industrial property laws only protect 'new' knowledge and that 'old' knowledge like herbal remedies that have been used for ages, may not be regarded as patentable. In yet another twist to the problem, delegates at the Nairobi conference argued that the following problems may impede the patenting of some traditional medicines: regional specificity and short duration of the patent rights, the issue of bio-piracy, the lack of official recognition of community rights (as distinct from those of an individual applicant), and the lack of emphasis on availability and access of local communities to medicinal plant resources (Richter 2003).

Based on historical precedents, and mistrust and suspicion of governments' intentions, traditional medicine practitioners are very sceptical of divulging their sources of knowledge, documenting it and sharing it. They fear (and with reason too) that once they divulge their knowledge and practices, the government would turn it into a gold mine for the modern physicians who consider them conservative, subjective, backward and unscientific. Practitioners, in the workshops held in

Kampala and Masindi, succinctly and emphatically argued for protection and granting of property rights to them for their products.

> If I take my herbal drug for testing, my name should be inscribed on it. If it is approved, I should be able to benefit from it. People have drugs, even those that can cure cancer. But they need to be given property rights or at least benefit twenty per cent from them.

Traditional healers also thought that their knowledge is worth being protected since it has withstood the test of time, having been passed on from generation to generation. In addition, it has allegedly been used to cure different ailments, even some that have proved a menace for western medicine such as cancer. The challenge then is to find ways through which indigenous people's intellectual property rights can be safeguarded, since in the absence of economic capital, their knowledge is the only pillar of refuge to lean on.

From the foregoing observations, it is evident that the model of integration being pursued by the Ministry of Health is not relevant and applicable to the development of traditional medicine and practice in Uganda. In the circumstances, it is not rash to propose that the Ministry consider another way of bringing traditional practitioners into the main fold of health service delivery in Uganda.

Some Empirical Evidence on the Challenges of Integrating Modern and Traditional Medicine

The experiences of integrating the public and private sectors in national health service delivery are many, and they manifest great differences in different parts of the world. However, they are even more problematic when we consider the traditional medicine sub-sector. For instance Birungi et al. (2001), from whom this paper has borrowed considerably, conclude thus: "[T]here has been no policy dialogue between policy makers, consumers and informal providers. Yet the latter constitute a significant source of care for both rural and urban poor.... while communities recognise and appreciate such providers, authorities continue to blame and ridicule them. By failing to recognise and consult with this category of provider, the integration policy seems not to be interacting, or catching up, with some of the realities of the Ugandan health care system'.

Boerma and Baya (1990) in *World Health Organisation Centre for Health Development* (2002) have noted that before commencing collaborative effort in health care between modern and traditional sectors, a careful assessment of potential benefits and obstacles should be made. The medical services utilisation patterns of the communities need to be ascertained and the specific role of the traditional health practitioners considered. In such efforts, the ideas of healers themselves about possible collaboration are crucial. Chi (1994) in WHO (2002) outlined six recommendations for effective integration. They are: promotion of communication and mutual understanding among different medical systems that exist in a society; evaluation of traditional medicine in its totality; integration at the theoretical and practical levels; equitable distribution of resources between traditional and modern western medicine; an integrated training and educational programme for both traditional and modern western medicine; and a national drug policy that includes traditional drugs.

Planning for the formalisation of traditional health services has many dimensions that need to be addressed, depending on the state of current sectoral development, level of political will, budget resources available, training infrastructure, the model of formalisation suitable to and preferred by the country, and the traditional health care community. It has been argued that underlying the general proposition for a mix of traditional and modern medicine is an agenda of incorporating the former into the political economic arena and cultural hegemony of bio-medicine (Morsy 1990, cited in Kagwanja 1997, also cited in WHO 2002). Clearly, if traditional medicine is to be given a formal place in national health care, this process needs to be done not only in close consultation with the traditional health sector, but taking direction from it as to appropriate models of partnership, formalisation and training.

A challenge to integrated health care is the need to conduct research to determine which illnesses are best treated through one approach rather than the other. In a study conducted in Zheijang, China, it was reported that simultaneous use of modern and traditional treatment is so commonplace that their individual contributions are hard to assess. Research to disaggregate the contributions of each medical system, in traditional medicine itself, and its integration is therefore, crucial (WHO 2002).

According to Chaudhury (1997), it is generally recognised that the regulation of traditional systems of medicine, the products used in these systems, and the practitioners of these systems, are weak in most countries. This leads to the misuse of the medicines by unqualified practitioners and loss in the credibility of the system. In traditional medicine, practitioners and manufacturers (particularly small ones) usually oppose any steps to strengthen regulation by health administration. Their fears are that regulation as applied to allopathic medicine is not suitable for traditional medicine and may stifle the ancient systems of medicine. Thus, they need to step up the systems themselves.

Important challenges to the integration of the two systems of medicine are the power differentials that occur after integration. Van Kirk, (1993) and Moffat and Herring (1999) as cited in Letendre (2002) have alluded to issues of a racial paradigm in relation to the health needs of the Aborigines of Canada and the fact that traditional medicine remains subject to the policies and regulations of Health and Welfare Canada. Western medicine has continuously demanded legitimisation from any other system of medicine and to see the scientific basis of medical care of the aborigines. The method of systematic recording of knowledge is in direct opposition to the philosophies of traditional medicine (Morse et al. 1991, Reynolds 1997, Shestowiski 1993 as cited in Letendre 2002). Furthermore, the complex structure of today's economic and political climate emphasises that accountability be outlined in measurable terms in line with the philosophies of western medicine, which conflict with traditional medicine.

A fundamental problem to integration is the way the two systems conceptualise illness prevention. While western medicine develops large programmes for illness prevention based on its medical models, and participates in activities directed toward this goal, this system is incompatible with that of traditional medicine. Traditional medicine emphasises the prevention of illness, but it is not known how traditional healers engage in this activity. For instance, among the Aborigines, illness prevention is not a meaningful concept; on the other hand, western medicine encourages patients to come for regular checkups to ensure normality (Morse et al. 1991 as cited in Letendre 2002).

Others (Myat 2004) have pointed to the disruption of traditional medicine systems by the colonialists and differences ingrained in the values and philosophies of the two models of health care. While traditional medicine approaches disease from a holistic point of view, taking into consideration multiple causal factors for a particular disease, modern medicine is disease oriented. In addition, traditional medicine practice encourages a close relationship between physicians and patient, which may not always be the case with modern medicine.

Should We 'Modernise' Traditional Medicine?

The response to the question posed by this paper is as daunting as understanding the dynamics and processes of traditional medicine and practice. However, to break the ice, this paper will take a firm but cautious path to discussing the issues at hand. The concept of 'modernisation' is not to be understood in its literal sense; instead, it is to be given a contextual meaning that implies a desire to reinforce the position of traditional medicine practitioners by granting them autonomy to develop their own knowledge systems, practices, capacities and capabilities through training, documentation, regulation, peer evaluation and monitoring systems, in the light of the diversity and unique circumstances that most practitioners find themselves in.

Conceptual Framework

This paper posits two sub-sectors within national health services - the modern (sector) and traditional medicine (sub-sector). Traditional health practices are grounded in the social and cultural milieu of the societies in which they are uniquely practised; in the beliefs, norms, values and healing philosophies of particular societies. On the other hand, the link between modern health services and socio-cultural context, especially in Africa and other continents where traditional medicine is very central to health care, is weak. In addition, the link between the two sectors, although vital, is also weak. Yet, for meaningful integration to take place, the relationship between government and the traditional sector, through the modern health sector, must be strengthened. Practitioners who took part in the study conducted in Masindi and Kampala argued that failure by government to popularise traditional medicine before crafting the National Health Policy was a glitch in the policy making process. Increasing knowledge and pledging support for the sector, they argued, could have increased its legitimacy as a knowledge system and healing practice. Besides, there are several outstanding challenges that stand in the way of meaningful integration (as reviewed in the previous two sections of this paper). For this reason, the paper proposes a new model, a new way of looking at the issue of cooperation between the traditional and modern health sectors - that of granting autonomy to traditional medicine practitioners to develop a future for the sector.

The new model - the model of 'modernisation' - is based partly on the challenges to integration referred to above, and on the desire to allow traditional medicine to grow as an independent system of healing with a unique and culturally relevant knowledge base and practice. However, it presupposes an active traditional medicine sector interested in cooperation with other actors not only in the health sector, but also other sectors of the economy (since health cuts across all sectors). This means that any efforts to improve it must take cognizance of this fact. 'Modernisation' of the traditional medicine sub-sector also implies that there will be an improvement in other sectors of the economy, in view of the linkages between health and other sectors. However, to 'modernise' the traditional medicine sub-sector requires that the actors (practitioners) in it take centre-stage, design the agenda and execute it themselves.

A model that seeks to 'modernise' traditional medicine within its context forsakes negative stereotypes that portray traditional medicine practitioners as backward, conservative and unscientific. It conceives healers as masters in their own field, and as individuals, groups and actors who have something to contribute to the development agenda. Therefore, to 'modernise' traditional medicine and practice requires efforts that increase practitioners' sensitivity to their place in the development agenda and health care, given the specific milieu of their communities.

This paper argues that to grant autonomy to traditional medicine practitioners, the village should be taken as a microcosm on which higher societal level organisation of the sub-sector should be based. This is because most of the key social processes on which traditional medicine practice are based stem from the way of life in the village. What may be observed at higher levels of social organisation may significantly differ from what takes place at the village level. Therefore if autonomy were to be granted, then the most appropriate starting level would be the village. In terms of operationalising the model, the following is proposed:

- A village in any district of the country could be selected as a pilot, and a specific area or 'speciality' of traditional medicine such as bone-setting selected. This would enable testing of the idea of autonomy for the 'modernisation' of traditional medicine. Although the idea of autonomy is emphasised, according to practitioners with whom the author had long discussions, it would work well within the general framework of the National Health Policy, a policy on traditional medicine and under stewardship of the Ministry of Health.[11] Autonomy is simply to evolve local solutions for local problems without much outside interference and programming - to give the practitioners a voice.

- An independent civil society organisation, preferably a local community-based organisation rather than government, could take on the onus of mobilising the bone-setters and initiate an association/network of bone-setters in that village. However, once the association takes off, this organisation could leave it to take its course and only make available its human resources for consultation.

- Through the network or association, the bone-setters could discuss issues pertaining to their practice so as to gain common ground of the similarities and peculiarities in their practice. The network would also act as a forum for setting an agenda for training, reporting, information dissemination, documentation of practices, evaluation, monitoring, research and development and regulation, which are the major components of this model. However, efforts must be expended to ensure that all these aspects of the 'modernisation' project of traditional medicine practice are as indigenous as possible, springing from the cultural milieu of the society, such as the sanctions, normative regulations and belief systems.

- A system of financing the activities of this association could be designed in such a way that the members of the association through their earnings finance the core activities of the network/association so created. Moreover, once the itinerary of the so-called modern world such as fancy cars and complicated gadgets are not built into the system from the beginning, the desire for resources to acquire such things does not arise and cannot be used as a basis for frustrating activities of the practitioners. The resources collected from the members can jointly be managed for the common good, like many local associations are doing.

In terms of political organisation, once this initial experimental group succeeds, there would be an opportunity for other groups to succeed too. It is therefore argued that for full scale 'modernisation' to take place, there would be need to horizontally and vertically scale up the model by encouraging similar associations to blossom at parish, sub-county, county and district levels and in other forms of traditional practice. It is envisaged that this model would, in terms of such organisation, replicate so fast since the country is already politically organised at the said levels. Therefore, traditional medicine structures would simply run parallel to formal local government structures as shown in the conceptual diagram.

Conceptual Diagram

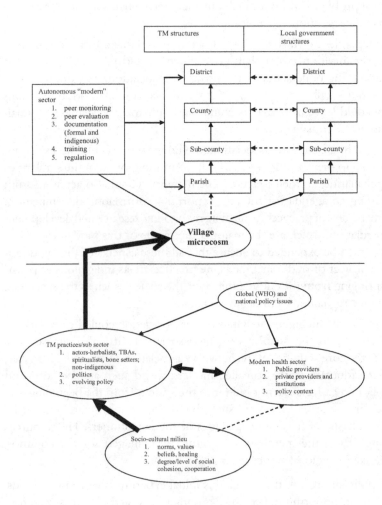

The proposed system of political organisation of the traditional medicine sector already exists within NACOTHA - one of the national umbrella organisations of traditional medicine (although yet to be formally recognised in the new dispensation). Therefore, these could be adopted in whole or with modification to please those who feel that NACOTHA is not legitimate.[12] From the structure of NACOTHA, it is evident that practitioners are capable of organising themselves and that they have already made important strides in the direction of autonomy. Probably what is needed (and as they rightly argue) is a policy within whose context autonomy could be operationalised. Thus the words of the Secretary General, NACOTHA become instructive in concretising our idea of autonomy. He said: 'We did all this without any support in terms of funding, we were self sustaining... we need support through a law and funding'. Therefore, autonomy is possible, since with minimal resources, practitioners were able to achieve a high level of organisation (in terms of establishing necessary governance structures).

Although the model may appear utopian at first sight, there is need to pay very close attention to its underlying arguments which include views on the role traditional practitioners play in health care delivery, cultural sensitivity, contextual relevance, emphasis on diversity and the centrality owed to traditional practitioners in solving their own problems. In the final analysis, the idea is to have a national movement of traditional medicine practitioners' associations/networks whose bargaining powers are greatly enhanced, whose practices and processes of health care delivery are improved through systematisation, and whose initiative to participate in development is bolstered, not by anybody but by and for the practitioners themselves.

The Main Tenets of the 'Modernisation' Model

(a) Autonomy

As mentioned above, it is envisaged that granting autonomy to traditional medicine practitioners would increase their self-awareness, highlight their central role in society, and enable them to exercise their rights as traditional practitioners and citizens. Autonomy would enable them to develop structures and institutions through which they could govern themselves and chart a path for their future. Through these structures, practitioners could confront issues of regulation and enforcement of the regulations that have proved to be a nightmare for the public health officials.

The model of 'modernisation' that this paper posits and whose central concept is autonomy is grounded (through this concept) in the contribution of Foucault to our understanding of government. To him, government is 'conduct of conduct'. However, the idea of autonomy encapsulates related ideas of self-policing, self-management and self-governance. However, government or 'conduct of conduct' can be seen in different perspectives. Borrowing from Foucault, this author takes the perspective of government as an ethical and moral enterprise. Thus autonomy, or self-government, becomes an ethical and moral endeavour on the part of traditional medicine practitioners concerned with the form of direction appropriate to their trade. Morality is understood as the attempt to make oneself accountable for one's own actions, or as a practice in which human beings take their own conduct to be subject to self-regulation.

To grant autonomy to traditional practitioners is to accept that there is a peculiar rationality surrounding the domain of traditional medicine, which only the traditional practitioners can exercise in their 'conduct of conduct'. Granting them autonomy is like giving them a stick to police and discipline themselves, which is opposed to the existing model of partnership where the public officials, through their own lens, are trying to govern traditional medicine and practice.

Governance of traditional medicine practice needs to go beyond individual conceptualisation of self-governance, to the governance of a society[13] - that is, there is movement from the governance of a multitude to the governance of a society and community - a society of traditional medicine practitioners. The idea is to have traditional medicine governed, but governed outside the public realm. This is because in the past the public officials have always emasculated the sector and demeaned it, regardless of the fact that it plays a crucial role in health care delivery.[14]

Granting autonomy to traditional medicine practitioners would have a number of advantages including the following: (i) it would not only enable them to govern themselves and channel their energies to improving their lot, but would also reduce their fear of being swallowed up, fear that has characterised interaction amongst themselves and between them and modern health services in the country to date. Commenting on the above, in the study conducted in Masindi and Kampala, practitioners cited power struggles, the politicisation of local associations, exploitation and connivance with local political leaders to extort money from them as key problems facing the sub-sector:

> The reason why TM is not developed stems from our associations. For example 'Uganda n'edagala lyayo' is like a political party. For one to stand for the post of chairperson, he has to use a lot of money. You must therefore recoup your expenses once you are voted into power. So you go to a computer person and make forms, which you sell expensively and arrest those who do not buy.

Self governance and autonomy through structures created by the practitioners themselves will help increase the bargaining power of the practitioners and predispose them well to constructively engage with government which has further advantages such as gaining a political niche, representation in national decision-making (parliament and executive), and lobbying, so as to increase resources going to the sector.

However, since autonomy cannot be secured while the sector is still fragmented, the starting point is mobilisation and organisation within the sector via the creation of local structures and institutions. Practitioners who took part in the studies conducted in Masindi and Kasese and Masindi and Kampala in 2004 and 2005 respectively strongly supported the formation of local associations of practitioners. For example in the first study, it was noted thus:

> If we can have a recognised association through which we can pass on our proposals, then the better, but today you find the assistance got is given to individuals... and if funding is given, it should not pass through our district because the officials there are corrupt, we can't get the assistance.

During the second study practitioners called for the formation of both local and umbrella organisations bringing together traditional medicine practitioners. The contributions of one participant are noted:

> We need to be one, just like a finger. You cannot split it. We were behind some years back, but when Museveni came - who depended on herbs during the war - he remembered us. I am asking that we get one way, one umbrella, one association of Masindi.

Therefore autonomy as envisaged in this model requires a number of pre-conditions and cannot be obtained cheaply. Rather, together with government, actors in both traditional and modern health sectors need to abandon hitherto cherished philosophical, colonial and practice oriented notions that provide the platform for the marginalisation of traditional medicine. But above all, lack of unity and infighting amongst practitioners, which strongly undermine them, need to be addressed urgently.

(b) Training

The 'modernisation' of traditional medicine will remain a wish unless training to improve traditional knowledge systems, practices, capacities and capabilities is carried out. While there is wide diversity in traditional medicine and practices in different parts of the country, it is still possible to undertake training in the different communities where traditional medicine is practiced. The need for training becomes more crucial given the fact that due to changes occurring in different countries, the young have increasingly migrated to the cities, leaving the old and infirm in the rural areas. The majority of the existing traditional medicine practitioners are aging and are likely to go to their graves with their knowledge. Capturing this knowledge before it is lost is very important and can be done only by those who own it. The million-dollar question is how this is to be done. How incentives are to be created to convince the old generation that their knowledge will not be 'stolen' and how to interest the young generation in a form of medicine that many consider archaic? Training is important also because of the need to create a critical mass of traditional medicine practitioners that can meaningfully engage with government and other actors in the health sector.

Training of traditional medicine practitioners could involve identifying diseases that can be effectively cured by traditional medicine, so as to avoid making traditional medicine appear to be a panacea for all illnesses. This would not only help to focus the activities of traditional medicine practitioners, but would also help in the development of knowledge systems and practices around these illnesses and develop comparative advantages in their management. Where there are national chemotherapeutic laboratories as in the case of Uganda, creating strong linkages between these laboratories and various institutions of traditional medicine practitioners would enhance training, research and development of appropriate cures for illnesses. Through such linkages, a national healing system based on traditional medicine is likely to evolve making actors in the traditional sector even more crucial and central in national health systems. However, for collaborative efforts between practitioners and national laboratories to succeed, practitioners should be assured of direct benefit from their products.

(c) Documentation

Probably one of the major weaknesses of traditional medicine in Africa and other parts of the developing world is that it is not documented. Evidence from countries such as China and India points to the fact that for traditional medicine to gain status in national health services, it must be documented. Documentation has a number of advantages, including making practices of traditional healers available for future generations, dispelling the false and imperialistic notions that traditional medicine is not scientific, showing evidence of the efficacy of traditional medicines and systematising the discourse. To date most of the traditional medicine practices in Africa in general and Uganda in particular are not documented. Accordingly, the Uganda National Council of Science and Technology (UNCST) in its draft Indigenous Knowledge Bill noted thus:

> ... whereas a traditional birth attendant may keep her record by tying knots around her waist, other people may not easily understand this form of record keeping. As a result of this, many IK bearers are dying with vital IK that could be useful in national development. Inadequate documentation of IK is attributed to secretive practice and low levels of education (illiteracy) of the practitioners (UNCST 2004:7).

However, it should be noted that some physicians such as Dr Jjukko trained in modern medicine in Uganda have crossed over to traditional medicine, and together with other colleagues have started documenting traditional medicine and its practice.[15]

It is important to note though, that for training and documentation to be possible, there is a need to offer basic education skills of writing and numeracy to practitioners for developing and systematising indigenous knowledge systems. In the case of Uganda, adult literacy education is a well developed and well supported aspect of the education sector from which traditional medicine practitioners can benefit.

(d) Peer Evaluation, Monitoring and Regulation

Pertinent in the agenda to 'modernise' traditional medicine are issues of monitoring, evaluation and regulation, which are very important to maintain standards and gauge whether practitioners are doing what they ought to be doing and how well they are doing it. The questions that arise from pondering these issues are: what is to be monitored, evaluated and regulated, who is to monitor, evaluate and regulate whom? How are evaluation, monitoring and regulation to be accomplished? Where are the evaluated, monitored and regulated to be found? These questions are both difficult and easy to answer; difficult because the traditional medicine project is very amorphous, but easy to answer because the project has its own experts.

Peer evaluation, monitoring and regulation may involve a one-on-one stewardship by actors in the traditional medicine sub-sector. The concept of stewardship is taken as an extension of the way that not only governments must be responsible for the welfare of the population, but also how individuals become responsible for the guidance, leadership, and direction of their peers. While this may not have direct welfare implications as in the case of government responsibility for its citizens, it may have serious consequences for the conduct of daily business, enhancing legitimacy, transparency and reinforcing the social contract. Through stewardship, traditional medicine practitioners may have the capacity to exert influence on each other, shape individual behaviour and restrain insatiable private desires that may threaten the practice of traditional medicine.

Unfortunately, stewardship in Africa is biased towards bio-medical systems as if these are the be-all and end-all of health care on the continent. Stewardship as deployed here gains its basis from the deeply entrenched though fast eroding African traditions. Such traditions could bolster a regulatory framework that would evolve into a situation where traditional medicine practitioners are granted autonomy. For example, in a locality such as a village, all practitioners involved in a certain specialty like traditional birthing could organise themselves into a network, choose their leaders, set standards of practice and regulations, and put in place a reporting system (for example, of the condition of their clients, births undertaken, problems encountered, colleagues defaulting etc.). Then a high premium for defaulting, bad practice, incompetence and reneging on the network springing from the cultural milieu of the society could be set. Compliance with such regulations could be secured through the deployment of the time-tested and strict negative social sanctions that are still relevant in many societies such as blacklisting, ostracism, and ridicule through songs. These social control mechanisms may not only make one an enemy of the people, but they could also threaten his or her citizenship and in all likelihood would be respected.

However, evaluation and monitoring as understood conventionally are difficult, if not impossible to achieve with traditional medicine and practice, because of the diversity of traditional medicine and the lack of initially set programme goals and objectives as may be the case with, for example, Early Childhood and Nutrition Programmes that are implemented in the modern health sector. Probably one way would be to have practitioners identify common practices related to certain illnesses in a particular cultural setting and evolve standards for these practices based on their values and philosophy. An objective way of assessing compliance to these standards could then be easily designed from which socially institutionalised monitoring and evaluation could be undertaken. Whatever the line of argument one may take, the most important aspects to keep in mind are the values of traditional medicine and practice, its philosophy, the cultural values, attitudes of social responsibility, and peer influence that traditional practitioners hold and how these can be translated into meaningful efforts on the ground.

Shortcomings of this Model

The question posed at the beginning of whether to 'modernise' traditional medicine, seems to linger on even after espousing a model that aims at empowering traditional medicine practitioners. The main challenge this 'modernisation' model faces, which raises new research questions, is how to control an informal sector that might develop in a 'modernised' traditional sector. The fear is that some actors who may not wish to be bound by a moral responsibility to fellow practitioners and their clientele might withdraw to the underworld where they will continue practising or even engage in harmful practices that may threaten the lives of their clients.

Another challenge relates to how the sector can be linked with other actors in health without necessarily jeopardising the autonomy and eroding the gains that would have been made. This is a particularly thorny issue that may need protracted negotiation; otherwise, the government may find it difficult to relinquish all manner of regulation of the activities of the sector to actors in that very sector. Sensing this, some traditional practitioners with whom the researcher interacted in Kampala suggested that the question of regulation was one to be handled by both government and the leadership of the practitioners. They argued for example that in the proposed bill, which provides for a practitioners board, bye-laws crafted by practitioners would be enforced by government in collaboration with the board, so as to avoid a role conflict that would threaten internal democracy if the council were to be both the lawmaker and enforcer. Contention may also arise on other issues such as human rights, property rights and funding that may complicate the operationalisation of the model.

Conclusions

The integration of traditional medicine as seen in the context of the discourse on public-private mix bespeaks of the paranoia that comes in the wake of the western donors' developmentalist notions, which not only assume that what can work in the West can work in the developing world, but also that what can work in one developing country can work in another. Within this skewed thinking, traditional medicine has been lumped under the same category with private modern medicine practitioners as part of the 'private sector' as if it shared any similarities with these actors other than healthcare provision. For those in the developing world, the struggle to de-colonise the mind and shrug off the huge blanket of ignorance and lack of depth of analysis that is a hangover from colonisation is called for here. Only then will we start making sense of our reality and adopt relevant, context specific solutions that can re-direct our societies on the road to development. While there is a need for the resources which the donors dispose of, we must not close our eyes to the realities that surround us.

It is difficult to integrate traditional medicine into national health services in societies where it has not developed into a unified system, that is, in societies where traditional medicine is practised disparately according to ethnic group and specific cultural settings. In such societies, trying to integrate traditional medicine and practices into national health services will only result in increasing the hegemony of the modern medical sector and seriously eroding the time-tested cultural medicinal practices. This is because traditional medicine is judged on the values, philosophies, accountability standards and efficiency measures of the Western model, which is just incompatible with local realities. In fact, trying out this model of integration, as is already the case in most developing countries, is as difficult to achieve as biting a bullet.

Therefore, it is imperative to consider the unique historical circumstances within which traditional medicine has evolved in Africa generally and in countries like Uganda, where it was outlawed, made inferior to modern medicine, and its practice shunned, ridiculed and castigated as backward. It is important to consider its diversity and context specificity in order to come up with policy options that give it the crucial 'space' and cutting edge it deserves in the national health systems of the country. In this breath, a model of 'modernising' traditional medicine through granting autonomy to the sector is suggested as discussed in the paper. Hopefully, through this, traditional medicine and its practice can find their place in the national health system.

Recommendations

A critical recommendation made by practitioners is that for any meaningful action to be taken in the sector (integration, autonomy or a public-private partnership), there is an urgent need to formulate and enact law and policy on traditional medicine and practice. According to practitioners, the policy would among others formally recognise traditional medicine, streamline leadership issues in the sector, provide for funding of the sector (under decentralised health service delivery funding for health comes from consolidated funding through the Primary Health Care grant), ensure representation of practitioners at all levels, attract necessary incentives for 'take-off' of the sector, and create appreciation for the environmental and socio-contextual circumstances in which traditional medicine practitioners operate.

To popularise traditional medicine and practice, it is important for government to undertake massive sensitisation of the public, including actors in the modern health sector who hold and cherish a negative and harmful colonial mentality about the activities of their counterparts. Short of this, the sector will remain operating in a context where actors are shunned by some during the day, but appreciated by the same people at night. There is a need to remove all negative attitudes of witchcraft that have been associated with the practice of traditional medicine, which in one way or the other encourages impostors to flourish.

Notes

1. The modern sector in Uganda is not based on purely bio-medical models and principles. Sometimes modern medicine has been practised in an informal/traditional manner, access is sometimes based on social networks and corruption, among others. These issues have been highlighted by Asiimwe et al., 1997 and Birungi et al., 2001.

2. Some practices in this sub-sector are at times similar to those of the modern sector. It is therefore difficult to talk about a purely modern sector or traditional sector.

3. 'Planning for Cost-Effective Traditional Medicine in the New Century. A Discussion Paper', WHO Centre for Health Development. Accessible at: http://www.who.or.jp/tm/research/bkg/3_definitions.html

4. The term 'integration' has come to be widely used to express the formalisation and official incorporation of traditional medicine into national health services.

5. The idea behind this partnership is to increase public participation in health care delivery. The PPP project implementing the partnership has categorised the different actors in the private sector into three categories: Private not for profit (PNFP) which comprises agencies that provide health services from an established/static health unit/facility and those that work in the community and other counterparts to provide non/facility based health services; Private health practitioners (PHP) who comprise all cadres in the clinical, dental, diagnostics, medical, midwifery, nursing, pharmacy, and public health categories which provide private health services outside the public and traditional and complementary medicine practitioners.

6. Traditional medicine may not necessarily be easily accessible and affordable. In fact, it may be socially very expensive and may not be accessible for social, geographical and economic reasons. A case in point is those people who are socially stigmatised for practising sorcery simply because they have visited a traditional healer.

7. Reporting the frustration some companies involved in the production of traditional medicine therapies for HIV/AIDS in South Africa are facing, Richter (2003) confirms the argument that mainstream medical organisations regard traditional medicine with much apathy or antipathy.

8. Richter also emphasises that it is important to take note of the fact that traditional healers, traditional medicine and beliefs of sickness and health, can vary from region to region and from clan to clan (p. 13).

9. Although the author cannot claim to give a thorough explanation of this form of healing, according to interaction he has had with various healers, this is a telepathic form of healing where a spirit medium intervenes between the afflicted party and the causes of his/her affliction. The healer simply aids the interaction between the patient and this supernatural power/medium since he is the only one endowed with the power to communicate with it.

10. While they may have another more structural meaning, especially from the point of view of traditional practices, these are generally considered to be spirits of departed members of the community which occasionally pay visits to the living. That is, they are the living-dead.

11. According to the practitioners, the Ministry of Health would not only attract experts from other countries to bolster efforts of local practitioners, especially in training, but it was in a better position to ensure government responsibility over the sector and continued support.

12. The organisational structure of NACOTHA starts at village to national level. From village to district level, the following offices exist: chairperson, vice chairperson, information secretary, youth secretary, treasurer, defence secretary, research officer, botanical section head, pharmacist section head, women representative, project manager and mobiliser. NACOTHA's structure, however, goes up to regional and national levels. At regional level, the following offices are provided for in the structure: regional chairperson, vice regional chairperson, inspector, treasurer, information secretary, women representative and secretary. At national level, the structure includes: Chairperson, vice chairperson, secretary women representative and secretary. At national level, the structure includes: Chairperson, vice chairperson, secretary general, treasurer, women representative, chief drug inspector, project manager, information officer, defence secretary, sanitation officer, secretary for youth, botanical section head, pharmacists section head, research officer, medical officer (western medicine), legal advisor and four committee members.

13. To take this notion of government/self-regulation is to accept Max Weber's thinking that 'there is no single Reason or universal standard by which to judge all forms of thought and that what we call Reason, is only the specific and peculiar rationalism of the west' (Dean 1999, p. 11). After Foucault, we know that even within western rationalism, 'there is a multiplicity of rationalities, of different ways of thinking in a fairly systematic manner, of making calculations, of defining purposes and employing knowledge' (ibid, p. 11).

14. The stifling of traditional medicine is not restricted to Uganda. In a review of the regulatory framework for traditional medicine in South Africa, Richter (2003) notes that the 'Traditional Health Practitioners Bill 2003' states that a person who 'diagnoses, treats, or offers to treat, or prescribes treatment or any cure for cancer, HIV/AIDS or such other terminal diseases as may be described, shall be guilty of an offence'. The question is; does modern medicine hold a sole preserve for curing these diseases? If so, why has it failed to end human suffering emanating from the same terminal diseases?

15. Jjuko and his colleagues have established a research centre at Kireka in Wakiso district near Kampala for conducting research in traditional medicine, and developing drugs and supplements from herbs. This group has also established a clinic for treating patients using drugs developed by the same group and a large botanical garden where they obtain the herbs necessary for the research. This garden also acts as a trial plot for herbs obtained from as far as India and China.

References

Abdol, K., Ziquba-Page, T. T., and Arendse, R., 1994, 'Bridging the Gap: Potential for a Health Care Partnership between African Traditional Healers and Biomedical Personnel in South Africa', *South African Medical Journal*, 84 s1-s16 as quoted by Colvin et al. in 'Integrating Traditional Healers into a Tuberculosis Control Programme in Hlabisa, South Africa', *AIDS Bulletin*, March 2002, p. 29.

Amai, C.A., 2002, 'Medicinal Plants and Bio-Diversity Report', Kampala, Ministry of Health.

Birungi, H., et al., 2001, 'The Policy on Public-Private Mix in the Ugandan Health Sector: Catching up with Reality', *Journal of Health Policy and Planning*, 16 (suppl 2): 79-86.

Bennet, S., 1996, 'The Public/Private Mix in Health Care Systems', in K., Janovsky ed., *Health Policy and Systems Development*, Geneva, World Health Organisation.

Chaudhury, R. R., 1997, 'Commentary: Challenges in Using Traditional Systems of Medicine', New Delhi, National Institute of Immunology.

Dean, M., 1999, *Governmentality: Power and Rule in Modern Society*, London, Sage Publications.

GoU, 1995, *Constitution of the Republic of Uganda*, Entebbe.

Hesketh, T. and Zhu, X. W., 1997, 'Health in China: Traditional Chinese Medicine: One Country, Two Systems', *British Medical Journal*, 315: 115-117.

Hutchison, P., 1998, 'Equity of Access to Health Services in Uganda: the Effects of Income, Gender, Proximity to Services and Quality of Care', Draft Report, World Bank, Uganda Resident Mission.

Letendre, D. A., 2002, 'Aboriginal Traditional Medicine: Where Does It Fit?', *Crossing Boundaries – An Interdisciplinary Journal*, Vol. 1, No. 2, Spring.

Mabirizi, F., 2001, 'The Technical Interface between Decentralised Development Planning and Structural Adjustment in Uganda', SPRING Research Series, No. 25, University of Dortmund.

MoH, 1999, *National Health Policy*, Kampala, Uganda.

MoH, 2000, *Health Sector Strategic Plan 2000/01-2004/05*.

MoH, 2004, 'Public-Private Partnership in Health (PPPH): Increasing Private Health Sector Participation in all Aspects of the National Health Programme, http://www.health.go.ug/part_health.htm, 2/02/04.

Mugisha, M., et al., 2004, 'Traditional Medicine Under Decentralized Health Service Delivery in Uganda: A Case Study of Masindi and Kasese Districts', Final Report Submitted to Network of Ugandan Researchers and Research Users (NURRU), under the National Policy Research (NPR) Agenda, Kampala.

Mugisha, M., et al., 2005, 'Building Consensus for Better Traditional Medicine Policy Formulation and Implementation Under Decentralized Health Service Delivery in Uganda', Excerpts from a Progress Report Submitted to Network of Ugandan Researchers and Research Users (NURRU), under the National Policy Research (NPR) Agenda, Kampala.

Nichter, M., ed., 1992, *Anthropological Approaches to the Study of Ethno-Medicine*, Arizona, Gordon and Beach Publishers.

Pannarunothai, S. and Mills, A., 1997, 'Characteristics of Public and Private Health Care in a Thai Urban Setting', in S., Bennet, B., McPake and A., Mills eds., *Private Health Care Providers in Developing Countries*, London, Zed Books.

Republic of Uganda, 1997, *Local Government Act*.

Richter, M., 2003, 'Traditional Medicines and Traditional Healers in South Africa', Discussion Paper Prepared for the Treatment Action Campaign and AIDS Law Project.

UNAIDS, 2000, 'Collaboration with Traditional Healers in HIV/AIDS Prevention and Care in Sub-Saharan Africa: A Literature Review', UNAIDS Best Practice Collection.

UNCST, 2004, 'National Indigenous Knowledge Policy for Uganda', (Draft for Finalisation), Kampala.

WHO, 2001, *Traditional Medicine Strategy*, 2001B-2005.

WHO, 2002, 'Planning for Cost-Effective Traditional Health Services in the New Century', Discussion Paper, Geneva.

17

Empowering Traditional Birth Attendants in the Gambia: A Local Strategy to Redress Issues of Access, Equity and Sustainability?

Stella Nyanzi

The Resource Gap in the African Health Care System

As an arena and a vector of power relations in society, the health system both embodies and conveys questions of access, equity, justice and sustainability that require to be followed through for a proper understanding of the functioning and functionality of the system... Amidst the crisis that has gripped the health sector, the decline in the overall health status of many Africans, the cut-back in the public health expenditure of the state, the various health emergencies facing the continent, and the challenges of reform that are posed, questions of access, equity and sustainability clearly arise both as important issues in their own right and as elements integral to the exercise of citizenship, democratic rights and the social contract. – (CODESRIA 2004:2).

The African continent, particularly the sub-Saharan region, has experienced several diverse natural and man-made calamities that widely devastated the physical infrastructure, social organisation, systems of governance and provision of public amenities. Civil wars, droughts, hunger, famines, epidemics, social upheavals, political unrest, dictates of international bodies, reform policies, dependency syndromes, corruption and multi-faceted poverty have gradually negatively impacted African communities; variously exhausting the existing limited resources which are critical to the establishment and sustenance of development efforts. Consequently, there exists a disproportionately high demand upon scanty resources, which is replicated in the health care system of sub-Saharan African countries.

The outbreak and persistence of epidemics of fatal diseases including HIV/AIDS, tuberculosis, malaria, ebola, cholera, and even preventable childhood diseases pose a major challenge to the meagre available resources. The effects of internal and foreign policies, specifically the Structural Adjustment Policies (SAPs) of the International Monetary Fund and the International Bank for Reconstruction and Development (IBRD), have amalgamated with economic and financial crises creating bigger debt burdens, more critical balance of payments deficits and depleted government revenues. These factors challenge the practicality of efforts to budget efficiently for appropriate and meaningful health care systems in sub-Saharan African (Birungi 1997). The health care system is further impoverished by severe brain drain as professionally trained, highly qualified and experienced health personnel not only die from the HIV/AIDS epidemic, but also either seek more fulfilling careers out of Africa due to several 'pull factors' in more developed countries, or they are forced out by inherent 'push factors' including political insecurity, natural disasters, sub-standard levels of amenities or diminishing returns from service. Furthermore, there is a disproportionate number of qualified health personnel (doctors, nurses, midwives, other paramedical manpower) to provide for a large population with ill-health, particularly in the rural areas because of limited training facilities, insufficient capacity building, and the few professional elite tend to congregate in the urban centres where the benefits accruing are relatively higher (Wallace 1990, Asghar 1999).

The Gravity of Reproductive Health in Africa

Fathalla (1988) defines reproductive health as 'the ability to live through the re-productive years and beyond with reproductive choice, dignity and successful child-bearing, and free of gynaecological disease and risk'. In this definition, con-cepts of choice (a woman's control over her reproductive processes), dignity (social and psychological well-being from the process of reproduction) and physical health of the reproductive organs, are integrated. However in sub-Saharan Africa, as in other developing areas, access to, equity over, and sustainability of repro-ductive health care are limited by several inherent factors including inequitable distribution of services, patriarchal cultural dictates, inequalities, diverse social cultural mechanisms, inadequate resources, economic disparities, the vicious circle of poverty, lack of drugs, misappropriation of public resources, poor governance, insufficient physical infrastructure, and limited numbers of professional health personnel. Although the fact that the lives of women in sub-Saharan Africa predominantly revolve around their reproductive functions, and despite the reported high fertility rates (Mayell 2001), the majority of women lack access to healthcare generally and specifically to the much needed reproductive healthcare. Consequently, sub-Saharan Africa is riddled with drastically low levels of repro-ductive health indicators.

According to WHO/UNICEF (1996), reproductive health problems account for over one-third of the total burden of disease in women. More than ninety-nine percent of the annual global estimates of 585,000 maternal deaths occur in developing countries; a women in sub-Saharan Africa who becomes pregnant is seventy-five times more likely to die as a result, than a woman in Europe (excluding Eastern Europe) or North America (Walraven et al. 2000). Estimates of maternal mortality rates in developing countries are at an average of about 450 per 100,000 live births (and this goes up to 2000 in some areas) compared to 30 per 100,000 live births in developed countries (WHO 1991, Paul 1993, Asghar 1999). Rates vary between different areas, regions and even within a country. For example Asghar (1999) reports a two-fold increase in maternal mortality in rural as compared to urban areas. An estimated 500,000 women die every year in developing countries as a result of complications of pregnancy and abortion (Mbizvo 1996, Fauveau 1993). The disabilities arising out of pregnancy, which drastically impair reproductive health functions of women and limit their economic activity, are often under-reported because they do not result in death. However, these are reported to be even more common: for example it is estimated for sub-Saharan Africa that for every maternal death, another fifteen women are disabled or permanently crippled by incontinence, uterine prolapse and infertility due to pregnancy or birth-related causes (Asghar 1999).

Between two and three million African women are left handicapped from obstetric complaints every year (Paul 1993). The most common causes of obstetric complications are prolonged obstructed labour, hypertensive disorders of pregnancy, haemorrhages, sepsis and unsafe abortions (Sibley 1997, Walraven et al. 2000).

Maternal mortality is also influenced by fertility rates. The fertility rates in rural sub-Saharan Africa are the highest in the world (Kirk and Pillet 1998, Ratcliffe et al. 2001, Ratcliffe, Hill and Walraven 2000). The demand for large families remains strong in most rural populations (Ware 1994, Oppong 1992). Modern family planning is uncommon in the rural areas and the continuing high levels of fertility are important contributors to the poor levels of reproductive health. Several social and cultural factors contribute to the high fertility rates, namely propagation of the family line, extension of the patrilineal clan, more children imply greater production due to more free labour, women's status in society is commonly established on the basis of reproductive performance particularly in virilocal marriage systems, religious factors, and the influence of the extended family (Bledsoe, Banja and Hill 1998, Caldwell, Orubuloye and Caldwell 1992, Oppong 1992). Cultural malpractices including female genital cutting, arranged marriages, early sexual debut, widow inheritance, levirate marriage, and ritual cleansing by sex with a virgin all exacerbate the injustices faced by African women through the abuse of their rights to reproductive health. Lastly, childhood mortality rates in sub-Saharan African are among the highest in the world (Blacker et al. 1985, UNICEF 1997). According to studies conducted in West Africa, the mortality of children aged 1-4 years is especially high (Hill et al. 1998, Leach et al. 1999).

Statement of the Problem

The reproductive health burden of African women is still a major challenge to African health systems that must of necessity be prioritised. In the light of depleted resources, shattered infrastructure and insufficient numbers of professionally trained health care personnel, traditional birth attendants (TBAs) offer a relatively low-cost, locally appreciated social group that could intervene to redress the gap in resources and improve African reproductive health.

Traditional Birth Attendants: Bridging the Gap?

According to the WHO Alma Ata definition, 'a traditional birth attendant (TBA) is a person - usually a woman - who assists the mother at child birth and who initially acquired her skills delivering babies by herself or working with other TBAs' (WHO 1978). Studies (*Maternal Neonatal Health* 2004) have classified three major types of TBAs. There is the TBA who is a full-time worker who can be called upon by anyone and expects to be paid either in cash or in kind. Secondly there is the TBA who is a woman's elderly relative or neighbour who does not make a living from the work and will only assist with the birth if the mother is a relative or a daughter or a daughter-in-law of a neighbour or close friend. This TBA assists in the birth as a favour and does not expect to be paid, but may receive a token or gift in appreciation. Lastly there is the family birth attendant who only delivers babies of close friends. In any society, the role of the TBA often reflects the culture and the social organisation.

Estimates indicate that sixty percent of births in the developing world occur outside a healthy facility and forty-seven percent are attended by a TBA (WHO 1997). In rural Africa, between sixty and ninety percent of deliveries are assisted by a TBA. High quality maternity care is often unavailable and home birth remains a strong preference for many (Butlerys et al. 2002). TBAs in many regions have been trained in midwifery and basic hygiene as part of the Safe Motherhood Initiative aimed at reducing maternal mortality. In resource-poor countries, this training has comparative advantages in attempting to provide professional health care for each birth (Walraven and Weeks 1999) because of the popularity of and easy access to TBAs who not only speak the local languages and allow traditional birthing practices, but also often have the trust of the local communities (Bij de Vaate 2002, Heeren 2001).There is a debate about the benefits of this form of empowerment of TBAs through education (De Brouwere et al. 1998).

This study investigated the role of TBAs in the health care of women in The Gambia. This paper discusses whether the empowerment packages provided to TBAs in The Gambia constitute a local strategy that redresses issues of access to, equity over, and sustainability of reproductive health.

Study Design and Methods

Library research was triangulated together with ethnography. Ethnographic fieldwork was conducted among sixty TBAs, 120 women who delivered in the presence of a TBA, twenty women who did not, and key informants including Divisional Health Team members, Village Development Committee members, and Community Health Nurses (CHNs). The research techniques included a literature review, a policy-statement review, ethnographic participant observation, participatory rural appraisal (PRA), ten focus group discussions and fifty-four individual in-depth interviews. The author participated in several birthing processes, and had babies named after her anthropological name at naming ceremonies in the study villages. Interviews conducted in the local languages of Wolof, Fula and Mandinka were recorded on audio-tape, transcribed verbatim, translated into English, entered into a computer and subjected to narrative analysis using Atlas.ti - standard computer software designed for the analysis of qualitative data.

Study Area and Population

Fieldwork was conducted in the hamlets, villages and urban centres surrounding Farafenni town, located in the North Bank of The Gambia, and approximately 200 kilometres from the capital Banjul. Geographically the area is flat Sudan savannah with wet season cultivation of rice, millet, sorghum and groundnuts. The study population is served by a hospital in Farafenni town and five dispensaries in nearby villages, and several 'trekking clinics'. Transportation is limited to walking or using bicycles, horse or donkey carts, or some bush taxis travelling on dirt roads (Greenwood 1990). Telephone services between Farafenni and the big villages were introduced in 1990. However, many of the smaller villages and hamlets still lacked telephone networks during the fieldwork period. Ambulance services are available to the main hospital. Eighty-eight percent of compounds have a reliable supply of safe water and most compounds have pit latrines (Hill et al. 1996). There are three predominant tribes: Mandinka (48 percent), Wolof (16 percent), and Fula (6 percent) (Walraven et al. 2000). The main income generating activity is subsistence farming, with a few petty traders. Education levels are mostly low for adults, with the majority of men having some basic Koranic school attendance. Islam is the predominant religion of The Gambia. The population is poor; in 1996 less than 10 percent of compounds owned bicycles, two thirds of compounds possessed a radio, 35 percent owned some form of cart, and less than half slept on iron or wooden beds (Hill et al. 1996). According to Walraven et al 2000, the total fertility rate was 7.5 births per woman, mean birth intervals were 33 months and just 9 percent of women were using either traditional or modern contraceptives. Polygamy is common with 51 percent of women with one or more co-wives, 56 percent of women aged 15-19 years are married and just over three percent of the women had attended school.

The Role of TBAs in the Health Care System in the Gambia

The Gambia adopted primary health care as the basis for national policy in 1978 (Ministry of Health 1993). This programme developed in the early 1980s and is now established countrywide. It includes classification of primary health care key villages based on size and population of 400 or more, so that they receive CHNs who are trained by the Medical and Health Department and paid from central funds. CHNs are the link between village-level primary health care services and referral health services available at dispensaries, health centres and hospitals. Each of the CHNs is responsible for the supplies, supervision and continuing education of the village health workers (VHNs) and trained TBAs in about five key villages.

TBAs are an integral part of the primary health care system in The Gambia. Before the establishment of this primary health care, several TBAs were already practising. In key primary health care villages, the community under the leadership of their development committees select two out of the existing TBAs to attend the centrally organised training as midwives. This generates resources within the community to contribute to the support of the village health system. In 1997 there were 460 trained TBAs and 52 assistant TBAs nationwide who conducted half of the deliveries (Gambia/UNICEF 1997).

All the TBAs in our study were illiterate. However, each of them had attended the initial training and more than half had attended at least one refresher course in the last two years. They reported that they gained immensely from the training sessions. Indeed there were reported differences particularly in the ability to identify complicated cases that needed immediate referral, better hygiene and sanitation practices during delivery and provision of more ante-natal monitoring and advice to pregnant women. The trained TBAs complained about some untrained women in the villages who were assisting in deliveries and often making blunders owing to ignorance because they lacked the basic training, thereby soiling the reputation of the good work of other trained TBAs. Likewise, some of the rural women stressed the fact that they valued the services of TBAs in their husband's clan because these elderly women were culturally attached to particular families. Thus they claimed in such cases it was irrelevant whether or not the TBA had received formal training. Culturally, preference was given to these familial ties. TBAs repeatedly requested more expanded programmes of training because it was impractical for an untrained TBA not to offer her services when she was urgently required to attempt to save the life of an unborn child and its mother.

Many TBAs were receiving supervision from their CHN, although a few reported they were disregarded by their CHN and two elderly women did not know who was supposed to supervise them. We observed good working relationships between the formal health care system and the primary health care system in cases where trekking, professionally trained, health personnel worked in close collaboration with the TBAs who mobilised pregnant women to attend mobile ante-natal clinics, jointly assisted in examinations of women, weighing of infants, summoned mothers and children for immunisation campaigns, referred complicated cases or even escorted them to the health facilities. However, there were instances of some TBAs discouraging women from using bio-medical medicine in preference to herbal concoctions, specifically in the case of women who needed 'softening of bones to aid delivery'. Others openly campaigned against modern contraception because it runs contrary to religious and cultural beliefs. There were few instances of reports from the TBAs of discrimination and disregard by medical personnel in hospitals, specifically when they travelled with critically complicated cases of women whose pregnancies had begun away from the hospital setting. In addition, some TBAs felt that their knowledge was despised as inferior by educated health persons, specifically if they were working with foreign-aided health centres. Furthermore, local women who initially went for ante-natal care at the TBA and then moved to the hospital towards the time of delivery reported that they were often ridiculed by hospital midwives for seeking unprofessional help, combining bio-medical drugs with traditional herbs or Koranic portions and sticking to the traditional health care system. They commented about the frequent contradictions between information from bio-medical health professionals and the indigenous traditional knowledge of the TBAs. Several TBAs lamented that pregnant women who went to the hospital were often subjected to caesarean section from the hands of foreign doctors because they over-looked some of the traditional birthing customs, rituals and practices which were effective at reducing this possibility. These disparities need to be addressed so that the gaps in information that TBAs hold can be addressed in the training and refresher courses. Furthermore, it is important that the politics of health care systems in which bio-medicine assumes supremacy as reflected by some professional health personnel is addressed through sensitisation about the need for mutual existence, support and collaboration so as to enhance the active participation of the TBAs and other lay village health workers.

Several TBAs were the sole providers of ante-natal care, delivery assistance, birth rituals, naming ceremonies or post-natal care for pregnant women in their areas. The majority of the women in the villages reported that they preferred to deliver with the help of a TBA, although the TBAs reported that some women waited until the last minute to notify them of their pregnancies, or only called them when they experienced complications. One woman revealed that she was shy and embarrassed of revealing her nakedness to another woman and thus resorted to seeking TBA assistance as a last resort when her labour was too long to bear. A few women (particularly those in the urban area) chose to deliver in hospital. There were disparities in reports about society's perception of TBAs: while some said they were still highly valued in their villages and rewarded for their services, some other TBAs lamented that they were fast becoming despised, over-worked with meagre or no reward, and sometimes even scorned for some of their traditional beliefs and practices. The majority of the TBAs emphasised the fact that the communal farm labour that the village is supposed to offer them on their rice fields was steadily becoming an ideal of the past. Decisions about whether or not a woman goes to a TBA, when, and how often she attends, are mostly made by the husbands. Husbands provided the money for all the women who had used the services of a TBA. The majority of the TBAs in the study did not support the use of modern contraceptives, even though they were trained about the benefits. There was evidence of widely held myths and misconceptions about the hazards of contraceptive use. TBAs provided more than reproductive health services in their villages. These TBAs were providing nutrition lessons, sanitation and hygiene information, health education against malaria, social role of leadership, collaborating in village development schemes, distributing herbal treatments, some bio-medical pain-killers, participating in income generation activities, and acted as society's gate-keepers who stored knowledge about sacred traditional norms, values and customs. The major challenges they face include lack of appropriate transport to facilitate referral of emergency cases, some resistance to collaboration with professionally trained health personnel, a shortage of refresher courses for all, and a heavy work-load for some who serve many villages and hamlets.

Conclusions

Empowering TBAs with training and support supervision backup by professionally trained health personnel bridges gaps in access to and equity of reproductive health care in The Gambia to a large extent. TBAs, although filling a big gap, may also be promoting inequity in the quality of the healthcare received by their clientele, specifically as they hold misconceptions about contraception, and believe in cultural nutrition taboos. They play a multiple role in the social, cultural, ritual, community development, and local leadership and are gatekeepers of the sacred traditional norms and values of their societies. Communities must be encouraged to support their TBAs in order to facilitate sustainability.

Acknowledgement

I acknowledge the support of Dr Gijs Walraven. Hawah Manneh, Emily Loppy, Yamundow Jallow, Ousman Bah, Sulayman Joof and Jarrai Bangoro who assisted with data collection, processing and entry. I am grateful to the MRC CHNs, CHNs, DHT, TBAs and women who participated in the study.

References

Asghar, R. J., 1999, 'Obstetric Complications and the Roles of Traditional Birth Attendants in Developing Countries', *Journal of Physicians and Surgeons*, Pakistan 9 (1): 55-57.

Bij De Vaate, A., Coleman, R., Manneh, H. and Walraven, G., 2002, 'Knowledge, Attitudes and Practices of Trained Traditional Birth Attendants in The Gambia in the Prevention, Recognition and Management of Postpartum Haemorrhage', *Midwifery*, 18: 3-11.

Bledsoe, C. H., Banja F. and Hill A. G., 1998, 'Reproductive Mishaps and Western Contraception: An African Challenge to Fertility Theory', *Population Development Review*, 23: 15-57.

Bledsoe, C. H., 2002, *Contingent Lives: Fertility, Time and Aging in West Africa*, Chicago and London, The University Of Chicago Press.

Butlerys, M., Fowler, M. G., Shaffer, N., Tih, P. M., Greenberg, A. E., Karita, E., Coovadia, H. and De Cock, K. M., 2002, 'Role of Traditional Birth Attendants in Preventing Perinatal Transmission pf HIV', *British Medical Journal*, 324: 222-225.

Caldwell, J. C., Orubuloye, I.O., Caldwell, P., 1992, 'Fertility Decline in Africa: A New Type of Transition?', *Population Development Review*, 18.

CODESRIA, 2004, Call for Abstracts, Institute for Health, Politics and Society in Africa. www.codesria.org.

Department of State for Health And Social Welfare, Gambia, 1998, *Public Expenditure Review of The Health Sector*, Banjul.

Dowling, S., 1983, 'Health for a Change', Children Poverty Action Group.

Fathalla, M. F., 1988, 'Research Needs in Human Reproduction', in E., Diczfulsi, P. D., Griddin and Khanna, P. D., eds., *Research Needs in Human Reproduction: Biannual Report 1986-1987*, Geneva, WHO 18.

Fauveau, V., 1993, 'Maternal Tetanus', *International Journal of Gynaecology and Obstetrics*, 40: 3-12.

Heeren, J. A., 2001, 'Knowledge Attitude and Practices in Postpartum Care in the North Bank East Division of The Gambia', Nijmegen, University of Nijmegen.

Hill, A. G., Hill, M. C., Gomez, P. and Walraven, G., 1996, 'Report of the Living Standards Survey Conducted in the Villages of the MRC Main Study Area, North Bank Division, Republic of The Gambia in June-July 1996', Farafenni, MRC.

Hill, A.G., Macleod, W.B., Joof, D., Gomez, P., Ratclifffe, A.A. and Walraven, G., 2000, 'Decline of Mortality in Children in Rural Gambia: The Influence of Village-Level Primary Health Care', *Tropical Medicine and International Health*, 5(2): 107-118.

Kirk, D. and Pillet, B. 'Fertility Levels, Trends and Differentials in Sub-Saharan African in The 1980s and 1990s', *Studies In Family Planning*, 29: 1-2.

Maternal Neonatal Health, 2004, 'Traditional Birth Attendants: Linking Community and Services', Www.Mnh.Jhpiego.Org/Best/Tba.Asp.

Mbizvo, M.T., 1996, 'Reproductive and Sexual Health', *Central African Journal of Medicine*, 42(3): 80-85.

Oppong, C., 1992, 'Traditional Family Systems in Rural Settings in Africa', in E. Berquo and P. Xenos, Eds., *Family Systems and Cultural Change*, Oxford, Clarendon Press, 69-86.

Paul, B. K., 1993, 'Maternal Mortality in Africa, 1980-1987', *Social Science and Medicine*, 37 (6) 745-52.

Ratcliffe, A. A., Hill, A. G. and Walraven, G., 2000, 'Separate Lives, Different Interests: Male and Female Reproduction in The Gambia', *Bulletin of the World Health Organisation*, 78: 570-579.

Ratcliffe, A. A., 2000, Men's Fertility and Marriages: Male Reproductive Strategies in Rural Gambia, PhD Thesis, Boston, Department of Population and International Health.

Ratcliffe, A. A., Hill, A. G., Harrington, D. P. and Walraven, G., 2002, 'Reporting of Fertility Events by Men and Women in Rural Gambia', *Demography*, 39 (3): 573-586.

Sibley, L., 1997, 'Obstetric First Aid in the Community - Partners in Safe Motherhood', *Journal of Nursing and Midwifery*, 42 (2): 117-121.

Wallace, H. M., 1990, *Health Care for Women and Children in Developing Countries*, Third Party Publishing Company.

Walraven, G. and Weeks, A., 1999, 'The Role of Traditional Birth Attendants with Midwifery Skills in the Reduction of Maternal Mortality', *Tropical Medicine and International Health*, 4 (8): 527-29.

Walraven, G., Telfer, M., Rowley, J., Ronsmans, C., 2000, 'Maternal Mortality in Rural Gambia: Levels, Causes and Contributing Factors', *Bulletin of the World Health Organisation*, 78 (5): 603-613.

Walraven, G., Scherf, C., West, B., Ekpo, G., Paine, K., Coleman, R., Bailey, R. and Morison, L., 2001, 'The Burden of Reproductive Organ Disease in Rural Women in The Gambia, West Africa', *The Lancet*, 357: 1161-1167.

Ware, H., 1994, 'Thoughts on the Course of Fertility Transition in Sub-Saharan Africa', in Looch, T., And V. Hertrich, eds., *The Onset of Fertility Transition in Sub-Saharan Africa*, Liege, IUSSP, 289-296.

World Health Organisation, 1978, *Report of the Alma Ata Conference on Primary Health Care*, Health for All Series, No. 1, Geneva, WHO.

World Health Organisation, 1990, *Integrating Maternal and Child Health Services with Primary Health Care*, Geneva, WHO.

World Health Organisation, 1991, *Essential Elements of Obstetric Care at First Referral Level*, Geneva, WHO.

World Health Organisation/ UNICEF, 1996, *Revised 1990 Estimates of Maternal Mortality*, Geneva, WHO/FRH/MSM/96.11.

VI

Conclusion

18

Social Context and Determinants of HIV Transmission: Lessons from Africa

Vinh-Kim Nguyen and Martyn T. Sama

Why Africa?

As Africa is the continent hit first and hardest by HIV, it is the social science research conducted on the epidemic on that continent that offers the most historical insight into the epidemic in developing countries. Research conducted in Africa mirrors and, to some extent, foreshadows research subsequently conducted elsewhere in the developing world and in the so-called 'second wave' countries, including China, India, and Russia. Until recently the dominant concern of social scientists has been to explain the prevalence rates in terms of African 'specificities'. When this research began, the epidemic was viewed through the prism of its Northern epidemiology (that is, as a disease mainly of gay men and intravenous drug users) and Africa seemed exceptional. HIV epidemics are heterogeneous, comprising diverse epidemics that wax and wane at different rates (Morison 2001). These differences were initially attributed to differing modes of transmission, leading to the early distinction between epidemics that were driven by sex between men in northern Europe and North America, and those that were spread by intravenous drug use in southern Europe. These Pattern 1' areas were distinguished from 'Pattern 2' zones, such as Africa, where the epidemic was viewed as predominantly heterosexually transmitted. Previous reviewers have also mentioned the lack of data exploring alternative routes of transmission (A. Ona Pela 1989, Schoepf 2001:429) but also concluded that the evidence does support predominantly heterosexual transmission accounting for the epidemic in Africa (Baylies 1997). This literature has essentially been concerned with identifying the primary determinant of the African epidemic. The previously widespread view that African culture was somehow responsible has been largely discarded with ongoing research which has pinpointed economic, and by extension political, factors that are particularly concentrated on the African continent. Specifically, widespread poverty and weak state capacity seem to offer a fertile ground for epidemics. This mirrors the controversy concerning the roots of gender vulnerability: are women vulnerable to HIV in Africa because of cultural constructions of femininity, or is vulnerability biological and exacerbated by interactions between sexuality and power exacerbated by economic circumstances? New directions for research concern the linkages between political ideologies, macroeconomic policy and both social and biological vulnerability to HIV. From an initial focus on gender and women's vulnerability, new approaches stress masculinities and sexualities as key sites that link broad-scale social forces with individual vulnerability. Increasing attention is being paid to violence, both within and without conflict situations, and how this may be fuelling HIV epidemics, which in turn links epidemics to geopolitical struggles. The following section traces the main developments in these controversies. Given the abundance of the literature, only the most relevant references are cited, with the most recent given preference.

Explaining the Epidemiology of AIDS in Africa: From Culture to Political Economy

Extensive epidemiological profiling of the epidemic in Africa was early on complemented by social science literature that described the social context of HIV transmission. This research initially sought to identify endogenous, social factors to explain the high HIV prevalence in Africa. As a result, cultural factors were the object of much scrutiny in the earlier years of the epidemic. Surveys of knowledge, attitudes, behaviours and practices (KABP) comprised the first wave of studies, and in epidemiologically important 'high risk' settings continue to be carried out (Ali 2001, particularly Fritz 2002, Mataure 2002). Although these yield useful data and insights they are subject to methodological limitations (Schopper 1993). Researchers also examined how representations of AIDS and its clinical syndromes related to local understandings of the body, sexuality and death (Ingstad 1990, Irwin 1991, Carton 2003), with an eye to developing 'culturally appropriate' interventions (Airhihenbuwa 1991, Schoepf 1992). Interestingly, initially this early research did not address the issue of stigma that was so prominent in social research and cultural theory about the epidemic in the North (Treichler 1991, Patton, 'Sex and Germs' 1985, Clatts 1989). Research also sought to identify 'cultural determinants' of risk (McGrath 1992), but relatively less attention was paid to the hypothesis that poverty might be a driving force, perhaps because of a few initial studies reporting higher rates in those better off (Dallabetta 1993). These results were likely spurious and the result of reporting bias. More recently, protective factors have also been sought in the realms of culture and religion (Lagarde 1997, Takyi 2003).

Although higher risk was subsequently found to be linked with poverty and associated phenomena such as migration (MacDonald 1996, Brockerhoff 1999), initial interest in exotic African 'sexual rites', such as the use of local preparations for vaginal douching and the application of leaves and powders prior to sexual intercourse for the purpose of enhancing the male sexual experience, has persisted (Runganga 1995, Gresenguet 1997, Kun 1998, Wijgert 2001). Non-sexual cultural practices were also investigated, with practices such as 'blood brotherhoods' and contact with non-human primates portrayed as cultural culprits in the expanding epidemic (Hrdy 1987), or female circumcision (Grisaru 1997). It was even claimed that the 'African sexual system' was characterised by promiscuity and therefore could explain the extent of the epidemic there (Caldwell 1989). Needless to say, the claim was spurious, being based on a selective reading of data (Le Blanc 1991). In an article that proved prescient, Epstein and Packard (Packard 1991) demonstrated parallels between social science research on AIDS and earlier studies of tuberculosis and other infectious diseases, warning that failing to engage with the political economic determinants that make the poor vulnerable would lead to research that essentially blamed the victims for circumstances over which they had no control. Such theories continue to be given credence because they conveniently blame those most vulnerable (Farmer 1992).

The slow demise of culturalism as an explanatory paradigm began in the second decade of the epidemic after a tide of research (Herrell 1991) that indicted poverty as the epidemic's primary social determinant. This research was the tip of an iceberg of literature and identified the mechanisms by which poverty led to vulnerability (for a review see Whiteside 2002). Poverty leads to riskier behaviour, either by favouring transactional sex, or by driving migration – an observation that helped develope the concept of vulnerability (Kalipeni 2000), in an effort to shift attention from individuals – who often have minimal control over their circumstances and must struggle just to get by - to social structures. Initially, however, little research sought to link everyday poverty to the broader political, social, and economic climate. This research was hampered by an excessively individualistic focus, invoking notions of a 'culture of poverty' that had been widely criticised decades earlier in social research on poverty (Geshekter 1995).

The habit of treating poverty as inevitable, rather than as a product of social processes, broke down with the publication of a critical article indicting structural adjustment programmes for creating conditions favourable to the epidemic by deepening poverty and cutting back health services at a time when the continent was already vulnerable to the scourge of infectious diseases (Lurie 1995). Lurie et al.'s controversial article stimulated critical thinking and its publication in a medical journal gave new respectability to the 'political economy of disease' thesis that was already well established in research on health in Africa. In this view, political ideologies are refracted through state and macro-economic policy to shape the disease environment, either directly through health care spending or indirectly in the way they allocate resources that can mitigate underlying health status (Turshen 1992, Bond 2003). Neo-liberal economic policy, often dictated to cash-starved African governments, has not only decreased access to curative health services but compromises public health by privatising basic necessities such as electricity and water (Fiil-Flynn 2001, McDonald DA 2002).

Lack of access to clean water and electricity can be hypothesised as leading to increased vulnerability to HIV by favouring the spread of diseases associated with poor hygiene, thus weakening the immune systems of the poor. Evidence for a more direct link exists. Epstein and Packard had warned that the early focus on sexual behaviour risked foreclosing other explanations for the epidemic in Africa, such as high prevalence of STIs and iatrogenic spread through unsafe use of injection equipment. Others pointed out the potential significance of STIs, which viewed in either an historical context (Jochelson 1991) or in the context of social change and urbanisation (Good 1991), and offered important lessons for AIDS prevention. These suspicions were widely shared by bio-medical researchers, and a solid body of research has now firmly established that STIs greatly enhance HIV transmission by up to 100-fold, in effect fuelling HIV epidemics. Effective diagnosis and treatment of STIs has been shown to decrease HIV incidence by as much as forty percent, indicating that lack of STI diagnosis and treatment services would be a significant determinant of HIV epidemics (Philpott 2002). This provides a direct link leading from macro-economic policies that reduce health expenditures to HIV epidemics.

Inadequate funding of health care may have fuelled iatrogenic spread of HIV by making unsafe use of injection equipment more likely. For instance, the privatisation of health services, when conjugated with the imposition of user fees in public health facilities, creates a market for unregulated injectionists. This hypothesis has yet to receive serious attention in social science literature. Iatrogenic spread is increasingly invoked to account for anomalies in the epidemiological paradigm, but has yet to receive serious epidemiological investigation (Gisselquist 2002, Gisselquist 2003). This is warranted, as it has important implications for future prevention programmes which, if iatrogenic spread is shown to be of epidemiological significance, would need to address determinants of unsafe injections.

Gender: From Women's Vulnerability to Masculinities and Sexualities

Unlike the epidemic in the North, epidemiological data from Africa from the beginning indicated that more women were infected than men. This was central to epidemiologists' assertion that the epidemic there was heterosexually spread, and also suggested that women were more vulnerable to HIV. It became quickly clear that while the reasons for that vulnerability were both biological and social, the latter was of prime importance. Since then, social scientists have viewed HIV transmission largely through the lens of gender, emphasising the vulnerability of women (Seidel 1993), a view that would explain findings that women with higher socio-economic status actually may be at increased risk of HIV (Chao 1994). This vulnerability is conditioned by a web of factors: cultural constructions of gender disempower women (Latre 1999) and make it more difficult for them to negotiate sexuality (Campbell 1995) and legitimise the economic disempowerment of women that makes them more dependent on transactional sex (Gysels 2002). Disempowerment is a continuum, extending from situations of sexual violence and slavery to more subtle forms of coercion (Ajuwon 2002). And it is a vicious cycle, as the epidemic has a disproportionate impact on women as they largely bear the burden of care (Upton 2003).

Disempowerment is often viewed in terms of individuals, downplaying the role of structural factors (poverty, violence, etc.) in conditioning vulnerability, which may occur even when women might be considered relatively empowered, for example, in the case of sex workers or wealthier women (Silberschmidt 2001). The importance of this distinction is underlined if we examine the female condom, which was thought to be a 'magic bullet' because it would give women control over protecting themselves. However, they may not work in situations where the social, economic and cultural context is otherwise not favourable (Susser 2000, Kaler 2001). Similarly, street youth may be empowered relative to other children, but this should not conceal the fact that selling sex is the easiest survival strategy (Swart-Kruger 1997). Understanding is thus moving away from more simple dichotomies of empowerment/disempowerment and agency/structure, and it is in the way gender is considered that this is most clear. Women, initially thought to be vulnerable and disempowered, are more pragmatic and participatory than previously thought, and this has drawn attention to the complexities inherent in sexuality and in masculinity (Davis 2000, Prazak 2000, Renne 2000, Stewart 2000). This mirrors a shift from health-education approaches to prevention to more participatory, community-based strategies (Campbell 2001). Social science research which has stressed the structural constraints of behaviour can be credited for developing prevention interventions that aim to change the gendered framework within which sexuality is negotiated (Campbell 1999, MacPhail 2001).

Increasingly nuanced views of gendered behaviour have led away from studies of 'risky' men, such as truck drivers (Gysels 2001), to focus on how masculinity is socially constructed and enacted (Campbell 1997). Ground-breaking studies in South Africa, for instance, have explored why men become abusive, while studies from Côte-d'Ivoire (Nguyen forthcoming), Senegal (Teunis 2001), Tanzania (Lockhart 2002), and Zimbabwe (Epprecht 1998) have shed light on the different contexts in which men have sex with women, showing that this may be driven by identity, circumstance, economic conditions, and emotional need, or a complex combination of all of these. Paradoxically, men can seem disempowered as well. Sex and violence appear to be refuges from expectations that can no longer be met in a deteriorating economy, and avowedly homosexual men feel obliged to marry and have children. The significance of political mobilisation to changing gender roles (Susser 2001) may reflect the ability of political processes to address these more distal, structural constraints to women's vulnerability. The relative empowerment of men compared to women has stimulated interest in developing interventions aimed at men, which may be more effective at changing sexual behaviour than developing women's skills at, say, negotiating condom use (Agha 1998).

Conflict and Violence: Linking the Macro and the Micro

Increasing attention is being paid to violence as an important co-factor in HIV transmission (Maman 2000, CADRE 2003). While initial studies indicated that gender roles that disempowered women relative to men made it more difficult for them to negotiate safer sex, further research suggests that sexual violence may be more widespread than previously thought (Jewkes 2003, Karanja 2003). While forced intercourse is believed to increase the risk of HIV transmission because of direct physical trauma, even in its absence the threat of violence - and the relative culture of male impunity that may favour easy resort to intimidation - could increase risk by constraining women into unprotected sexual relations when they would otherwise refuse (Wojcicki 2002). Two situations have emerged as being of particular concern. First, in South Africa, several studies of masculinity have indexed the legacy of apartheid, noting that the social emasculation of men under apartheid, which continued as liberation failed to bear economic fruit for most black South Africans, could be correlated with constructions of masculinity that stressed virility (Campbell 1997, Niehaus 2000). Recently, an 'epidemic' of rape - including child rape - has been the focus of much sensational media attention in South Africa, crystallising a 'national scandal of masculinity' (Posel 2003). Sexual abuse of children has been identified elsewhere in Africa as a cause of STIs (Pitche 2001). Secondly, war-affected populations are more vulnerable to HIV - not only because they are more vulnerable to gender-based violence, but also because of displacement and lack of access to prevention services as well as STI diagnosis and treatment (McGinn 2000) (Ward 2002). HIV is more prevalent in military personnel than in the general population (Martin Foreman 2002), power differentials between military and civilians are greater, military are often away from their wives and high HIV prevalence rates make soldiers a particularly high risk group (Heinecken 2001) and conflict situations potentially explosive for HIV (Sarin 2003). More worryingly, evidence from war-torn countries such as Sierra Leone and the Congo (Melby 2002, Wakhweya 2002) indicates the use of rape as a weapon of war, and has raised concerns that HIV may have been deliberately spread in Rwanda (Elbe 2002) as well as in South Africa by the apartheid regime. If such 'weaponisation' of HIV is indeed occurring, this would mark a worrisome development.

Several Pathways Explaining How War Fuels HIV Epidemics

Warfare displaces civilian populations, increasing vulnerability the same way it does for migrants - by broadening sexual networks and increasing the chance of exposure to the virus (Holt 2003). Displaced populations generally have less access to medical services and constitute, in effect, a 'complex medical emergency' (Khaw et al. 2000) with its own particular ecology of disease (Kalipeni 1998). And warfare, of course, results in significant troop movements, bringing high risk groups into contact with new populations. Of even more concern are 'low intensity' conflicts where the main strategy is the terrorising of civilian populations - particularly efficient at triggering and spreading epidemics. These situations are notorious for the prevalence of rape and other forms of gender violence. These concerns have been borne out epidemiologically. An HIV-2 epidemic was associated with the war of independence from Portugal in Guinea-Bissau (Lemey 2003) and, more recently, with the Congolese civil war.

Wars can be considered symptomatic of a more generalised phenomenon, which is the conjugation of weak states, generalised availability of firearms, and mounting social inequality, with the result that state breakdown is occurring in many parts of the world and in Africa in particular (Joseph 2003). HIV epidemics are thus fuelled by state breakdown but, in turn, can feed it as the social fabric is impacted by the epidemic (see below) (Ostergard 2002).

Beyond Social Determinants

Clear determinants of HIV epidemics are difficult to discern from the complex tangle of social factors cited in the literature. While culture, poverty, gender relations, social inequality, and violence are all identified as facilitators of transmission, none has demonstrated a robust, linear relationship to HIV prevalence. There does not appear to be a relationship between risk and social capital (Campbell 2002, Djamba 2003), although further studies are clearly warranted. Recently, state capacity has been cited as another potential determinant (Joseph 2003), and is a hypothesis that also bear further investigation as it holds broad geographical interest in the light of emerging epidemics in Central Asia. In contrast, biological factors have been identified which clearly amplify HIV epidemics. While the role of STIs is most cited, there is some evidence that other infections may make immune systems more vulnerable to HIV.

The recent controversy over the historical origins of the AIDS epidemic suggests another direction of study. The hypothesis that polio vaccine trials, conducted in the former Belgian Congo, may have inadvertently triggered the epidemic by inoculating hundreds of thousands of Africans with biological matter potentially contaminated by HIV's chimpanzee ancestor virus, SIVCPZ, was widely publicised. Molecular epidemiologic methods were used to shed light on the issue. The HIV epidemic stems from a zoonotic event, when human populations were infected with an ancestral retrovirus derived from the Simian Immunodeficiency Virus present in wild chimpanzee populations in the Congo River basin (Yusim 2001). Molecular methods were used to calculate when HIV and SIV strains diverged. This divergence occurred in the inter-war period (Chitnis 2000), at a time of significant social upheaval in the Belgian Congo (Headrick 1994). This social context lends credence to the hypothesis that zoonotic spread led to the divergence of HIV and SIV. These social transformations, driven by colonial labour policies, were ultimately to lead to the death of an estimated ten million Congolese from starvation and epidemics of trypanosomiasis (Lyons 1992). These social and ecological changes suggest that humans would have been more exposed, or vulnerable to chimpanzee viruses (Lemey 2003). The origins of the epidemic were thus neither purely biological nor social, but were entangled from the beginning. While numerous others have pointed to the need for bio-social approaches, there are few examples in the literature.

Bio-social interactions include societal (that is, social, cultural, political and economic) responses to epidemics. These change both social relations and disease ecologies, with important implications for public health. For instance, colonial public health efforts aimed at containing infectious diseases throughout Africa, being the aspect of colonial government most widely experienced by Africans, were to profoundly shape African social life and politics with implications for future epidemics, including HIV (Dozon 1991). The efficacy of bio-medical treatments for infectious diseases became obvious with the introduction of parenteral anti-infectives after the Second World War. As a result, injectable treatments were widely sought-after. Re-use of needles in treatment and vaccination campaigns have been implicated in the emergence of blood-borne epidemics on the continent including HIV (Marx 2001). Reluctance to confront the epidemic in its early years on the continent can be attributed to suspicions lingering from the colonial era when notions of 'diseased natives' were used to enforce segregation. This story underlines that bio-medical responses to disease ecologies are, by their very nature, very powerful at shifting those disease ecologies and need to be part of the picture in understanding how epidemics evolve. Causes and determinants of epidemics are bio-social, and understanding them must include examination of the responses to epidemics.

The Response to the Epidemic

Africa has become a veritable laboratory for HIV prevention – and now treatment programmes – and has been fertile ground for an increasingly sophisticated civil society, active in combating the epidemic. The first generation of prevention programmes concentrated on mass information, education and communication ('IEC') campaigns to raise awareness, and social marketing to increase condom availability. A second generation stressed translating knowledge into behaviour change through interpersonal strategies, such as peer education and testimonials by PLWHIV. These have had limited results, probably because the ability of individuals, particularly the poor, to effect change in their circumstances is actually quite low. This indicates that behavioural change to reduce HIV transmission risk is unlikely to be achieved without addressing structural determinants. Increasing the visibility of people living with HIV created a strategic imperative to achieve greater involvement of PLWHIV in the fight against the epidemic. This imperative fuelled initiatives to foster self-help and empowerment amongst PLWHIV, particularly by supporting self-help groups and disseminating techniques to encourage individuals to testify publicly. These were an important tool for building awareness and contributed to growing activism on the part of African people with HIV/AIDS. However, until now, these have largely been 'cookie-cutter' campaigns fashioned out of standardised strategies and interventions applied throughout the world, often by the same consortia of NGOs and international aid donors.

Emerging Challenges to the Consensus

Compared to a wealth of technical documents, critical social science literature on the response to the epidemic is sparse (with the exception of South Africa, which will be discussed below). Since an early rejection of the epidemic as a purely biomedical or public health problem, the consensus has been that the epidemic is a problem of development (Hemrich 2000), and not just a health issue, and that as a result broad multi-sectoral responses are required, essentially calling for technical solutions (Haddad 2001). The legacy of the late Jonathan Mann (former Director of the WHO's Global Programme on AIDS in the early years of the epidemic) has been to enshrine human rights as an anchoring principle of the response: specifically, HIV testing must be voluntary and confidential, and risk groups and people living with HIV must not be stigmatised (Leslie 2002). More pragmatically, this has translated into widely, if not necessarily explicitly adopted, affirmative action policies that call for greater involvement of people living with HIV, and communities affected by HIV, in the response to the epidemic (UNAIDS 2000). This is the cornerstone of a range of widely agreed-upon strategies that seek to empower those most vulnerable. Much of the 'rights and empowerment' response, however, has remained confined to the discursive realm (Seidel 1993), although there is evidence that, as funding is ramped up, meaningful changes are occurring on the ground (Nguyen 2002, Simon-Meyer 2002).

In the face of ever-rising HIV rates, with few successes to cite, cracks in the consensus have emerged, with dissenting views coming from field workers, public health quarters, and political activists. Those writing from the front lines point out that while the notion of vulnerability provides a useful framework within which to develop and assess these responses (Delaunay 1999), it may be disconnected from the realities in the field where scarce resources must first be directed to the most valuable rather than the most vulnerable. Rationing has largely escaped attention, (for an exception, see Kenyon 2003), although the use of 'selection criteria', particularly in deciding who gets scarce treatment, indicates that this is the case (Nguyen 2003). From the standpoint of public health and social justice, the 'rights and empowerment' approach has recently been challenged (Cock 2002). By undermining classical approaches to epidemic control, it is argued that 'AIDS exceptionalism' - especially as concerns voluntary testing as opposed to universal screening, is in effect 'promoting an African holocaust' (Alcorn 2001). While activists have long been vocal in the demand for more resources, in the past years they have clearly linked this to the problem of third-world debt (Dely 1999). Without debt relief (Cheru 2000), and indeed structural reform as well as changes to the global order (Poku 2002), the AIDS crisis will only get worse. Neo-liberal prescriptions, which advocate decreasing the role of the state and privatising services, increase vulnerability even as they decrease the ability to respond to the epidemic (Odhiambo 2003). These challenges to the consensus raise fundamental concerns about the efficacy of the current response as it now stands. Presumably, if the development, rights and empowerment approach does not address the root causes or is at cross-purposes with the reality on the ground, the responses it advocates should be ineffective. What does the literature tell us?

Improving the Response: From Learning Lessons to Best Practices to Critique

The most substantial body of research concerned with the impact of the response has been understandably concerned with directly improving that response as quickly and as broadly as possible, and the bulk of it forms a voluminous literature of technical reports and evaluations. Epidemiological evaluations are rarer, as this entails time-consuming randomised-control trials that are not only difficult and expensive to perform, but often do not translate into results that are valid in the 'real world'. While the interventions that have been scientifically evaluated are briefly reviewed below, this should not be taken to imply that these are the only, or even the best, available. Most often, it is only interventions where there is some controversy or lack of clarity that are submitted to full scientific evaluation.

The bulk of the evaluation of the response has been a blend of qualitative and quantitative insights summarised and disseminated as lessons learnt through a broad range of grey literature. Considerable attention has been devoted to systematising these lessons in order to identify 'best practices', initially defined by UNAIDS as 'anything that works whether fully or in part and that provides useful lessons learnt' (Funnell 1999). Best practices have been identified for practically every conceivable issue raised by HIV/AIDS, and these are easily consultable via the web-sites of UNAIDS, FHI, the International HIV/AIDS Alliance, and other organisations. However, even if a programme 'works' in delivering intended outputs, the chain of causality from these to broader socio-behavioural outcomes - including decreased HIV rates - is difficult to evaluate. The sheer complexity of intervening variables and circumstances means that successes, or failures, must be explained after the fact. For example, the explosive HIV epidemic in South Africa has been attributed to highly specific local circumstances. These include the legacy of apartheid, particularly in how the economic system of apartheid and the struggle against the regime shaped masculinities (Campbell 1997, Niehaus 2000), concurrent epidemics of STIs (particularly herpes, Chen C. Y., 2000), the political 'distraction' of the post-apartheid transition to democracy (Marais), as well as poverty and social inequality (Delius 2002). Conversely, the apparent success that has met some AIDS control programmes has been attributed to political will, an ill-defined and under-researched concept that is argued to have been behind existing efforts (Boone 2001). Complex social phenomena cannot be reduced to a handful of variables, indicating that further understanding of the impact of the response will require scrutiny from more qualitatively oriented approaches. In addition to surveys and focus groups, ethnography has been crucial to developing an understanding the relationship between social change and epidemics. Newer methods include developing 'scenarios' to predict what the epidemic will look like in twenty years (UNAIDS 2003).

Quantitative Evaluations of Specific Interventions Exist, Particularly in the Arena of Prevention

Change in sexual behaviour has been the major goal of these programmes. While behaviour change has been shown to result in decreased HIV incidence at the population level (Kamali 2000), the ability of prevention programmes to change behaviour has been limited. Epidemiological high-risk groups are priority targets for intervention, as it is here that interventions are likely to have the most impact and are therefore most easily measured. The best evidence for efficacy comes from studies of interventions promoting condom use done with commercial sex workers. In a landmark study, Laga and colleagues demonstrated that condom promotion and STI treatment decreased incidence of HIV in sex workers in Kinshasa (Laga 1994). Surprisingly little research has evaluated prevention interventions aimed at other traditional high risk groups: youth, men and migrants, although these are the focus of increasing attention (see, for example, Campbell 2001). Of a range of potential 'structural interventions' – that is, interventions aimed at changing the environment rather than behaviour – only condom distribution programmes have been formally evaluated (Rosenfield 2001). This represents a significant gap, which may reflect the persistence of the tendency to assume epidemiological risk is solely attributable to individual behaviour, the difficulty of developing, implementing and evaluating 'structural' interventions and, finally, that many interventions either never get documented or there is a time lag inherent in documenting interventions.

The point was made early on by anthropologists and cultural critics that behaviour is embedded in and enacts meanings that are context-dependent, explaining why appeals to abstract rationality do not universally translate into behaviour change (Parker 1995). 'Culturally appropriate' awareness-raising campaigns have since become the mainstay of prevention campaigns. The difficulties in evaluating these campaigns likely explain why so few of these have been examined. On the basis of published studies, the results are mixed. While some studies have shown campaigns are effective at raising knowledge (Rogers 1999, Stadler 2002, Tambashe 2003) this does not appear to reliably translate into behavioural change (Yoder 1996, Snell 2002). Similarly, research neither supports nor contradicts the notion that behaviour change will result from 'putting a face' to HIV by encouraging positive people to 'come out' (MacIntyre 2001, Camlin 2003).

In the arena of treatment, the literature on best practices for treatment is still relatively sparse for developing countries relative to the wealth of research conducted in the North. The clinical efficacy of anti-retroviral drugs and drugs to prevent opportunistic infections has been established in African settings (Laurent 2002). However, these initial studies, as well as others currently underway, are being conducted in (relatively) resource rich clinical settings under highly structured circumstances, making it difficult to evaluate what obstacles to successful treatment outcomes will be encountered in the 'real world' of urban clinics or rural primary health care centres, and what the most effective measures for addressing them will be.

The availability of data on the efficacy of interventions makes them subject to cost-efficacy analyses. This allows interventions to be ranked, usually by the cost per infection averted and eventually comparing these to the cost of treatment (Marseille 2001, Hutton 2003). Cost efficacy studies have come under fire by activists for putting a price on human life that inevitably discriminates against the poor (Boelaert 2002) and constituting a barrier to action (Nelson 2002). In response, it has been argued that priorities must be set and that economic tools are important in making rational decisions (Brunet-Jailly 1999).

In summary, the literature indicates that while there is solid evidence for achieving meaningful outcomes for a handful of interventions, for the rest the tangle of variables makes it difficult to demonstrate quantifiable efficacy. While the programme evaluation literature has been vital to improving the response and has improved our understanding of the epidemic and its context – it is often in the context of the evaluation of an intervention that previously unsuspected but important information may be gleaned – it is necessarily concerned with pro-gramme outputs rather than broader social impacts of programmes. Arguably, it is to these complex phenomena that social science is poised to add value. The surprising lack of studies so far indicates that this will be important to improving future responses.

Lessons – and Questions – from South Africa

South Africa, as examples already cited indicate, has been an exceptional case. In addition to the recent historical context of apartheid and the transition to democracy, it has also had the fastest growing epidemic - mushrooming from less than one percent of the population in 1990 to over twenty percent ten years later (Abdool Karim 2002, Williams 2001). It also has the most resources to respond to the epidemic - and to document it - as the most developed country on the continent. Its strong research capacity is reflected by the quantity and quality of research produced there. As a result South African experience dominates the literature on HIV/AIDS in Africa in general, and on the response in particular. The literature on HIV/AIDS in South Africa is exceptionally broad and deep compared to elsewhere in Africa, and offers a treasure-trove of insights into the conjugation of politics and the epidemic. The relevance of the socio-economic context to understanding both the dynamics of HIV transmission, as well as its impact and the response to it, has been confirmed for the South African epidemic. There, the legacy of apartheid, particularly in the form of steep gradients of socio-economic inequality, has been identified as the driving force behind the epidemic and challenges neo-liberal assumptions that the epidemic can be explained in terms of individual behaviour (Schneider 2002).

In the New South Africa's vibrant democracy, HIV and the adequacy of the government's response has been widely debated (Vliet 2001). The debate has become increasingly politicised, driven by an active civil society with grassroots skills honed in years of struggle against the apartheid regime. After the advent of effective therapy for HIV in 1996, it was here that the issue of access to treatment was brought to the foreground of the international stage in 2000 (Bass 2000). The first ever International AIDS Conference, held in Durban that year, provided a dramatic stage for a confrontation between the pharmaceuticals industry, the South African government, and a coalition of activists from South Africa and around the world. The confrontation was carried out in a series of court battles between the government and the industry (around the right to import generic drugs) and the government and the activists (around the need to supply treatment to prevent transmission from mother to child). President Mbeki's comments to the effect that HIV did not cause AIDS only served to fan controversy (Fassin 2003). Both court battles were settled in favour of expanding access to treatment and, at the time of writing, the government is rolling out an even more ambitious treatment programme after losing a subsequent case against the activists.

The cost of ensuring access to treatment highlighted the glaring funding gap in the response to the epidemic, even in comparatively wealthy South Africa. While early attention focussed on the cost of treatments, increasing attention is being paid to health systems. The direct impact of the epidemic on health services, as staff either fall ill themselves (Goudge 2000) or 'burn-out' (Raviola 2002), when conjugated with the chronic under-funding of public health systems in Africa, has dealt a devastating blow to the ability of existing health systems to respond to treatment needs. South Africa's comparatively functional health care system paradoxically makes these problems more visible there. Worsening child health directly and indirectly due to HIV infection has strained resources further and only added to the psychological burden of staff who must deal with unprecedented child morbidity and mortality (Pillay 2001, Walraven 1996). This happens even when most morbidity and mortality occurs outside of health care institutions, as is the case elsewhere in Africa (Ngalula 2002) – raising the concern that improving health care systems may only increase the burden they have to bear, in effect shifting it out of the domestic realm into the public sector, with potential impact on other diseases. The potential flow of resources into HIV/AIDS care and treatment raises major concerns about health equity (Ntuli 2003). Health sector reform will clearly need to respond to the realities of both containing the epidemic – through better diagnosis and treatment – and its multiple impacts (see above), although there has been relatively little discussion of this in the research literature. While the role of primary care needs to be rethought (Petersen 2002), broader, political issues will need to be addressed.

It is difficult to imagine that any meaningful reforms can be undertaken without reallocation of international debt, as debt servicing decreases health expenditures (Cheru 2002). The political nature of these issues poses the related question of governance – who will decide, and how (De Waal 2003). This issue is particularly complex in an era of globalisation, where aid donors and transnational corporations have greater financial clout than most African states (Poku 2002) and where local factors clearly play an important role in shaping both the epidemic and the response to it. The need for a concerted international response is clear (Thurman 1999), but risks becoming mired in American domestic politics (Brainard, 2003:776, Gow 2002) and while some Americans have been optimistic, claiming that 'a new institutional order is emerging in the global fight against HIV/AIDS' (Morrison 2003), the experience of the New Partnership for African Development (NEPAD) is not encouraging (De Waal 2002).

Three questions emerge from this largely South African literature. South Africa's experience shows that the response to the epidemic, and the impact of that response, is eminently political, and that politics is rooted in local histories of engagement and struggle. This suggests that it may be difficult to 'graft' political responses onto terrains that do not have the same history of engagement and struggle. South Africa's case militates against the consensus that universal, technical 'development' solutions will work equally well everywhere. This question requires further study. A second and related question concerns the issue of governance – what are the best mechanisms for making decisions about how to respond to the epidemic? If authoritarian solutions are more effective, as has been argued by some and as the case of Cuba would suggest, who is to decide? How? Finally, it is impossible to consider the response in isolation from the impact, as the case of health systems tells us. Social transformations wrought by HIV/AIDS, from changes in knowledge and attitudes to illness, affect those who must respond directly. This can be a vicious cycle, or it can be an opportunity for an effective politics of solidarity.

Summary and Gaps Identified

The literature reviewed in this paper indicates that the role of social and biological factors in facilitating the spread of HIV epidemics has been well described and that, for some of these, sufficient epidemiological evidence exists that we may speak of determinants - that is, factors that play a robust, quantifiable role at the population health level. However, what still remains poorly understood is why epidemics 'take off' in certain areas and not in others. The literature suggests that specific, local interactions between social and biological factors determine epidemiological pathways.

Significant gaps exist in our understanding of the relationship between HIV epidemics and social change. Understanding the impact of the response to the epidemic is quite narrow, with studies largely limited to measuring factual knowledge and behaviour change. Recently more attention has been paid to the impacts of the epidemic on specific parts of society: population structure, labour, the economy, the health sector, population health. The literature strongly suggests that the aggregate effects of these impacts will transform society. Social transformations due to the epidemic and the response to it are likely to shape the bio-social environment within which HIV epidemics wax or wane, and therefore are of considerable importance to future efforts to curb its spread and impact.

A striking overall finding has been the lag between the bulk of mainstream social science research and reports from organisations engaging in front-line HIV prevention. For instance, the relationship between HIV and gender, sexuality, conflict and violence was first widely documented in non-academic sources. On the other hand, critical social science - some of it still largely unpublished – early on warned against overly reductionist explanations and sought to explore the link between the epidemic and the broad political ecology of disease in Africa. This suggests that a more fruitful dialogue needs to be engaged between academic researchers, and evolving communities of practice being constituted around the front lines of the epidemic.

What Drives HIV Epidemics?

Specific findings are that while a number of biological and social co-factors have been identified, evidence for a determining epidemiological effect exists for STIs, with strong evidence for lack of male circumcision, and younger age of first intercourse for women while a number of social conditions are identified as increasing vulnerability to HIV, none individually has emerged as a robust determinant of HIV prevalence.

Indications that interactions between biological factors and these social conditions (gender, migration, poverty and social inequality) can provide the necessary conditions for epidemics to 'take off' suggest a broader hypothesis: that local configurations of biological and social co-factors explain how epidemics are generated, and their subsequent growth and scope. These bio-social interactions

are locally contingent and dynamic; that is, they evolve over time, thereby shaping
the ebb and flow of epidemics over regions. Understanding of these bio-social
interactions requires that historical, political, economic, social, cultural data are
considered alongside bio-medical and epidemiological evidence. This hypothesis
maps out a research agenda that will require that social scientists and biologists
work together to better understand how HIV epidemics evolve, how they may
be contained, and the intended and unintended consequences of the social response.

Gaps and Priorities

Little is known about the epidemiological role of sexual violence, men who have
sex with men (MSM), and common unregulated injection and surgical practices,
such as those used to treat infectious diseases or interrupt unwanted pregnancies.
(Of these new epidemiological pathways, MSM will likely receive the most attention, given the difficulties in studying sexual violence and the controversy that
surrounds the iatrogenic hypothesis.)

Even less is known about how Structural Adjustment Policies, which
compromised public health care on the continent from the 1990s onwards, may
have shifted disease ecologies to favour HIV transmission. The relationship between
macro-economic policy, social inequality, poverty and health also bears further scrutiny.

Is the Response Working?

Specific findings are that social changes that occur upstream from the demographic
impact can mitigate its impact. These changes reflect the multifaceted, societal
response to the epidemic. The response may be consciously orchestrated as a
matter of government or aid policy, occur more spontaneously as families and
communities respond to awareness-raising campaigns or an illness at home, or
emerge from discourses in the media, popular culture, and everyday discourse.
These changes are part and parcel of cultural processes stemming from urbanisation, and democratisation.

The response can result in significant changes in sexual behaviour, as has been
documented by decreasing sero-prevalence rates in some countries and groups.
Even where prevention efforts have not translated into decreased sero-prevalence,
countless surveys have demonstrated shifts in knowledge, attitudes, behaviour
and practices. Children and youth are becoming increasingly sexually literate, and
may be delaying onset of sexual activity in response to HIV prevention messages.
These index the social and cultural ramifications of the epidemic, although little
else is known about these.

Empirical evidence suggests that in many places responses to AIDS are
extremely local; as suggested above, this may lead to new of forms of bartering,
or other informal relations that reconfigure local hierarchies or governance structures. Other impacts may restructure sexual economies in ways that alter transmission dynamics. General explanations of such phenomena may benefit from

explicitly considering cognitive or behavioural responses to aspects of the pandemic – at the individual level – that could cumulate in institutional transformations. Here the key point is that the societal impacts of HIV/AIDS are not a linear function of infection or prevalence rates; rather, infection, fear of infection, or responses to infection may disrupt the foundations on which social, political, or economic institutions and relations are built.

Gaps and Priorities

Capturing the broader societal impact of these has been notoriously difficult. And yet, evidence suggests that HIV/AIDS is a motor of social change in Africa, much of that mediated through international prevention and treatment efforts. Concerns that behaviour change may not be sustained in the long-term, that prevention programmes may have unwittingly driven men to 'protect' themselves by selecting young girls as sexual partners, or that treatment programmes may stigmatise their beneficiaries, highlight the need for critical assessments that examine longer-term societal changes and their impact on social relations, culture, politics and economies. This social change has been difficult to capture as it falls outside of the indicators of prevention programmes. For instance, sophisticated AIDS prevention campaigns in the media have problematised the category of the adolescent, in effect making it available as an identity to young Africans in unprecedented ways; similarly, the culture of sexual openness that has permeated even out-of-the-way places in Africa on the heels of AIDS groups has created social spaces within which it has been possible to organise a homo-social sphere and, now, openly gay and lesbian groups. These phenomena point to a rapidly shifting social landscape that needs to be taken into account in continually refining our response to the epidemic – a lesson that is being learned now in the North, where HIV is now resurgent in communities where it had been controlled.

The vigorous and sustained response that exists within the households and communities that continue to bear the brunt of the consequences and care for the ill and those that survive them has remained largely off the radar screen. Better understanding of this grassroots response, particularly in high prevalence countries, would be an important step in developing strategies to support this endogenous response.

Practical experience in fighting AIDS is extraordinarily difficult to get. There is clearly a rich body of experience fighting the epidemic that exists throughout Africa at the community level. The bulk of care, for instance, is carried out by households and early research suggests that there has been an extraordinary robustness in the ability of communities to respond to the orphan crisis in southern Africa. However, much of this experience remains undocumented or, at best, relegated to anecdotal accounts within reports. There is a substantial 'grey' literature, which concerns programme and project implementation, often written for donor agencies. As a result, and understandably, this literature has been jargon-filled and often lacks relevance with respect to the issues facing communities and societies struggling against AIDS. What has been documented is not being used. This difficulty has been acknowledged of late, with a growing emphasis on producing 'toolkits' and manuals that can assist in project design and implementation. Organisations like the Population Council, the International HIV/AIDS Alliance, FHI, and so on, are actually quite good at disseminating what they produce. The problem is that grassroots practitioners are too overwhelmed to produce any documentation whatsoever. The existence of this gap is borne out by programmes like Population Council's 'Horizons' project that aim to bridge it with operations research.

Important gaps remain in our knowledge about how HIV prevention, treatment, and advocacy efforts to shift disease ecologies (for example by reducing prevalence of sexually transmitted infections), create and sustain new forms of community, and catalyse a new political activism around health. Critical research to address these gaps can play an important role in harnessing HIV-driven social transformations to address broader issues in public health and social justice. Lack of understanding of these social transformations potentially compromises the success of continued HIV prevention and treatment efforts in Africa and globally.

Including communities, NGOs, activists and researchers in this dialogue will certainly help to improve sharing of lessons and disseminate 'best practices'. While these are short-term goals, they are nonetheless vital precisely because we are in the midst of an epidemic that is largely out of control. However dialogue can also be made to work towards broader, long-term goals. The sheer scope of this epidemic means that we should not forget that academic institutions will train generalists and specialists who must become leaders in the fight against AIDS throughout the continent – whether they be health care personnel, teachers, lawyers, engineers, mineworkers and so on (what Mary Crewe has called 'mainstreaming HIV/AIDS'). Just as the epidemic is transforming Africa, it should be transforming higher education globally. Evidence-based and theoretical research can add enormous value to the response to the epidemic. Just as an example, I would like to cite the Treatment Action Campaign, which this week successfully lobbied to make ARV treatment available to South Africans with HIV in their country. TAC's campaign drew on a practical history of social mobilisation (against the apartheid regime), but also on a blend of theoretical approaches developed in the social sciences.

Mobilising, and benefiting from that experience, will require critical dialogue between academic institutions and NGOs (including the activist groups that have done so much to challenge mainstream thinking about AIDS in Africa of late), as well as with the myriad community-level organisations (i.e. church based groups, youth clubs, self-help groups and so on) that actually bear the brunt of the epidemic and carry out the most critical aspects of prevention and care. Without this community voice, and in the absence of an institutional platform for developing critical *and* engaged research, it has been difficult to develop perspectives that think outside, or are even critical of, how programmes are implemented in the field. As a result, much of the existing research is of little help to communities that engage with the difficult realities and critical choices that must be faced, and it has not been an inspiration for developing innovative approaches to addressing the challenges of the epidemic.

References

Abdol, K., Ziquba-Page, T. T. and Arendse, R., 1994, 'Bridging the Gap: Potential for a Health Care Partnership Between African Traditional Healers and Biomedical Personnel in South Africa', Supplement, *South African Medical Journal*, 84 s1-s16 as quoted by Colvin et al., in 'Integrating Traditional Healers into a Tuberculosis Control Programme in Hlabisa, South Africa'.

Abel-Smith, B., 1986, 'Health Insurance in Developing Countries: Lessons from Experience', *Health Policy and Planning*, 7(3), 215-226.

Abel-Smith, B., 1993, 'Financing Health Services in Developing Countries: The Options', *NU Nytt om U-landshälsard*, 2/93, vol. 7.

Adam, P. et Herzlich, C., 1994, *Sociologie de la maladie et de la médecine*, Paris, Nathan, Coll Sociologie, 128.

Adebayo, A., 1990, *Structural Adjustment for Socio-Economic Recovery and Transformation: The African Alternative*, Ethiopia, UNECA.

Adjanohoon, E., *Médecine traditionnelle et pharmacopée, contribution aux études ethnologiques et floristiques au Mali*, Paris, Acet, 1979.

Aguercif, M., Aguercif-Meziane, F., 'Le système de santé publique en Algérie: évaluation 1974-1989 et perspectives', in *Les Cahiers du CREAD*, n° 35/36, 1993, pp. 97-102.

Ahluwalia, R., Mechin, B., 1979, *La médecine traditionnelle au Zaïre, fonctionnement et contribution potentielle aux services de santé*, Ottawa, CRDI.

Ahrin, D. C., 1995, 'Health Insurance in Rural Africa', *The Lancet*, 345, pp. 44-45.

AIDS Bulletin, 2002, March, p. 29.

Ake, C., 1996, *Democracy and Development in Africa*, Washington, DC, Brookings Institution.

Akin, J., Birdsall, N. and de Ferranti, D., 1987, *Financing Health Services in Developing Countries: An Agenda for Reform*, Washington DC, The World Bank.

Akinkugbe, O. O., Olatunbosun, D. and Folayan Esan, G. J. eds, 1973, *Priorities in National Health Planning*, Proceedings of an International Symposium, Caxton Press.

Alam, M. M., Huque, A. S. and Westergaard, K., 1994, *Development Through Decentralization in Bangladesh: Evidence and Perspective*, Dhaka, University Press Ltd.

Alesina, A., Bagir, R. and Easterly, W., 1993, 'Public Goods and Ethnic Divisions', *Quarterly Journal of Economics*, 114 (4):1243-84 November.

Amai, C. A., 2002, 'Medicinal Plants and Bio-diversity Report', Kampala, Ministry of Health.

Amin, A. A., 1995, 'The Problem of Decreasing Incomes and Increasing Cost of Health Care in Cameroon', *Les Camers d'OCISCA*, no. 23, Yaoundé.

AMPPF, 1992, 'Enquête de Base IEC à Bamako auprès des populations', 69 pages.

Anderson, J., 1975, *Public Policy Making*, Nelson, London.

Antoine, P. et Bâ, A., 1993, 'Mortalité et santé dans les villes africaines', Afrique Contemporaine', n° 168, octobre-décembre, pp. 138-146.

Antrobus, P., 1989, 'Women and Development: An Alternative Analysis', *Journal for International Development*, 1.

Appadurai, A., 2001, *Après le colonialisme, les conséquences culturelles de la globalisation*, Paris, Payot.

Arndt, C. and Lewis, 2000, 'The Macroeconomic Implications of HIV/AIDS in South Africa: A preliminary Assessment', *South African Journal of Economics*, vol 68:5, pp. 856-87.

Asghar, R. J., 1999, 'Obstetric Complications and the Roles of Traditional Birth Attendants in Developing Countries', *Journal of physicians and surgeons*, 9 (1): 55-57.

Atchley, R. C., 1976, *The Sociology of Retirement*, New York, Wiley & Sons.

Atelier National sur la Définition d'une Politique Nationale de Communication pour le Développement au Mali, 1993, PNUD, FAO, TCP/1357, novembre, pp. 107.

Atim, C., 1998, *The contribution of Mutual Health Organisations to Financing, Delivery and Access to Health Care: Synthesis of Research in Nine West and Central African Countries*, Abt. Assocs/PHR, Bethesda, MD.

Atim, C., 1999, 'Social Movements and Health Insurance: a Critical Evaluation of Voluntary, Non-profit Insurance schemes with Case Studies from Ghana and Cameroon', *Social Science and Medicine*. 48, 881-896.

Azougli, I., 1988, Système de santé en Algérie : perceptions de l'institution médicale dans deux quartiers d'Alger, Thèse de doctorat en Sociologie, Paris, EHESS.

Baile, S., 1990, 'Women and Health in Developing Countries', *The OECD Observer*, December 1989/January 1990, pp. 18-20.

Baniafouna, C., 2001, *Congo démocratie*, vol 4. *Devoir de mémoire. Congo - Brazzaville* 15 octobre 1997-31 décembre 1999, Paris, l'Harmattan.

Banque Mondiale, Sénégal, 1994, *Evaluation des conditions de vie*, Washington.

Bardhai, P. and Mookherjee, D., 2000, 'Capture and Governance at Local and National Levels,' *American Economic Review*, 90 (2): 135-39, May.

Baszanger, I., 1986, 'Maladies chroniques et leur ordre négocié', *Revue française de sociologie*, Vol. XXVII, Janvier-Mars, pp. 3-27.

Becker, G. S., 1979, 'Corruption and Punishment: An Economic Approach', *Journal of Political Economy*, 76, 169-217.

Becker, G. and Stigler, G. J., 1974, 'Law Enforcement, Malfeassance, and the Compensation of Enforcers', *Journal of Legal Studies*, III: 1-19.

Bennet, S., 1996, 'The Public/Private Mix in Health Care Systems', in Janovsky, K., ed., *Health Policy and Systems Development*, Geneva, World Health Organisation.

Bennett, F. J., ed., 1979, *Community Diagnosis and Health Action: A Manual for Tropical and Rural Areas*, London, Macmillan.

Benoist, J., 2002, *Petite bibliothèque d'anthropologie médicale*, Paris, AMADES.

Bergstrom, T. C. and Goodman, R. P., 1973, 'Private Demands for Public Goods', *American Economic Review*, 63 (3): 280-96, June.

Berman, P. A., 1997, 'National Health Accounts in Developing Countries: Appropriate Methods and Applications', *Health Economics*, Vol. 6, pp. 11-30, 1997.

Besley, T. and Burgess, R., 2002, 'The Political Economy of Government Responsiveness: Theory and Evidence from India', *Quarterly Journal of Economics*, 117(4):1415-51, November.

Besley, T. and S. Coate, 1999, 'Centralized versus Decentralized Provision of Local Public Goods: A Political Economy Analysis', NBER Working Paper No. W7084.

Besley T. and McLaren J., 1993, 'Taxes and Bribery: The Role of Wage Incentive', *The Economic Journal*, Vol.103, 1196, 1- 41.

Betancourt, R. and Gleason, S., 2001, 'The Allocation of Publicly-provided Goods to Rural Households in India: On some Consequences of Caste, Religion and Democracy', *World Development*, 28 (12), pp. 2169-82, December.

Bidounga, N., 1990, 'Prise en charge de la tuberculose et évaluation du programme à Brazzaville', Mémoire de fin de cycle au Centre Inter-Etat de Santé publique d'Afrique Centrale, Brazzaville.

Bij de Vaate, A., Coleman, R., Manneh, H. and Walraven, G., 2002, 'Knowledge, Attitudes and Practices of Trained Traditional Birth Attendants in The Gambia in the Prevention, Recognition and Management of Postpartum Haemorrhage', *Midwifery*, 18, pp. 3-11.

Bijlmakers, L., 2003, *Structural Adjustment: Source of Structural Adversity*, Leiden, African Studies Centre.

Bijlmakers, L. A., Basset, M. T. and Sanders, D. M., 1996, 'Health and Structural Adjustment in Rural and Urban Zimbabwe', Research Report No. 101, Nordic African Institute.

Birungi, H. et al., 2001, 'The Policy on Public-Private Mix in the Ugandan Health Sector: Catching up with Reality', *Journal of Health Policy and Planning*, 16 (supplement 2): 79-86.

Bledsoe, C. H., 2002, *Contingent lives: Fertility, time and aging in West Africa*, Chicago and London, The University of Chicago Press.

Bledsoe, C. H., Banja, F., Hill, A. G., 1998, 'Reproductive Mishaps and Western Contraception: An African challenge to fertility theory', *Population Development Review*, 23, pp. 15-57.

Bloom, G. and Shenglan, T., 1999, 'Rural Health Prepayment Schemes in China: Towards a more active role for government', *Social Science and Medicine*, 48, pp. 951-960.

Bonnel, R., 2000, 'HIV/AIDS and Economic Growth: A Global Perspective', *Journal. of South African Economics*, Volume 68: 5, pp. 820-55.

Breton A., Wintrobe, R., 1975, 'The Equilibrium Size of a Budget Maximizing bureau: A Note on Niskamen, *Journal of Political Economy*, 83, 193-20.

Brooks, D. D., 2002, *L'eau, Gérer localement*, CRDI, 80p.

Brownlee, A., 1993, 'La recherche sur les systèmes de santé: un outil de gestion', Ottawa, CRDI.

Brox, J. A., Kumar, R. C. and Stollery, K. R., 2003, 'Estimating Willingness to Pay for Improved Water Quality in the Presence of Item Non-response Bias', *American Journal of Agricultural Economics*, 85 (2), pp. 414-428.

Bryant, J., Charles Boelen and Buz Salasky, eds., 2001, 'Managing a Successful TUFH Project', (WHO), Mini-Symposium Report.

Butlerys, M., Fowler M. G., Shaffer N., Tih, P. M., Greenberg, A. E., Karita, E., Coovadia, H. and De Cock, K. M., 2002, 'Role of Traditional Birth Attendants in Preventing Perinatal Transmission of HIV', *British Medical Journal*, 324, pp. 222-225.

Caldwell J. C., Orubuloye I. O., Caldwell, P., 1992, 'Fertility Decline in Africa: A New Type of Transition ?', *Population Development Review*,18.

Carley, M., 1981, *Social Measurement and Social Indicators: Issues of Policy and Theory*, George Allen and Unwin.

Carria, G. and Politi, C., 1996, 'Exploring the Health Impact of Economic Growth, Poverty Reduction and Public Health Expenditure', Macroeconomics, Health and Development Series, WHO Technical Paper No. 18.

Carrin, G., 1987, 'Community Financing of Drugs in Sub-Saharan Africa', *International Journal of Health Planning and Management* 2, pp. 125-145.

Cartier-Bresson, J., 1992, 'Eléments d'analyse pour une économie de la corruption', *Revue du Tiers Monde*, vol. XXXIII, n° 131, 581-609.

Cartier- Bresson, J., 1998, 'Les analyses économiques des causes et des conséquences de la corruption: quelques enseignements pour les PED', *Mondes en Développement*, Tome 26, 102-25.

Centre international de l'enfance, 1976, *La santé de la famille et de la communauté*, Dakar, Saint-Paul.

Chabot, J., Boal, M., Da Silva, A., 1991, 'National Community Health Insurance at Village Level: The Case from Guinea Bissau', *Health Policy and Planning*, 6 (1), pp. 46-54.

Chaudhury, R.R., 1997, 'Commentary: Challenges in Using Traditional Systems of Medicine', New Delhi, National Institute of Immunology.

Chavundika, G. L., 1994, *Traditional Medicine in Modern Zimbabwe*, Mount Pleasant, Harare, University of Zimbabwe Publications.

Cichon, M., Gillion, C., 1993, 'Le financement des soins de santé dans les pays en développement', *Revue internationale du travail*, Vol. 132, n° 2, pp. 193-208.

CODESRIA, 2004, 'Call for abstracts: Institute for health, politics and society in Africa', www.codesria.org.

Collier P. , Dercon, S. and Mackinnson, J., 2002, 'Density versus Quality in Health Care Provision: Using Household Data to make Budgetary Choices in Ethiopia', *The World Bank Economic Review*, Vol. 3.

Collins, D., Quick, J. D., Musau, S. N. and Kraushaar, D. L., 1996, 'Health Financing Reform in Kenya: The Fall and Rise of Cost-Sharing, 1989-94', Management Sciences for Health and U.S. Agency for International Development, Stubbs Monograph Series, No. 1, Boston.

Constitution de la République du Congo adoptée au référendum de janvier 2002.

Constitution of The Federal Republic of Nigeria, 1999, Federal Government Press, Lagos.

Constitution of the Republic of Uganda, Entebbe.

Creese, A., Bennett, S., 1997, 'Rural Risk-Sharing Strategies in Health', Paper presented to an International Conference sponsored by the World Bank, Innovations in Health Care Financing, March 10-11, Washington, DC.

Cresson, G., 1991, 'Le travail sanitaire profane dans la famille: analyse sociologique', Paris, Thèse de doctorat, ehess.

Cresson, G., 1995, *Le travail domestique de la santé*, Paris, Harmattan, coll. Logique sociale.

CRDI, 2003, *Population et santé dans les pays en développement*, vol.1: *Population, santé et survie dans les sites du réseau*, INDEPTH, Réseau.

Criel, B., 1998, *District-based Health Insurance in sub-Saharan Africa*, Part I and II, Studies in health services organization and policy, Antwerp.

Criel, B., van der Stuyft, P. and van Lerberghe, W., 1999, 'The Bwamanda Hospital Insurance Scheme: Effective for Whom? A Study of its Impact on Hospital Utilization Patterns', *Social Science and Medicine*, 48, pp. 897-911.

Cuddington, J., 1993, 'Modelling the Macro-economic Effect of Aids with an Application to Tanzania', *The World Bank Economic Review*, vol. 7, no. 2.

Cuddington, J., Hancock, T. and Rogers, A., 1994, 'A Dynamic Aggregative Model of the AIDS Epidemic with Possible Policy Interventions', *Journal of Policy Modelling*, vol. 16: 5, pp. 473-96.

Dahlgren, G., 1990, 'Strategies for Health Financing in Kenya - The Difficult Birth of a New policy', *Scandinavian Journal of Social Medicine*, Supplement 46, pp. 67-81.

Daubrée, C., 1995, *Marchés parallèles et équilibres économiques: expériences africaines*, Paris, Editions l'Harmattan.

De Bethume, X., Alfani, S. and Lahaye, J.P., 1989, 'The Influence of an Abrupt Price Increase on Health Service Utilization: Evidence from Zaire', *Health Policy and Planning*, 4 (1), pp. 76-81.

De Ferranti, D., 1985, 'Paying for Health Services in Developing Countries. An Overview', World Bank Staff Working Paper, no. 721.

De La Moussaye, Eric et Jacquemot, P., 1993, 'Politique de santé: les trois options stratégiques', *Afrique Contemporaine*, n° 166, avril-juin, pp. 15-26.

Delaunay, V., 1996, 'Santé de la reproduction et changement socio-économique dans un milieu rural sénégalais: Cadre conceptuel d'un programme de recherche', ORSTOM, Paris.

Deolalikar, A. N., 1997, 'Cost and Utilization of Health Services in Kenya', Mimeo, August.

Department Denmark, 1995, 'Structural Adjustment in Africa: A Survey of the Experiences', Report Prepared by the of State for Health and Social Welfare.

De Rosny, E., 1981, *Les yeux de ma chèvre*, Paris, Plon.

Desgrées du Loû, A., 1994, 'Santé de la reproduction et effets du SIDA', Ministère de l'Emploi et de la Solidarité, Paris.

Desgrées du Loû, A., 1998, 'Santé de la reproduction et SIDA en Afrique subsaharienne: Enjeux et défis', *Population*, 1998, No. 4, pp. 701-730.

De Wikdeman, E., 1935, *A propos de médicaments indigènes congolais*, Bruxelles.

Diamond, P. A. and Jerry, A. H., 1994, 'Contingent Valuation: Is Some Number Better than No Number?', *Journal of Economic Perspectives*, 8(4), 45-64.

Dillinger, W., 1993, *Decentralization and Its Implications for Urban Service Delivery*, The World Bank, Washington DC.

Diop, F. P., 1994, *Evaluation of the Impact of Pilot Tests for Cost Recovery on Primary Health Care in Niger*, Technical Report No. 16, Bethesda, MD, Health Financing and Sustainability (HFS) Project.

Direction de la Statistique et de la Comptabilité Nationale, 1998, 'Enquête Budget Camerounaise Auprès des Ménages: Synthèse Méthodologique, Opérations sur le Terrain et Exploitations des Données', Yaoundé, Ministry of Plan and Regional Development.

Dixon, S., McDonald, S. and Roberts, 2001, 'HIV/AIDS and Development in Africa', *Journal of International Development*, Vol. 13, No. 4, pp. 391-409.

Dmytraczenko, et al., 2003, 'Health Sector Reform: How it Affects Reproductive Health', Population Research Bureau, Policy Brief.

Dowling, S., 1983, 'Health for a Change', Children Poverty Action Group.

DSCN, 2002, *Conditions de vie des populations et profil de pauvreté au Cameroun en 2001: Premiers résultats*, Direction de la Statistique et de la Comptabilité Nationale, Mai, Yaoundé.

Dujardin, B., 2003 *Politiques de santé et attentes des patients: Vers un dialogue constructif*, Paris, Karthala.

Dunn, K., 2000, 'Tales from the Dark Side: Africa's Challenge to International Relations Theory', in Isaacs, Harold, ed., *Journal of Third World Studies*, Vol. XVII, No. 1, Spring.

Dutour, O., et al., 1989, 'Aspects anthropologiques du diabète sucre', *ECOL Hum.*, Paris, Vol II, No. 1.

Egrot, M. et Taverne, B., 1990, 'Interventions sanitaires et contexte culturel: Actes de la deuxième journée d'anthropologie médicale de l'AMADES', Marseille 28 avril.

El Harti, A., 'Le système de santé au Maroc entre les contraintes financières et les exigences sociales', *Afrique et Développement*, Vol. XIII, n° 2, 1988, pp. 5-27.

Ela, J. M., 1991, 'Luttes pour la santé de l'homme et royaume de Dieu dans l'Afrique d'aujourd'hui', *Iteco, peuples et libérations*, n°117, Bruxelles, janvier, pp. 38-45.

Evans, R. G. and Stoddart, G. L., 1994, 'Producing Health, Consuming Health Care', in R. G. Evans, M. L. Barer and T. R. Marmor, eds., *Why Are Some People Healthy and Others Not?: The Determinants of Health of Populations*. Hawthorne, NY: Aldine De Gruyter.

Evans-Pritchard, E. E., 1937, *Witchcraft, Oracles and Magic among the Azande*, Oxford, Oxford University Press.

Estrella, M., et al., 2005, *L'évaluation et le suivi participatifs: Apprendre du changement*, Paris, Karthala, CRDI (Economie et développement).

Fairhead, J. et Leach, M., 1994, 'Représentations culturelles africaines et gestion de l'environnement', *Politique Africaine*, n° 53 mars, pp. 11-24.

Fall, A., 1996, 'Prévalence élevée des cas de tuberculose dans le district sanitaire de Mbacké (Sénégal)', Mémoire de fin de cycle, Institut de santé et développement.

Fassin, D., 1996, 'Les effets sociaux des maladies graves', Paris, Erasme, Décembre.

Fassin, D. (dir.), 2001, *Critique de la santé publique*, Balland.

Fassin, D. et Defossez, A., 1992, 'Une liaison dangereuse. Sciences Sociales et santé publique dans les programmes de réduction de la mortalité naturelle en Equateur', *Cahiers des Sciences Humaines*, vol. 28, n° 1, pp. 23-36.

Fathalla M. F., 1988, 'Research Needs in Human Reproduction', in E., Diczfulsi, P. D., Griddin, P. D., Khanna, eds., *Research Needs in Human Reproduction*, Biannual report 1986-1987, Geneva, WHO 18.

Fauveau V., 1993, 'Maternal Tetanus', *International Journal of Gynaecology and Obstetrics*, 40, pp. 3-12.

Flores, N. E. and Richard, T. C., 1997, 'The Relationship Between the Income Elasticities of Demand and Willingness to Pay', *Journal of Environmental Economics and Management*, 33 (3), 287-95.

Foner, A. and Schwak, K., 1981, *Aging and Retirement*, Monterey, Brookes/Cole.

Foster, A. D. and Rosenweig, M. R., 2001, 'Democratisation, Decentralization and the Distribution of Local Public Goods in a Poor Rural Economy', Research Paper.

Foster, G. M., 1976, 'Disease Aetiologies in Non-western Medical Systems', *American Anthropologist*, 78, pp. 773-782.

Frankl, V., 1984, *Man in Search of Meaning*, 3rd edition, Pocket Books.

Friedrich, H., et al., 1987, 'Faire face à une maladie chronique', *Sciences Sociales et Santé*. Vol. V, No. 2, Juin, pp. 31-44.

Frykblom, P., 1998, 'Questions in the Contingent Valuation Method, Five Essays', PhD Thesis, Acta Universitatis Agriculturae Sueciae Agraria, 100, Swedish University of Agricultural Sciences, Uppsala.

Gabriel, T., 1991, *The Human Factor In Rural Development*, Belhaven Press.

Gautier, A., 2000, 'Les droits reproductifs, une nouvelle génération de droits?', *Autrepart*, No. 15, pp. 167-180.

Gilson, L., 1988, 'Government Health Care Charges: Is Equity Being Abandoned?', EPC Publication No. 15. London.

Giorgis, B.W., 1991, 'The Integration of Gender Analysis in Health Research', CODESRIA Workshop on Gender Analysis and African Social Science, Dakar.

Good, C. M., 1987, *Ethnomedical Systems in Africa: Patterns of Traditional Medicine in Rural and Urban Kenya*, New York, Guildford Press.

Government of Kenya, 1965, Sessional Paper No. 1 of 1965, *African socialism and its Application to Planning in Kenya*, Nairobi, Government Printer.

Government of Kenya, 1979, *Development Plan 1979-83*, Nairobi, Government Printer.

Government of Kenya, 1986, Sessional Paper No. 1 of 1986, *Economic Management for Renewed Growth*, Nairobi, Government Printer.

Government of Kenya, 1993, *Strategic Action Plan for Financing Health Care in Kenya*, Nairobi, Government Printer.

Government of Kenya, 1995, 'Guidelines for District Health Management Boards', Nairobi, Government Printer.

Government of Kenya, 1995, *Kenya Health Policy Framework Paper*, Nairobi, Government Printer.

Government of Kenya, 1996, *Health Sector Reform Programme: Annual Summary Report*, Nairobi, Health Sector Reform Secretariat (HEROS).

Green, E. C. and Makhubu, L., 1984, 'Traditional Healers in Swaziland: Toward Improved Cooperation between the Traditional and Modern Health Sectors', *Social Science and Medicine* (18), pp. 1071-1079.

Grenier, L., 1998, *Connaissances indigènes et recherche. Un guide à l'intention des chercheurs*, CRDI.

Griffin, C. C., 1989, 'Strengthening Health Services in Developing Countries Through the Private Sector', Washington, DC, International Finance Corporation Discussion Paper 4.

Gros, J., ed., 1998, *Democratization in Late Twentieth-Century Africa: Coping With Uncertainty*, Westport, CT, Greenwood Press.

Gruat, J. V., 1990, 'Social Security Systems in Africa: Current Trends and Problems', *International Labour Review*, 129 (NE4), pp. 405-421.

Heeren, J. A., 2001, *Knowledge Attitude and Practices in Postpartum Care in the North Bank East Division of the Gambia*, Nijmegen, University of Nijmegen.

Henrad, J. C., 1988, 'Maladies chroniques invalidantes', *Sciences Sociales et Santé*, vol VI, No 2, Juin, pp 25-30.

Henry, W. E., 1974,. 'The Role of Work in Structuring the Life Cycle', *Human Development*, 14.

Herzlich, C., 1970., *Santé et maladie (Analyse d'une représentation sociale)*, Layahe, Mouton, Coll. Les textes sociologiques.

Hesketh, T. and Zhu, X. W., 1997, 'Health in China: Traditional Chinese Medicine: One Country, Two Systems', *British Medical Journal*, 315, pp. 115-117.

Hill, A. G., Hill, M. C., Gomez, P. and Walraven, G., 1996, *Report of the Living Standards Survey Conducted in the Villages of the MRC Main Study Area, North Bank Division, Republic of the Gambia in June-July 1996*, Farafenni, MRC.

Hill, A. G., Macleod, W. B., Joof., D., Gomez, P., Ratclifffe, A. A. and Walraven, G., 2000, 'Decline of Mortality in Children in Rural Gambia: The Influence of Village-Level Primary Health Care', *Tropical Medicine and International Health*, 5 (2), pp. 107-118.

Holme, T. H. and Rahe, R. H., 1967, 'The Social Readjustment Rating Scale', *Journal of Psychosomatic Research*, 11, pp. 213-218.

Houdégbé, J., 1998, *Rentabilité Economique des Politiques de Conservation des Aires Protégées au Bénin: cas de la Zone cynégétique de la Djona*, Thèse de Doctorat en Economie Rurale, Cires-Université d'Abidjan.

Hours, B., 1992, 'La santé publique entre soins de santé primaires et management', *Cahiers des Sciences Humaines*, Vol. 28, n° 1, pp. 123-140.

Hours, B., 2001, *Systèmes et politiques de santé: de la santé publique à l'anthropologie*, Paris, Karthala.

Hutchison, P., 1998, 'Influence on Self-Assessment of Health: Expanding Our View Beyond Illness and Disability', *Journal of Gerontology*, 55B (2), pp. 107-116.

Idachaba, F. S., 1985, *Rural Infrastructures in Nigeria*, Ibadan, Ibadan University Press.

Jaffré, Y. et Olivier de Sardan, J., 1995, « Tijiri, la naissance sociale d'une maladie », *Cahiers des Sciences Humaines*, Vol. 31, No. 4, p. 773-795.

Janzen, J., M., 1978, *The Quest for Therapy in Lower Zaire*, Berkeley, University of California Press.

Janzen, J., M. et Arkinstall, W., 1995, *La quête de la thérapie au Bas-Zaïre*, Paris, Karthala.

Jordan, E., 1994, 'Differences in Contingent Valuation Estimates from Referendum and Checklist Questions', *Journal of Agricultural and Resource Economics*, 19 (1), 115-128.

Journée d'étude, 1999, *Epidémiologie des cancers solides en Algérie*, Juillet.

Jungmenn, O. and Philimeon, 1999, 'Retirement Can Spark Depression', *BBC Online*.

Kahneman, D. and Knetsch, J. L., 1992, 'Valuing Public Good: The Purchase Of Moral Satisfaction', *Journal of Environmental Economics and Management*, 30, pp. 57-70.

Kala, R., 1985, « Considération épidémiologique à propos de l'étude rétrospective des tuberculeux à l'Hôpital Général de Brazzaville », Thèse de doctorat de médecine, INSSA, Brazzaville.

Kamara, E., 2000, *The Effects of Structural Adjustment Programmes on Women's Health in Kenya*, ed., *Africa in Transformation*.

Kanbur, R., 1990, 'La pauvreté et les dimensions sociales de l'ajustement structurel en Côte d'Ivoire. Les dimensions sociales de l'ajustement structurel en Afrique sub-saharienne', *Document de travail*, No. 2, Washington DC, Banque Mondiale.

Kaufman, A., 1989, 'Les malades face à leur cancer', in Aïch, P., et al., *Vivre une maladie grave: analyse d'une situation de crise*, Paris, eds. Méridiens Klincsieck, Coll, Réponses sociologiques.

KDHS, 1998, *Kenya Demographic Health Survey, 1998*, Nairobi, Government Printer.

KDHS, 2003, *Kenya Demographic Health Survey, 2003,*. Nairobi, Government Printer.

Kenya, Republic of, 1986, *The Seventh National Development Plan 1994–1996*, Nairobi, Government Printer.

Kenya, Republic of, 1992, *Women and Children in Kenya: A situational Analysis*, Government of Kenya and UNICEF, Nairobi, Mangra Phics.

Kenya, Republic of, 1994b, *Kenya's Health Policy Framework*, Ministry of Health, Nairobi, Government Printer.

Kenya, Republic of, 1996, *Economic Reforms for 1996–1998, The Policy Framework Paper,* Government of Kenya, IMF, World Bank, 16th February.

Kenyatta National Hospital Audit Reports Nos. KNH/1A/57/51 and KNH/FIN/35 2003.

Kimani, V., 1995, 'African Traditional Health Care: The Place of Indigenous Resources in the Delivery of Primary Health Care in Four Kenyan Communities', PhD Thesis, Department of Community Health, University of Nairobi.

Kimathi, W. and Omiya, P. J., 1994, *The Growing Burden of Poverty on Women and its Effects on their Reproductive Health Rights, an Analysis of the Kenyan Case*, Sexual and Reproductive Health and Rights of Women, An IPPF Discussion Paper.

Kirchgässler, K. et Matt, E., 1987, 'La fragilité du quotidien', *Sciences Sociales et Santé*, Vol. V, No. 1, Février, pp. 93-113.

Kirk, D., Pillet, B., 'Fertility Levels, Trends and Differentials in Sub-Saharan African in the 1980s and 1990s', *Studies in Family Planning*, 29: 1-2.

Klimek, C. Y. et Peters, G., 1995, *Une politique du médicament pour l'Afrique: contraintes et choix*, Paris, Karthala.

Klitgaard, R., 1988, *Controlling corruption*, Berkeley, CA, University of California Press.

Korte, R., Richter, H., Merkle, F. and Gorgen H., 1992, 'Financing Health Services in Sub-Saharan Africa: Options for Decision Makers During Adjustment', *Soc. Sci. Med.*, Vol. 34, No. 1, pp. 1-9.

Kriström, B., 1993, 'Comparing Continuous and Discrete Contingent Valuation Questions', *Environmental and Resource Economics*, 3, 63-71.

Kutzin, J. and Barnum, H., 1992, 'Institutional Features of Health Insurance Programs and Their Effects on Developing Country Health Systems', *International Journal of health Planning and Management*, 7, pp. 51-72.

Last, M. and Chavundika, G. L., eds., 1986, *The Professionalisation of African Medicine*, Manchester, Manchester University Press.

Li, C.-Z. and Fredman, P., 1994, 'On Reconciliation of the Discrete Choice and Open-Ended Responses in Contingent Valuation Experiments', in Li, C.-Z., *Welfare Evaluations in*

Contingent Valuation - An Econometric Analysis, PhD Thesis, Umea Economic Studies No. 341, Department of Economics, Umea University.

Loi 121/92 portant mise en place du Plan National de Développement Sanitaire (PNDS).

Mabirizi, F., 2001, 'The Technical Interface Between Decentralised Development Planning and Structural Adjustment in Uganda', SPRING Research Series, No. 25, University of Dortmund.

Macgregor, J., 1991, 'Towards Human-Centered Development: Primary Health care in Africa', *African Insight*, Vol. 21, No. 3.

Mafouana Nsala, M. P., 1998, *La prévalence de l'infection à VIH chez les tuberculeux hospitalisés au service de pneumo-phtisiologie du CHU-B*, Mémoire fin de cycle en Santé publique.

Marga Institute, 1984, *Intersectoral Action for Health-Sri Lanka Study*, Marga Institute.

Maslow, A. H., 1968, *Towards the Psychology of Being*, 2nd Edition, New York, Van Nostrand Reinhold.

Master Plan of Operations: Country Programme of Cooperation Document (1997-2001), Federal Government of Nigeria and UNICEF.

Maternal Neonatal Health, 2004, 'Traditional Birth Attendants: Linking Community and Services', www.mnh.jhpiego.org/best/tba.asp

Mbiti, D., Mworia, F. and Hussein, I., 1993, 'Cost Recovery in Kenya', *The Lancet*, 341, 376.

Mbizvo, M.T., 1996, 'Reproductive and Sexual Health', *Central African Journal of Medicine*, 42 (3), pp. 80-85.

McFadden, P., 1992, 'Health as a Gender Issue', Nairobi, Center for African Family Studies (CAFS).

Mebtoul, M., et al., 1998, 'Les significations attribuées à la prise en charge de deux maladies chroniques', Université d'Oran.

Mein, G., Higgs, P., Ferre, J. and Standford, S. A., 1998, 'Paradigms of Retirement: The Importance of Aging in Whitehall Study', *Social Science Medicine*, 47 (4), 535-545.

Michel, Henry, 1979, Pour une éducation africaine de la santé. Essai d'un manuel pédagogique adapté à l'Afrique, Thèse d'Etat, Université de Dakar.

Miguel E. and Gugerty, M. K., 2002, 'Ethnic Diversity, Social Sanctions and Public Goods in Kenya', Mimeo, Berkeley, University of California.

Mills, A., 1983, 'Economics Aspects of Health Insurance', in K., Lee, A., Mills, eds., *Health Economics in Developing Countries*, Oxford University Press.

Mills, A. V., Smith, J. P., et al., 1990, *Health System Decentralization: Concepts, Issues and Country Experiences*, Geneva, World Health Organisation.

Ministère de la Santé et de la Population, 1998, *Système national de santé : éléments de réflexion, Assises nationales de la santé*, 27 et 28 mai.

Ministry of Public Health, 1997, 'National Health Management Information System', Annual Activity Report, Yaoundé.

Mitchell, R. C. and Carson, R. T., 1986, 'Using Surveys to Value Public Goods: The Contingent Valuation Method', Washington DC.

MoH, 1999, *National Health Policy*, Kampala, Uganda.

MoH, 2000, *Health Sector Strategic Plan 2000/01-2004/05*, Kampala, Uganda.

MoH, 2004, 'Public-Private Partnership in Health (PPPH): Increasing Private Health Sector Participation, in all Aspects of the National Health Programme', http://www.health.gov.ug/part_health.htm, 2/02/04.

Moley, D. and Lovel, H., 1986, *My Name is Today*, London, Macmillan.

Munasinghe, M., 1996, 'Environmental Economics and Sustainable Development', *World Bank Environmental Paper* No. 3, Washington, DC.

Mwabu, G. M., 1992, 'A Framework for Analyzing Health effects of Structural Adjustment Policies', Paper presented for International Science and Medicine Africa, Network (SOMA-NET) Nairobi, 10th-14th August.

Mwabu, G. M., 1993, 'Health Sector Reform in Kenya 1963-93: Lessons for Policy Research', Paper Presented at the Conference on Health Sector Reform in Developing Counties, 10-13 September, New Hampshire, USA.

Mwabu, G. M., 1993, 'Quality of Medical and Choice of Medical Treatment in Kenya: An Empirical Analysis', Working Paper No. 9, African Technical Department, Washington DC., The World Bank.

Mwabu, G. M., 1995, 'Health Care Reform in Kenya: A Review of the Process', *Health Policy*, 32.

Mwabu, G. M. and Wang'ombe, J., 1995, 'User Charges in Kenya Health Service Pricing Reform: 1989-93', International Health Policy Program, Working Paper, February.

Mwanzia, J., Omeri, I. and Ong'ayo, 1993, 'Decentralization and Health Systems in Kenya: A Case Study', Nairobi.

N'Diaye, S., Diouf, P. et Ayad, M., 1995, *Santé Familiale et Population*. Région de Thiès: Résultats de l'Enquête Démographique et de Santé au Sénégal. EDS-II, 1992/93. Dakar: Division des Statistiques Démographiques, décembre.

N'guessan Coffie, F. J., 1997, *Estimation de la demande des soins de santé antipaludéens et des Méthodes Préventives en Milieu Rural Ivoirien: le cas des villages de Memni et Montezo*, Thèse de Doctorat en Economie Rurale, Cires-Université d'Abidjan.

Nasirumbi, H., 1995, *Health Policies as they Affect Gender and Development in Kenya: A Case Study of HIV/AIDS Policies*, Mimeo, July.

Ndi-Ndi, J., 1998, *Prise en charge des malades tuberculeux à l'hôpital Jamot de Yaoundé*, Mémoire fin de cycle de santé publique, Université de Yaoundé.

Neill, H. R., Cummings, R. G., Ganderton, P. T., Harrison, G. W. and MacGuckin, T., 1994, 'Hypothetical Surveys and Real Economic Commitments', *Land Economics* 70, 145-154.

Ngetich, K., 2004, 'The Utilization of Traditional and Modern Medicine in the Urban Settings: A Case Study of Nairobi City', PhD Dissertation, Kenyatta University.

Ngugi, R., 1999, *Health Seeking Behavior in the Reform Process for Rural Households: The Case of Mwea Division, Kirinyaga District, Kenya*, Nairobi, African Economic Research Consortium.

Nichter, M., ed., 1992, *Anthropological Approaches to the Study of Ethno-medicine*, Arizona, Gordon and Beach Publishers.

Noterman, J. P., Criel, B., Kegels, G. and Isu, K., 1995, 'A Prepayment Scheme for Hospital Care in the Masisi District in Zaire: A Critical Evaluation', *Social Science and Medicine*, 40 (NE7), 919-930.

Ntangsi, J. V., 1996, 'An Analysis of Health Sector Expenditure in Cameroon Using a National Accounts Framework'.

Nuyens, Y., 1988, 'Health Systems Research in the WHO Global Strategy for Health for All', in *Methods and Experience in Planning Health: The Role of Health Research Systems*, Nordic School of Public Health Report No. 4, [x2] Götenborg, pp. 50-70.

Oates, W., 1972, *Fiscal Federalism*, New York, Harcourt Brace Jovanovich.

Odera, O. A., 1995, 'Retired Person's Adjustment to New Roles And Implications for Social Work. A Case Study of Pensioners in Njikoka Local Government Area of Anambra State', Unpublished Masters Project, Nsukka, Department of Sociology and Anthropology, University of Nigeria, Nsukka.

Okwemba, A., 2004, 'KNH Raises Fees Amid Graft Claims', *Daily Nation*, 4 March, pp. 23-25.

Olenja, J. M., 1991, *Women and Health Care in Siaya*, in S. Gideon, ed., *Development in Kenya: Siaya District*, Nairobi, Institute of African Studies.

OMS, 1975, 'Comment répondre aux besoins sanitaires fondamentaux des populations dans les pays en voie de développement', Genève.

OMS, 1981, 'Elaboration d'indicateurs pour la surveillance continue des progrès réalisés dans la voie de la santé pour tous d'ici 2000', Genève.

OMS, 1982, 'Rôle des centres de santé dans le développement des systèmes de santé des villes', Genève.

OMS, 1990, 'La médecine par les plantes: réalité ou fiction'.

OMS, 1992, 'Economie hospitalière et financement des hôpitaux dans les pays en développement', Genève.

OMS, 1993, *Les accoucheuses traditionnelles*, OMS Genève.

OMS, 1996, *La tuberculose en Afrique: un continent 46 pays un combat incertain couronné de succès*, AFRO, Brazzaville.

OMS, 1997, *Guide pour la surveillance de la résistance bactérienne aux médicaments antituberculeux*.

OMS, 1998, 'Crossroads: WHO Report on the Global Tuberculosis Epidemic,' Geneva.

OMS, 1998, 'Prendre en charge la tuberculose au niveau nationale', Genève.

OMS, 1998, 'Rapport sur la santé dans le monde', Genève.

OMS, 1999, 'Recherche concernant les maladies tropicales, progrès',

OMS, 2000, 'Les principes méthodologiques généraux pour la recherche et l'évaluation relatives à la médédecine Traditionelle'.

OMS, 2001, *Observation de la santé en Afrique*, Volume 2, N° 1.

OMS, 2003, 'Rapport sur la santé dans le monde (façonner l'avenir)'.

OMS, 2003, 'Accélérer l'action contre le Sida en Afrique'.

ONU-SIDA, 1997, *Tuberculose et SIDA. Point de vue*.

Oppong, C., 1992, 'Traditional Family Systems in Rural Settings in Africa', in E. Berquo and P. Xenos, eds., *Family systems and cultural change*, Oxford, Clarendon Press, 69-86.

ORSTOM, Abidjan, CIV, ed., 1995, GIDIS-CI, Groupement Interdisciplinaire en Sciences Sociales Côte d'Ivoire, Abidjan, CIV (ed.); Groupe de Partenaires 'Transition de la Fécondité et Santé de la Reproduction', ed., Santé de la reproduction dans les pays à croissance démographique rapide: approches méthodologiques, ORSTOM; GIDIS-CI, Abidjan (CIV); Abidjan (CIV), 1995, 'Santé de la Reproduction dans les Pays à Croissance Démographique Rapide: Approches Méthodologiques', *Atelier*, 10-13 mai.

Oufriha, F. Z., 'La difficile structuration du système de santé en Afrique: Quels résultats?', *Les cahiers du CREAD*, n° 35/361993, pp. 7-58.

Oufriha, F. Z., 1988, 'Essai sur le système de soins en Algérie', *Economie Appliquée et Développement*, n° 13, 1er trimestre, pp. 60-75.

Owino, P. S. W., 1993, 'The Impact of Structural Adjustment on the Production and Availability of Pharmaceutical Products in Kenya', PhD Thesis, University of Sussex.

Owino, P. S. W., 1997, 'Public Health Sector Efficiency in Kenya: Estimation and Policy Implications', IPAR Discussion Papers.

Owino, P. S. W., 1998a, 'Enhancing Health Care among the Vulnerable Groups: The system of Waivers and Exemptions', IPAR Discussion Paper.

Owino, P. S. W., 1998b, 'Public Health Care Pricing Practices: The Question of Fee Adjustment', IPAR Discussion Papers.

Owino, P. S. W. and Munga, S., 1997, 'Decentralization of Financial Management System: Its Implementation and Impact on Kenya's Health Care Delivery', IPAR Discussion Papers.

Owour, C., 1999, 'The Position of Traditional Medicine in Health Care Delivery: The Kenya Case', *Mila*, 4, pp. 27-36.

Packer, C. A. A., 2002, 'Using Human Rights to Change Tradition: Traditional Practices Harmful to Women's Reproductive Health in Sub-Saharan Africa', Utrecht University, Institute for Legal Studies.

Pannarunothai, S. and Mills, A., 1997, 'Characteristics of Public and Private Health Care in a Thai Urban Setting', in Bennet, S, McPake, B., and Mills, A., eds., *Private Health Care Providers in Developing Countries*, London, Zed Books.

Parsons, T., 1995, 'Structures sociales et processus dynamique : le cas de la pratiquez médicale moderne', in Bouricaud, F., *Eléments pour une sociologie de l'action*, Paris, Plon.

Pathmanathan, I., 1993, 'Gestion de la recherche sur les systèmes de santé : un outil de gestion', Ottawa, CRDI.

Paul, B. K., 1993, 'Maternal Mortality in Africa, 1980-1987', *Social Science and Medicine*, 37 (6), pp. 745-52.

Pearce, T. O., 1982, 'Integrating Western Orthodox and Indigenous Medicine', *Social Science and Medicine*, 16, pp. 1611-1617.

Pedinelli, J. L., 1988, 'Conduite et représentation des familles et des patients atteints de maladies graves et soumis à des thérapeutiques de suppléance', Paris, CNRS.

Piaget, J., 1974, *Le structuralisme*, Paris, PUF.

Dozon, J., et al., 1997, *Le sida en Afrique, recherche en Sciences de l'homme et de la société*, Paris.

Pillsbury, B. K., 1982, 'Policy and Evaluation Perspectives in Traditional Health Practitioners in National Health Care Systems', *Social Science and Medicine*, 16, pp. 1825-34.

Plan Stratégique 2001-2005, AMPPF.

PNUD, 2002, *Rapport national pour le développement humain*, Brazzaville.

PNUD, 2001, 'Rapport national sur le développement humain au Sénégal: gouvernance et développement humain', New York.

Prescott-Allen, R., 2003, 'Le bien-être des nations. Indice par pays de la qualité de vie et de l'environnement', Eska/CRDI.

Programme national de lutte contre la tuberculose, 2000, *Analyse épidémiologique de 1992à 1994,* Brazzaville, Congo.

Qaim, M. and De Janvry, A., 2003, 'Genetically Modified Crops, Corporate Pricing Strategies, And Farmers' Adoption: The Case Of BT Cotton In Argentina', *American Journal of Agricultural Economics,* 85 (4), pp. 814-828.

Quick, J. D. and Musau, N.S., 1994, 'Impact of Cost-sharing in Kenya-1989/93, Kenya Health Care Financing Project', Nairobi, MoH, Kenya.

Rae, G. O., Manandu, M. and Mondi, F. V., 1988, 'Health Care Delivery', in A. B., Ayako and J. E. O., Odada, eds., Report of Proceedings of the Workshop on the Impact of Structural Adjustment Policies on the Well-being of the Vulnerable Group in Kenya, Nairobi, 3-5 November.

Rakotomanana, F., et al., 1999, 'Profil des malades perdus de vue en cours de traitement dans le programme national de lutte contre la tuberculose à Madagascar', *Cahier de la santé,* vol. 9, n°4, juil.- août, pp. 225-229.

Rakotomizao, J. R., et al., 1998, 'Facteurs d'abandon du traitement antituberculeux à Antananarivoville et Antsirabe', *Int J. Tuber Lung Dis 2,* pp. 891-892.

Randall, A., Hoehn, J. P. and Tolley, G. S., 1981, 'The Structure of Contingent Markets: Some Results of a Recent Experiment', Paper presented at the American Economic Association Annual Meeting, Washington D C.

Rappaport, H. and Rappaport, M., 1981, 'The Integration of Scientific and Traditional Healing', *American Psychologist,* 36 (2), pp. 774-781.

Ratcliffe, A. A., 2000, 'Men's Fertility and Marriages: Male Reproductive Strategies In Rural Gambia', Thesis, Doctor of Science, Department of Population and International Health, Boston, Massachusetts.

Ratcliffe, A. A., Hill, A. G., Harrington, D. P. and Walraven, G., 2002, 'Reporting of Fertility Events by Men and Women in Rural Gambia', *Demography,* 39 (3): 573-586.

Ratcliffe, A. A., Hill, A. G. and Walraven, G., 2000, 'Separate Lives, Different Interests: Male and Female Reproduction in The Gambia', *Bulletin of the World Health Organisation,* 78: 570-579.

Rathonina, 1998, « Etude épidémiologique et la lutte contre la tuberculose de la circonscription, médicale de Vakinakotia à Madagascar », Mémoire de fin de cycle, Ecole de santé publique, Madagascar, les cahiers de l'IGRAC, No. 1, 2005.

Razakazo, 1999, « Situation épidémiologique de la tuberculose à Madagascar », Mémoire de fin de cycle, Ecole de santé publique, Madagascar, les cahiers de l'IGRAC, No. 1, 2005.

Report of the International Symposium on Urban Management and Urban Violence in Africa, 1994, IFRA, Ibadan.

Republic of Cameroon, 2000, *Interim Poverty Reduction Strategy paper,* Cameroon, August 23.

Republic of Kenya, 1962, The Witchcraft Act, Cap. 67 (1925, Revised in 1962 and 1981).

Republic of Kenya, 1996, *National Development Plan 1997-2001,* Nairobi, Government Printer.

Republic of Uganda, 1997, Local Government Act.

République du Sénégal, Ministère de la santé, 1989, 'Programme de développement intégré du secteur de la santé', avril.

Richter, M., 2003, 'Traditional Medicines and Traditional Healers in South Africa', Discussion paper prepared for the Treatment Action Campaign and AIDS Law Project.

Rivers, W. H. R., 1924, *Medicine, Magic and Religion*, New York, Harcourt Brace Press.

Roberts, C., 1979, 'Mungu na Mitishamba: Illness and Medicine Among the Batabwa of Zaire', Doctoral Dissertation, University of Chicago.

Rondinelli, D. A., Nellis, J. R. and Cheema, G. S., 1983, 'Decentralization in Developing Countries: A Review of Recent Experiences', World Bank Staff Working paper No. 581, Washington DC, The World Bank.

Rose-Ackerman, S., 1978, *Corruption: A study in political economy*, New York, Academic Press.

Salem, G., 1998, *La santé dans la ville*, Karthala/Orstom.

Sama, M., 2004a, 'Malaria Intervention in Central Africa: A Health Systems Challenge', A Paper Presented at the CODESRIA's Governing African Health Systems Institute, 8 March-2 April.

Sama, M., 2004b, 'Health Sector Reform Process: Decentralization', A paper presented at the CODESRIA's Governing African Health Systems Institute, 8 March–2 April.

Schneider, P., Diop, F. P. and Bucyana, S., 2000, *Development and Implementation of Prepayment Schemes in Rwanda*, Technical Report No. 45, Bethesda, MD, Partnerships for Health Reform (PHR) Project.

Seaward, B. L., 1994, *Managing Stress: Principles and Strategies For Health and Well Being*, London, Jones and Bartlett.

Seck, M., 1991, 'Une stratégie de promotion de la santé', *Vie et Santé*, n° 6, pp.3-5.

Selye, H., 1956, *The Stress of Life*, New York, McGraw Hill.

Shepard, D., Vian, T. and Kleinau, E. F., 1990, 'Health insurance in Zaire', Policy, Research and External Affairs Working Papers, WPS 489, Washington DC, Africa Technical Department, The World Bank.

Shepard, D. S., et al., 1998, 'Household Participation in Financing of Health Care at Government Health Centres in Rwanda', in A., Mills and L., Gilson, eds., *Health Economics for Developing Countries*, London School of Hygiene and Tropical Medicine.

Shleifer, A. and Vishny, R., 1993, 'Corruption', *Quarterly Journal of Economics*, pp. 599-617.

Titi Nwel, P., 1999, 'La corruption au Cameroun', Fondation Friedrich Ebert Stiftung.

Sibley L., 1997, 'Obstetric First Aid in the Community - Partners in Safe Motherhood', *Journal of Nursing and Midwifery* 42 (2), pp. 117-121.

Sindiga, I., 1995, 'Traditional Medicine in Africa: An Introduction', in I. Sindiga, C. Nyaigoti-Chacha and M. Kanunah, eds., *Traditional Medicine in Africa*, Nairobi, East African Educational Publishers, pp. 1-15.

Smith, G. and Naim, M., 2000, *Mondialisation, souveraineté et gouvernance*, CRDI.

Smyke, P., 1980, *Women and Health*, Zed Books, London.

Société des nations (SDN), 1923, *Rapport provisoire sur la tuberculose et la maladie du sommeil en Afrique équatoriale*, Genève.

Sow, I., 1987, *Les structures anthropologiques de la folie en Afrique noire*, Paris, Payot.

Stigler, G., 1970, 'The Optimum Enforcement of Law', *Journal of Political Economy*, 78, pp. 526-536.

Stover, et al., 1996, *Report on Status and Observations on Cost-sharing: Issues in Supervision and Decentralization*, Nairobi, Ministry of Health, August.

Strauss, A., 1992, *La trame de la négociation (Sociologie qualitative et interactionnisme)*, Paris, Editions l'Harmattan.

Sy, A. B., 1991, 'Quelle santé pour l'Afrique?', *Afrique-Espoir*, No. 2, 1991, pp. 2-7.

Tanzi, V., 1995, 'Fiscal Federalism and Decentralization: A Review of Some Efficiency and Macroeconomic Aspects in Development Economics', Annual World Bank Conference Washington DC, The World Bank.

Tchicaya, C., 1992, *Intégration du dépistage et de la prise en charge de la tuberculose: service de soins de santé primaires*, Mémoire, Brazzaville, INSSA.

The Guardian, Lagos, 2000, 'Lamentations of Pensioners Amid Government Palliatives', 22 June.

The Guardian, 2003, 'The Pension Crisis', 2 October.

The Guardian, 2004, '50 Retired Teachers Die Waiting for Pension', 29 January.

The Guardian, 2004, 'WHO's Ranking of Nigeria's Health System', 7 January.

Thebeaud, A., 1977, 'Besoins de santé et réponse de l'institution sanitaire en Algérie, *Cahiers de Sociologie et de Démographie médicale*, No. 4, octobre-décembre, pp. 170-183.

Thiam, S., 1989, 'Prise en charge des enfants tuberculeux à Dakar', Mémoire de fin de cycle, Dakar, Institut de Santé et développement.

Tinga, K., 1998, 'Cultural Practice of the Midzichenda at Crossroads: Divination, Healing, Witchcraft and the Statutory Law', *Afrikanische Arbeitpapiere* (AAP), 55: 173-184.

Tshinko, B. L., Constandriopoulos, A. P. et Fournier, P., 1995, 'Plan de paiement Anticipé des Soins de Santé de Bwamanda (Zaïre). Comment a-t-il été mis en place?', *Social Science and Medecine*, 40 (8), 1041-1052.

Twumasi, P., 1984, 'Professionalisation of Traditional Medicine in Zambia', Nairobi, IDRC.

UN Development Program, 1998, *Human Development Report 1998*, New York, Oxford University Press.

UN Development Program, 2003, *Human Development Report 2003, Millenium Development Goals*, New York, Oxford University Press.

UNAIDS, 2000, 'Collaboration with Traditional Healers in HIV/AIDS Prevention and Care in Sub-Saharan Africa: A Literature Review', UNAIDS Best Practice Collection, p.10.

UNICEF, 1990b, *The State of the World's Children*, Oxford University Press.

Unschuld, P. U., 1976, 'Western Medicine and Traditional Healing Systems: Competition, Cooperation or Integration?', *Ethics in Science and Medicine*, 3, pp. 1-20.

Vimard, P., 1997, 'Modernisation, crise et transformation familiale en Afrique subsaharienne', *Autrepart*, No 2, p. 143-159.

Vimard, P., 2000, 'Politique démographique, planification familiale et transition de la fécondité en Afrique', *La Chronique du CEPED*, No. 36, 4.

Vogel, R. J., 1990b, 'Health Insurance in Sub-Saharan Africa: A Survey and Analysis', Policy, Research And External Affairs Working Papers, WPS 476, Washington DC, Africa Technical Department, The World Bank.

Vogel, R. J., 1990a, 'An Analysis of Three National Health Insurance Proposals in Sub-Saharan Africa', *International Journal of Health Planning and Management*, 5, pp. 271-285.

Waddington, C. J. and Enyimayew, K. A., 1989, 'A price to pay. Part 1: The Impact of User Charges in Ashanti-Akim District, Ghana', *International Journal of Health Planning and Management*, 5, pp. 287-312.

Waissmen, R., 1995, 'Interactions familiales et impact de la technologie dans la gestion d'une maladie chronique', *Sciences Sociales et Santé*, Vol XIII, No 1, Mars, pp. 81-100.

Wallace, H. M. and Kanti, G., 1990, *Health Care for Women and Children in Developing Countries*, Oakland, Third Party Publishing Company.

Walraven, G., Scherf, C.,   West, B., Ekpo, G., Paine, K., Coleman, R., Bailey, R. and Morison, L., 2001, 'The Burden of Reproductive Organ Disease in Rural Women in The Gambia, West Africa', *The Lancet*, 357, pp. 1161-1167.

Walraven, G., Telfer, M., Rowley, J. and Ronsmans, C., 2000, 'Maternal Mortality in Rural Gambia: Levels, Causes and Contributing Factors', *Bulletin of the World Health Organisation*, 78 (5), pp. 603-613.

Walraven, G. and Weeks, A., 1999, 'The Role of Traditional Birth Attendants with Midwifery Skills in The Reduction of Maternal Mortality', *Tropical Medicine and International Health*, 4 (8), pp. 527-29.

Walt, G., 1994, *Health Policy: An Introduction to Process and Power*, Johannesburg, Witwatersrand University Press.

Ware, H., 1994, 'Thoughts on the Course of Fertility Transition in Sub-Saharan Africa', in Looch T., and V. Hertrich, eds., *The Onset of Fertility Transition in Sub-Saharan Africa*, Liege, IUSSP, pp. 289-296.

Warren, D. M., 1974, 'Bono Traditional Healers', in Z. A. Ademunwagun, J. A. Ayoade, I. E. Harrison, eds., *African Therapeutic Systems*, Los Angeles, Crossroads Press, pp. 120-124.

Wasikama, T. M. C., 1998, « Utilisation alternative des terres: une analyse économique de la préservation des forêts tropicales primaires (cas du Parc national de Taï, sud-ouest de la Côte d'Ivoire) », Thèse de Doctorat en Economie Rurale, Cires-Université d'Abidjan.

Werner, D., 1994, 'The Economic Crisis, Structural adjustment and Health Care in Africa', *Third World Resurgence*, No. 42/43, pp. 10-17.

Whittington, D., 1998, 'Administering Contingent Valuation Surveys in Developing Countries', *World Development*, 26:21-30.

Whittington, D., Briscoe, J., Mu, X. and Barron, W., 1990, 'Estimating the Willingness to Pay for Water Services in Developing Countries: A Case Study of Contingent Valuation Surveys in Southern Haiti', *Economic Development and Cultural Change*.

WHO, 1985, 'Report of the Consultation on Approaches of Policy Development for Traditional Practitioners, Including Traditional Birth Attendants', Geneva, WHO Publication.

WHO, 1986, 'Ottawa Charter for Health Promotion', Paper presented at the First International Conference on Health Promotion: The Move Towards a New Public Health. Ottawa, 17-21 November, Ottawa.

WHO, 1988, *The Challenge of Implementation: District Health Systems for PHC*, Geneva, World Health Organisation.

WHO, 1999, *World Health Report, 1998*, Geneva, World Health Organisation.

WHO, 2001, 'Traditional Medicine Strategy', 2001B-2005.

WHO, 2002, 'Planning for Cost-Effective Traditional Health Services in the New Century', A Discussion Paper, Geneva.

WHO, 2002, 'WHO Traditional Medicine Strategy 2002-2005', Geneva, WHO.

WHO, 2003, *World Health Report 2003, Shaping the Future*, Geneva, World Health Organisation.

WHO and UNICEF, 1978, 'Alma Ata: Primary Health Care. Report of the International Conference on Primary Health Care', Alma Ata, USSR, 2-6 September, Geneva, WHO.

Wone, I., 1984, 'Médecine et développement au Sahel, indicateurs de santé', *Cahier Medesahel*, n° 1.

World Bank, 1987, *Financing the Health Sector: An Agenda for Reform*, Washington DC, The World Bank.

World Bank, 1987, *World Development Report*, New York, Oxford University Press.

World Bank, 1990, *World Demographic and Health Survey*, Washington DC.,: The World Bank

World Bank, 1993, *Report of the World Bank Africa Technical Department: Better Health in Africa*, Human resources and poverty division, Washington, The World Bank.

World Bank, 1993, *World Development Report*, New York, Oxford University Press.

World Bank, 1994, *Better Health in African Experience and Lessons Learned*, Washington DC., The World Bank.

World Bank, 1994a, 'Cameroon Diversity, Growth and Poverty Reduction', Working draft, Human Resources and Poverty Division, African Region.

World Bank, 1994b, *Adjustment in Africa: Reforms, Results and the Road Ahead*, Washington DC, World Bank.

World Bank, 1994c, *World Development Indicators*, Washington DC, World Bank.

World Bank, 1997, *The State in a Changing World – World Development Report 1997*, Oxford, Oxford University Press.

World Health Organisation, 1978, *Report of the Alma Alta Conference on Primary Health Care*, Health for all Series no 1, Geneva, WHO.

World Health Organisation, 1990, *Integrating Maternal and Child Health Services with Primary Health Care*, Geneva, WHO.

World Health Organisation, 1991, *Essential Elements of Obstetric CareaAt First Referral Level*, Geneva, WHO.

World Health Organisation, 1993, *Planning and Implementing Health Insurance in Developing Countries: Guiding Principles. Macroeconomics*, Health and Development Series, Geneva.

World Health Organisation, 2000, *The World Health Report 2000. Health Systems Improving Performance*, Geneva, WHO.

World Health Organisation/ UNICEF, 1996, *Revised 1990 Estimates of Maternal Mortality*, Geneva, WHO/FRH/MSM/96.11.

Yoder, P. S., 1982, 'Biomedical and Ethnomedical Practice in Rural Zaire', *Social Science and Medicine*, 16, pp. 1851-1857.

Young, A., 1975, 'Magic as a Quasi-Profession: The Organization of Magic and Magical Healing Among the Amhara', *Ethnology*, 14, pp. 245-265.

Young, A., 1983, 'The Relevance of Traditional Medical Culture to Modern Primary Health Care', *Social Science and Medicine*, 17 (16), pp. 1205-1211.